THE PROVINCE OF AFFLICTION

AMERICAN BEGINNINGS, 1500–1900

A Series Edited by Edward Gray, Stephen Mihm, and Mark Peterson

ALSO IN THE SERIES:

Trading Spaces: The Colonial Marketplace and the Foundations of American Capitalism
by Emma Hart

*Urban Dreams, Rural Commonwealth: The Rise of
Plantation Society in the Chesapeake*
by Paul Musselwhite

Building a Revolutionary State: The Legal Transformation of New York, 1776–1783
by Howard Pashman

Sovereign of the Market: The Money Question in Early America
by Jeffrey Sklansky

National Duties: Custom Houses and the Making of the American State
by Gautham Rao

Liberty Power: Antislavery Third Parties and the Transformation of American Politics
by Corey M. Brooks

The Making of Tocqueville's America: Law and Association in the Early United States
by Kevin Butterfield

Planters, Merchants, and Slaves: Plantation Societies in British America, 1650–1820
by Trevor Burnard

*Riotous Flesh: Women, Physiology, and the Solitary
Vice in Nineteenth-Century America*
by April R. Haynes

Holy Nation: The Transatlantic Quaker Ministry in an Age of Revolution
by Sarah Crabtree

A Hercules in the Cradle: War, Money, and the American State, 1783–1867
by Max M. Edling

Frontier Seaport: Detroit's Transformation into an Atlantic Entrepôt
by Catherine Cangany

Beyond Redemption: Race, Violence, and the American South after the Civil War
by Carole Emberton

A complete list of series titles is available on
the University of Chicago Press website.

THE PROVINCE OF AFFLICTION

Illness and the Making
of Early New England

BEN MUTSCHLER

THE UNIVERSITY OF CHICAGO PRESS

CHICAGO AND LONDON

The University of Chicago Press, Chicago 60637
The University of Chicago Press, Ltd., London
© 2020 by The University of Chicago

Published 2020
Printed in the United States of America

29 28 27 26 25 24 23 22 21 20   1 2 3 4 5

ISBN-13: 978-0-226-71442-4 (cloth)
ISBN-13: 978-0-226-71456-1 (e-book)
DOI: https://doi.org/10.7208/chicago/9780226714561.001.0001

Library of Congress Cataloging-in-Publication Data

Names: Mutschler, Ben, author.
Title: The province of affliction : illness and the making of early New England /
   Ben Mutschler.
Other titles: American beginnings, 1500–1900.
Description: Chicago : University of Chicago Press, 2020. | Series: American
   beginnings, 1500–1900 | Includes bibliographical references and index.
Identifiers: LCCN 2020000791 | ISBN 9780226714424 (cloth) | ISBN 9780226714561
   (ebook)
Subjects: LCSH: Diseases—Social aspects—New England—History—18th
   century. | Diseases—Social aspects—New England—History—19th century. |
   Public health—New England—History—18th century. | Public health—New
   England—History—19th century. | New England—History—18th century. |
   New England—History—19th century.
Classification: LCC RA446.5.N48 M87 2020 | DDC 362.10974—dc23
LC record available at https://lccn.loc.gov/2020000791

♾ This paper meets the requirements of ANSI/NISO Z39.48–1992
(Permanence of Paper).

TO THE MEMORY OF MY PARENTS,

PHYLLIS HALEVY MUTSCHLER

AND

LOUIS HENRY MUTSCHLER

CONTENTS

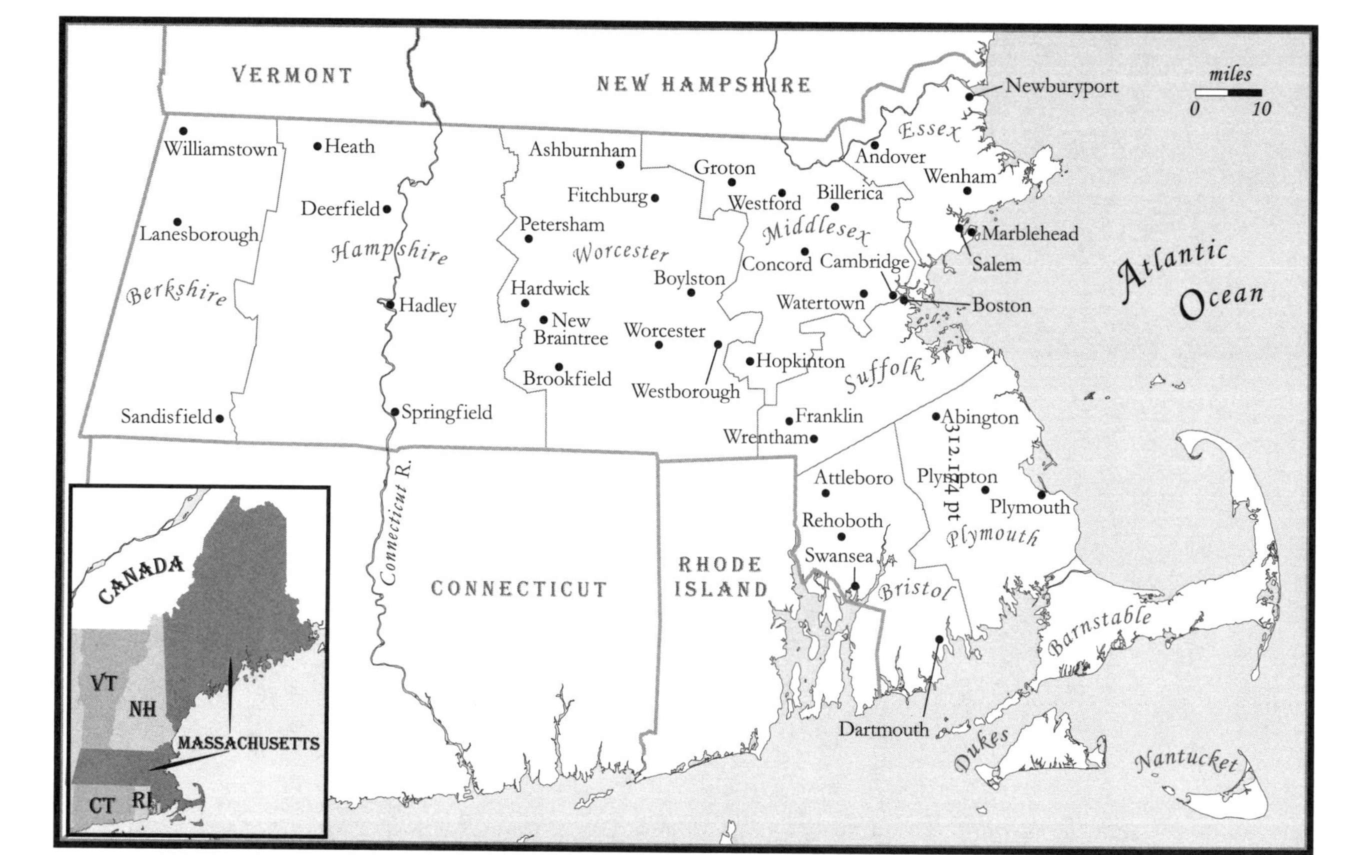

miles
0   10
VERMONT
NEW HAMPSHIRE
Newburyport
Essex
Williamstown
Heath
Ashburnham
Groton
Andover
Wenham
Fitchburg
Westford
Billerica
Deerfield
Petersham
Middlesex
Marblehead
Lanesborough
Hampshire
Worcester
Concord
Cambridge
Salem
Berkshire
Hardwick
Boylston
Watertown
Boston
Hadley
New
Braintree
Worcester
Suffolk
Sandisfield
Brookfield
Westborough
Hopkinton
Springfield
Franklin
Abington
Wrentham
Connecticut R.
Attleboro
Plympton
312.1174 pt
Rehoboth
Plymouth
CONNECTICUT
RHODE
ISLAND
Swansea
Plymouth
Bristol
Barnstable
Atlantic
Ocean
Dartmouth
Dukes
Nantucket
CANADA
VT
NH
MASSACHUSETTS
CT   RI

Introduction

On a late summer day among one of Philadelphia's leading families, when the thick heat in the city could rival places well to the south, young Henry Drinker happily chomped through a piece of watermelon until he ate "too close to the Rine." It was an innocent enough mistake for a six-year-old to make. But as his mother surmised in her diary, that moment of youthful exuberance had been costly, the cause of Henry's "vomiting and disordered bowels" and the beginning of a serious sickness. Between late August and October 1777, Elizabeth Drinker kept a vigilant record of her son's precipitous decline and slow recovery. Henry voided "3 large Worms, and vomited one alive." He was unable to eat for nearly two weeks, "reduced almost to a Skelaton," and ran a constant fever. While there were promising signs of recovery by September 6, when Henry's appetite began to return, his mother judged his illness "to be an inviterate Bloody and white flux," a worrisome condition. She confessed, "I cant help being happrehensive [*sic*] of his falling into a Consumption," which would be chronic and finally fatal. Henry had lived through earlier bouts of worms and bloody, mucous-laden stools—and in his sufferings and recovery, he was typical of many children of his time—but his mother had seen enough illness in her family to fear the worst. At age forty-two, Elizabeth Drinker had already lost three children, two girls and a boy. The first "little Henry," named after his father, had died as an infant in 1769.[1]

Drinker viewed young Henry's progress in the coming weeks with a mixture of optimism and restraint. A promising morning was followed by a discouraging night; Henry's appetite continued to increase but his fever remained; and his bowels could come "down in a frightfull manner," as they had on September 15, when they appeared "red, Bloody and inflam'd" and cast a "bitter" smell through the room. There were continuous "calls to the Pot," a steady administration of "clysters" (enemas) and other physic that Drinker appears to have applied both on her own and in consultation with physicians, and, above all, a good deal of careful watching and waiting. Finally able to have his britches put on and walk across the room with the help of a servant who had been charged with carrying him about the house, Henry suffered another setback at the end September, "taken off his feet again" by pains in his "hams" and a cold brought on by the autumn chill. It was not until October 26, two months after his initial sickness, that Elizabeth Drinker could signal Henry's full return to daily affairs. On that day, Drinker joined her sister, her three healthy children, and Henry at Quaker meeting, noting with relief "the first time of our little Henrys going since his recovery."[2]

The troubles had all started, in Elizabeth Drinker's mind, with a few errant bites of melon. As in so many other incidents in early modern life, the thin membrane separating the workaday world and a world of perils had been all too easily punctured.

∾

The origins of this book lie in Henry Drinker's unfortunate encounter with that watermelon rind, in its evocation of the closeness of danger and the possibility of sudden change in everyday affairs. Elizabeth Drinker's remarkable diary, one of the richest accounts we have of daily life in eighteenth-century America, was my first window onto the ubiquity of sickness and other misfortunes in the period. But I subsequently found that while Drinker's diary is perhaps more insistent than other sources in its recording of illness, it is by no means exceptional.

Almost any source from the period reveals a world riddled by affliction. Letters contain polite inquiries into health and offer running accounts of the status of family, friends, and acquaintances. Newspapers and almanacs feature all manner of information about sickness: the spread of epidemics ravaging distant lands and neighboring colonies and towns, the arrival of infected goods and persons subject to quarantine and cleansing, and the sale of enslaved persons whose bodies are advertised as "healthy" and as already having weathered smallpox. Sermons seize on severe sickness as a warning that death might strike at any moment and as an inducement to examine the diseased state of one's soul. The acts and resolves of colonial assemblies depict a staggering range of afflictions besetting early modern folks. War veterans and their families ask for restitution for medical care; towns press for relief in the wake of epidemics; the injured, infirm, and simply unlucky plead for special licenses and exemptions from taxes, fees, or other public obligations. Government itself is subject to diagnosis and cure, the "republican remedy for the diseases most incident to republican government" in *Federalist* No. 10 being the most prominent example of many prescriptions penned by political physicians. From the minute accounts of persons feeling unwell to the grand metaphors of a diseased society and politics, sickness has left its impress on the records of early American life.

There was nothing new, of course, in finding the regular presence of sickness in early America; widespread illness and the pain and suffering that accompanied it are often identified as key elements of the early modern world.[3] But if sickness is easily detected in the records of the past, its influence on the rhythms, tempo, tenor, and structures of daily life is not readily apparent. I was less intrigued by the immediate ways in which illness was addressed through different modes of healing, or managed through public health measures, or experienced by sufferers—topics on which there is already a rich body of scholarship—than by a more general question: How did sickness figure in the larger scheme of daily affairs?

The evanescence of illness makes this sort of question difficult to answer. Sickness manifests itself in the historical record as a problem that waxes and wanes at any given moment, sometimes surging forward and trumping other concerns, sometimes fading into the background. We have the easiest time in seeing illness and thinking about its significance when it comes to the fore in spectacular epidemics, in the traumatic and swift sicknesses that devastate the stricken and alarm those around them, in the "final illnesses" that the living seize upon as a means of narrating the end of life. But there are many other moments when illness, though noted, sits quietly in the background, taking its place alongside many other stories. Even dramatic accounts of sickness may be mixed together with enough other kinds of information—the mundane comings and goings of neighbors, a brief note of work accomplished, accounts of the weather, and the like—that it is difficult to know how to interpret their importance. The often repetitive and terse references to persons being unwell, sprinkled through everything from letters and diaries to public records, lose meaning in their diffusion. What we lack is a sustained way of thinking about how the manifest disturbances of illness figured in daily life.

I conceived of a book that would offer a portrait of early American society and government with illness at its center. Ultimately, I decided to locate the study in New England. This would mean losing some wonderful materials, Drinker's diary among them, and revisiting a much-studied region. But the rich primary sources in New England—including diaries, correspondence, petitions, newspapers, institutional archives, and town, church, and court records—spoke directly and in intriguing ways to the question that interested me most profoundly: the continuous, often vexed interplay between the workaday world and the world of illness.

From the earliest years of European settlement until well into the eighteenth century, New Englanders experienced an ongoing tension between a "work ethic" Protestantism and the providentialism that undergirded daily life. On the one hand, they felt the compulsion toward steady, sober work and resisted the delays and stoppages caused by illness. On the other hand, they believed that afflictions—not only illness, but other misfortunes such as accidents and fires—were Man's fate to accommodate and endure. They were to act, in John Winthrop's words, as a "community of perils," in which the infirmities and misfortunes of one would be shared by all. The sick could expect the help of the good neighbor and townsperson versed in the ways of affliction but could also expect some pressure to muscle through their malaise.[4]

Equally important, the distinctive political economy of New England, and particularly of Massachusetts, offers a unique purchase on early modern social welfare. Recent scholarship has shown that, for all of its distinctive characteristics, the region was well-integrated into the Atlantic world of the early modern era. Indeed, in its provision for the poor and in its public health regulations, New England carried forward cutting-edge developments that had their origins in sixteenth- and seventeenth-century England. Town, province, and state governance became deeply integrated into matters of misfortune, offering succor (however spare to modern eyes) and demanding adherence to public health laws that privileged community welfare over the individual. Such developments were elusive elsewhere in British North America, and the generosity and intensity of social provision point to the region as being at the vanguard of social welfare provision.[5]

How did New Englanders negotiate the tension between the world of work, of striving and industry, muscle and motion, and the world of sickness, of absence, delay, and excuse, of tasks done shabbily or left undone altogether? Their struggles to manage that conflict fill the pages that follow.

◦∞◦

The Province of Affliction sets out to explore the ways in which illness shaped the contours of society and government in New England's "long eighteenth century," from roughly 1690 through 1820. Decades of work by medical historians and other scholars investigating New England and other regions of the Atlantic world now offer many revealing angles of vision on disease and its influence on early modern life. Grand narratives map tectonic changes in world history that can be attributed in no small degree to disease, including most spectacularly the demographic catastrophe visited upon Native Americans that opened the way to European conquest.[6] Studies of public health offer insight into the early development of medicine and public authority.[7] Explorations of the boisterous and competitive "medical marketplace" reveal negotiations between patients and their practitioners.[8] And examinations of the sick themselves—their encounters with public and private charity, their interior lives—illuminate the boundaries within which the subjective experience of illness emerged.[9] All of these studies help us to see sickness and healing not apart from larger social, political, and cultural contexts, but rather deeply implicated within them.

This study builds on and extends this work by further integrating the history of disease into a broader narrative of early American social and political development. The central objects of study are not diseases, nor healers, nor even patients in and of themselves, but rather the social and governmental entities of early America—family, household, town, colony, state, and finally national government—as they engaged with the problems presented by disease.

Eighteenth-century New Englanders tended to refer to their ailments not as specific diseases but rather as generic fevers, agues, and disorders, or else simply noted that they were unwell, ill, or dangerously sick. This book examines the problems routinely presented by the condition of being sick, whatever the cause—the disruptions it created, the pressures it placed on the afflicted and those who cared for them. There were questions of organization to be addressed: Who would tend the sick and perform work in their stead? What tasks would be sacrificed in the name of care? And there were questions of limitation and threshold: When could sickness count as an excuse for shoddy or incomplete work? What special allowances would be granted the ailing and those who cared for them in a society accustomed to sickness?

The book explores the ways in which the authority and urgency of illness—its ability to arrive suddenly and contort the lives of the sick and those around them for a time before vanishing—shaped and strained the ligaments of society and government in early New England. The ideal vision of the social and political order was one in which family, church, and commonwealth were integrated into an interlocking, mutually reinforcing whole. Illness could be the occasion that showed the very best that New Englanders had to offer in this regard, a shining example of what even staunch critics of the colonial world writing later in the nineteenth century would call an admirable spirit of "cooperation": families tending their ill, neighbors pitching in and visiting, the church offering prayers and collections for the afflicted, the protective hand of government helping when disaster struck. But the burdens of illness exposed significant tensions as well. Illness imbued daily life with a radical sense of contingency. Like accidents, natural catastrophes, and sudden changes in the economy, sickness was understood to be a force of downward mobility. The threat not only of death, but of suffering and impoverishment, made illness an occasion to make demands on family, neighbors, and finally governing bodies at all levels. In the process, the turmoils of domestic life circulated through the social world and bubbled up into civic affairs.

After offering overviews that introduce readers to key themes and persons in the book (chapters 1 and 2), the following two sections elaborate a spectrum of responses to illness, ranging from accommodations for those who were well-positioned in community life, on the one hand, to provisions for the sick poor, on the other. While attentive to changes over time and space—particularly the precocious institutional responses to the sick that arose in the ports—these chapters focus on the durable patterns of daily life that held firm until the last third of the eighteenth century.

Even for the well-connected, illness could present serious challenges to their efforts to achieve and maintain a "competency," or a middling level of subsistence. Because no farm was entirely self-sufficient, the achievement of a competency inevitably required farm households to engage in interdependent relations with their neighbors, or to produce surplus goods for sale in local and distant markets to gain the cash necessary to buy what could not be found locally. Although such strategies made farmers beholden to others, they were performed in the name of preserving a sturdy independence.[10]

A consideration of illness within families (chapter 3) and households (chapter 4) helps us see more clearly the physical labor that the term "competency" itself could elide: it was able-bodied labor that made land valuable through improvements or a crop successful through careful attendance. Illness meant the inability of workers to perform as they normally did, illuminating the extent to which physical ability was bound up in the achievement of the competency ideal. Moreover, a focus on illness—and on the severe disruptions to labor caused both by the absence of workers and by the secondary loss of those taken away from other household chores to care for the ill—highlights the collective, familial, and household basis of competency. Success required the good fortune of maintaining an able-bodied household, particularly wives, daughters, and female servants whose work in the domestic economy of cooking, cleaning, and dairying was immediately missed in its absence.

As New Englanders struggled to address the needs of the ill and manage the social and financial costs of care in support of a competency, the relations between neighbors and within families and households were defined and tested. At what point in an acute or chronic sickness did a family exceed the limits of the social credit economy that brought neighbors as nurses into their houses and workers into their fields? At what point was a son or daughter, having fallen ill while serving abroad as a helper, apprentice, or hired laborer, no longer a parent's responsibility? And when did failures of the worker's body dissolve the bonds of protection and benevolence that held master to servant? Both custom and law left ample room for negotiation and debate.

At the other end of the spectrum from the competent lay the sick poor and a wide assortment of persons brought into dependency through affliction. Dependency was the moral foundation of social and political relations in this world before the Revolution, something more important than the simple deference that one owed superiors and the condescension that superiors graciously bestowed on subordinates.[11] But during and after the Revolution, those espousing the ideal of dependency faced a host of new challenges, particularly as superiors confronted what they took to be the insubordination of those beneath them in station.[12]

Illness lets us see another set of problems confronting patriarchal authority within the matrix of dependency, by highlighting the difficulties and vulnerabilities that attended the *fulfillment* of patriarchal obligation. If one side of patriarchal rule was underwritten by the customary and legal access that men had to women's bodies, labor, and property, the other side of patriarchal rule was premised on the patriarch's protection of subordinates. It is here that we see the vulnerabilities of the patriarchal order. As protectors of their families, husbands and masters also assumed enormous liabilities, something we see clearly in times of affliction and most especially during epidemic (chapter 5) and war (chapter 6).[13]

War removed healthy persons from households and returned them injured, desperately ill, or chronically infirm. Epidemics of diseases like smallpox cut through towns where they not only killed, but also left a bevy of survivors to pay for the immense social response deemed necessary to curtail contagion. In the aftermath of war and epidemic, sick individuals and their families could be burdened with costs that were beyond their means to pay and forced to negotiate with government for help. The book explores the assumptions embedded in the narratives of affliction that ordinary people laid before government and examines the ways in which officials sorted through their stories, placing a price on suffering. In the petitions presented to the Massachusetts General Court, we see the final expression of the centrifugal force that illness as an engine of dependency exerted on society and government throughout much of the eighteenth century. The social and political costs of illness radiated outward from the afflicted to their families and towns and connected them, finally, to the highest levels of government. Protection called for no less.

The final section of the book brings the idea of agency to bear on the question of the public accommodation of the sick. Emerging most forcefully after the Revolution, the notion of agency, or the exercise of will that enabled autonomous action, implied that in a free society, the ultimate sign of liberty was one's ability to shape his or her own destiny.[14] The idea that persons might act autonomously had the potential to cast the ill, and particularly the sick poor, in a new and often unfavorable light. We see in the institutional response to the sick, in pension applications for war veterans (chapter 7) and in state provision for the sick poor (chapter 8), critical ways in which earlier patterns of accommodation began to wither or were severed altogether in the early republic.

In the 1790s, the federal government tried to remove illness as a legitimate cause for Revolutionary War veterans to receive an invalid pension. Promoters of the new criteria for "decisive disability" argued that there was no way for the government to determine whether illness had been caused by constitutional debility or the poor habits of the aging soldiers themselves. At the same time, the Massachusetts General Court developed policies to address the needs of a growing class of "state paupers"—former Loyalists, free blacks, newly arrived immigrants, wandering laborers, widows and single mothers—none of whom had acquired legal settlement in post-Revolutionary Massachusetts. Next to legislators' salaries, the pauper accounts soon became the single most expensive recurring item on the budget and were eventually cut across the board. The book argues that the "protections" formerly offered subjects in the monarchical world, their ability to place personal stories in front of their governors and ask for compassionate consideration, lay at the heart of this bureaucratic turn in governance in the early republic. The force of those earlier assumptions of monarchical protection, and their potential to expand after the Revolution, made cost-minded government officials anxious to limit the scope of individual claims to relief.

An epilogue carries the story into the 1820s. Major changes to poor relief (both at a local and state level) and the opening of the Massachusetts General Hospital (1821) created a new medical landscape in the early national period, which increasingly distinguished between the "worthy" and "unworthy" ill. Despite the championing of the almshouse by reformers as the most humane and efficient means of treating the poor, advocates for the hospital pointed to the dangers that the worthy ill faced in receiving public relief. Reformers argued that young men and women who had left behind family and community in pursuit of social advancement might find themselves bereft of the local institutions traditionally responsible for their welfare should they fall ill. The hospital and other related charities for the sick poor were designed to step into that breach, saving the worthy from the moral contagion that they would face amidst the assorted mass of unfortunates who populated the almshouse—the foreign poor, the sturdy beggar, the free African American, and the supposedly idle and dissolute. With the ability to discriminate between who was worthy of care and who could be left to the public poor laws, the hospital and other charities offered a new institutional means of restoring social order. The failures of charitable reform reflected the ongoing challenges carried over from the eighteenth century, but those enduring problems were increasingly focused on the sick themselves.

In considering the ways in which competency, dependency, and agency framed the problem of illness in early New England, a key insight from the interdisciplinary field of disability studies is especially useful: while we all labor under various shades and intensities of impairment—from those with slight nearsightedness to the totally blind, for example—it is society, through its response to those impairments, that creates categories of persons who are considered "disabled." Illness is not quite the same thing as physical impairment, although chronic illness, discussed in the final section, shades into something quite close to lasting debility. But thinking about illness as a problem of ability and disability helps us to investigate the interplay between expectation and allowance that lay at the center of many negotiations and conflicts through much of the eighteenth century, and highlights subtle changes in what could be asked both of the sick and government in the early republic.[15]

PROVINCE AS PLACE AND METAPHOR

The word "province" in the book's title does double duty within these pages. The first two sections of the book focus most sharply on Massachusetts during the provincial period, from 1691 until the Revolution; the final section carries the work into the early republic. The extended time frame is necessary both to trace durable patterns of illness, carried forward from the seventeenth century and elaborated in the eighteenth, and to appreciate the ways in which the persistence of those patterns in the early republic created significant tensions, particularly in the political accommodation of illness.

If the time frame is expansive, the geographic range of the study is restricted. While I consider other places within New England and further afield for the sake of comparison and to engage especially illuminating material, the book sets its deepest roots in Massachusetts. The limited geographic focus is necessary for both practical and conceptual reasons. Illness was pervasive enough to become subject to legislation in a variety of domains—public health regulations, poor laws, the law of household governance, and provisions for soldiers and their families—and a focus on a single place makes it more feasible to follow significant changes in law in these areas over time. But more importantly, the accommodation of illness itself became deeply implicated in questions of territorial rights and obligations, making the boundaries of colony and state not simply manageable units of study, but rather essential parts of the story. While illness could arrive from outside the borders of the colony or state—in the body of the sick sailor landing in port, the beleaguered soldier returning from the theater of war, or the weary transient looking for work—the accommodation of illness was a local affair. Families, towns, and commonwealths were asked to care for their own, which led to struggles over just who rightfully belonged to these entities and what, if anything, could local society provide the "stranger" or "foreigner" in distress.

A second, metaphorical meaning of province employed in this book draws our attention to the aesthetics of illness in everyday life, the ways in which the experience of being ill set a tone, created a texture, and shaped essential rhythms in daily affairs. Perhaps more than any other element of the experience of illness, those aesthetic considerations have been lost to us. We may feel that we know intuitively something about the lives of historical subjects laboring under illness, something more immediate and visceral than we learn from reading their journals and books with their marginalia, or touching the objects they have left us, or gazing at their portraits: we know what it means to suffer with a fever, to vomit, to be sidelined by illness. We have embodied critical elements of their experience. Yet historians of the body have rightly tried to help us "unlearn" some of these thoughts, warning that the conception of the body—even the notion of a body as something that is discrete and contained—is an historical development. The fluid and porous early modern body is distanced in important ways from our own.[16] Though we continue to cope with the problems presented by illness in our lives and those of family, friends, and acquaintances, we have no ready way to grasp the social and political meanings that early Americans attached to being sick, no ready frame of reference for the prevalence, intensity, and duration of their ills in early America. Likening the experience of illness to life in a cultural province can speak to just this problem, conveying something of the curiously blended ways of life created by the common but not continuous presence of disease.

A cultural province lies outside a metropolitan center, close enough to emulate life in the metropole, distant enough that its own customs and rituals emerge of necessity. The regular presence of illness in New England opened up a social and political space in daily life that can be thought of as a cultural province, a province lying outside but still close to a state of health and of relations that depended on healthy and functioning persons to succeed. Located on the periphery of health, the cultural province of affliction in this sense resembles other cultural provinces in the eighteenth century, especially in its creativity in negotiating a world where high ambitions clashed with stark limitations, in this case imposed by illness.[17]

We might sharpen this second conceptual frame for thinking of illness in early modern life by contrasting it with a very different way that sickness has been conceived of in our time. Writing as a cancer survivor, Susan Sontag opens her *Illness as Metaphor* (1978) with a metaphor of her own, the distant and lesser "kingdom" of illness in which we will all, at some point, be forced to live in painful isolation.[18] In early New England, the notion of illness as a foreign country or kingdom does not work well. The experience of illness was too common, too much a part of daily affairs. Between 10% and 30% of New England's children did not live through their first year; those who weathered childhood diseases could expect to encounter another onslaught in their teens; although few women died in childbirth, the regularity of pregnancy was often a cause of indisposition and worry; and any individual might find that the diseases that they had undergone earlier in life turned chronic in old age.[19]

Yet if early modern illness was not foreign, neither can it be viewed as a norm that affected everyone at all times, particularly in New England. Compared to the death traps found in London, the sugar and rice fields of the West Indies and the Carolina Lowcountry, and the malarial swamps of the Chesapeake, New England was considered refreshingly healthful, especially in the seventeenth century when its isolated and thinly populated towns largely escaped the ravages of epidemic disease. By the 1720s, new concentrations in the population and more steady communication between places throughout the region and in the broader Atlantic world created an environment in which epidemics could violently erupt with deadly and terrifying force. Sailors from New England's ports, subject to tropical diseases on their voyages, could die at astonishing rates. But even when we take into consideration those years punctuated by epidemic and the bleak mortality rates for young men in the ports, demographers have found that New England's population was not eroded by disease in the manner of places where endemic maladies steadily claimed lives.[20]

New England was a place where the fortunate could survive illness, not avoid it. In this respect, New England was not that different from other places in the early modern world, especially as compared with the developed world today. Historians of morbidity and mortality have suggested that the kinds of diseases that have sickened and killed humankind have changed over the course of history. Like other places in the developed world, America has undergone an "epidemiological transition," from a preponderance of acute and infectious diseases of the early modern period to the chronic, degenerative maladies more characteristic of modern societies. In the eighteenth century, disease was less a constant presence in any individual's life than an episodic one. While a person stood an excellent chance of becoming ill at any given moment, those afflictions most often resolved quickly, leading to either death or relatively rapid recovery. For any given person, the chance of *falling* ill was greater than the chance of *being* ill. This is not to say that New Englanders did not have their share of chronic ailments; the elderly, in particular, who existed in greater number in New England than elsewhere, presented the problem of more steady infirmities. Injuries, too, could lead to chronic impairment and the need for constant treatment. But the picture of society as a whole is one of continual confrontation with episodic disease that moved through families, neighborhoods, and towns. Children and the elderly were known to be especially vulnerable. But when, where, and whom sickness would strike and with what intensity were open questions. In the meantime, other dimensions of daily life continued of necessity.[21]

Because it resided neither at the fringes of daily life nor at the center of it, illness in New England created, in our second meaning of the word, a province of affliction, a place in between, where health was common enough to fuel expectation and sickness common enough to beg for allowance; where vital activity coexisted with lethargy and incapacity; where the venerable aged, having outlived their peers, would recall many seasons of distress. It is this creative tension that flourished at the intersection between illness and health, the ongoing interplay between the prerogatives of the sick and those of the well, that interests me most profoundly.

BODIES IN A STATE OF BECOMING:
SOCIAL AND POLITICAL IMPLICATIONS

The medical historian Charles Rosenberg has suggested that the early modern body was "always in a state of becoming—and thus always in jeopardy." He reminds us that early moderns did not consider their bodies to be static, but rather constantly changing. Health was continually altered by a person's interaction with the natural environment, the "non-naturals" that she might partake in (including food, drink, exercise, and rest), and her success in moderating intake, processing, and outgo. Health consisted in a body in perfect balance but was fragile, easily disrupted, and in need of continuous adjustment and correction.[22] *The Province of Affliction* is, in a sense, an extended exploration of the social and political implications of Rosenberg's insight as they played out in individual lives and in the larger organization of and response to illness.

On one level, I hope to illuminate, by focusing on a small cast of characters, the personal plight of sick persons and the everyday, lived experience of inhabiting a world in which bodies were always in a state of becoming—the unsteadiness of their lives, the sudden changes that could come on, their own descent into illness, and the decline of those around them. Beginning with chapter 1 and continuing through the first two sections of the book, readers will become well-acquainted with Massachusetts residents Ebenezer Parkman (1703–1782), minister and farmer in Westborough; Ashley Bowen (1728–1813), sailor, ship rigger (and sometime soldier, dreamer, and artist) of Marblehead; and Elizabeth Porter Phelps (1747–1817), goodwife and good neighbor of Hadley. Here are three generations, representing three areas of Massachusetts, and three of the best diaries we have from the period. Of these, Parkman dominates: the temporal span of the diary, the depth and consistency of his entries, and his abiding interest in the illnesses of family, household workers, and flock make his journal invaluable for this study. In addition to these individual accounts, I have explored stories of affliction as revealed in petitions to general assemblies, which fortunately exist in large numbers. Here one finds the sentiments of the elderly, the middling and poor, the widow, the soldier and veteran, the Indian, and, less often, the free African American.

On another level, I aim to shed light on the societal implications of these stories of affliction. The book focuses on four recurring problems that illness presented routinely, not just for the sick and those immediately implicated in their illnesses, but for also townsfolk, selectmen, commissioners, reformers, and officials at all levels of government. I refer to these problems, sketched below, as extremity, locality, protection, and social suffering.

That the early modern body was always in a state of becoming helps us understand why the sick were able to command attention. There was, in the first place, the fear that even seemingly innocent difficulties could be transformed into something dire. Death was always a possibility, one that New Englanders seem to have taken to heart. As Maris Vinovskis, Daniel Scott Smith, and J. David Hacker have pointed out, New Englanders were convinced that mortality in the region was far greater than what modern demographers have found. It is not difficult to understand why. The high incidence of infant and childhood death (10–30% of children did not survive the first year of life), the rituals of death (at least 10–25 funerals per year in a small village), and the emphasis placed on the uncertainty of life in funeral sermons all encouraged New Englanders to think of life as fragile, even as survivors of the diseases of childhood and youth could live into their sixties and seventies. We can see in the fine-grained language used to describe serious conditions—those who were "poorly," "very poorly," "dangerous," "exceedingly dangerous," and so on—the sense that the body in a state of becoming could move swiftly toward its end.[23]

The possibility that one might fall ill—that one might be healthy today and ailing tomorrow—imbued daily life with a sense of radical contingency, which included the fear of death, but went well beyond it. Letter writers were careful, in making plans for future visits, to add the refrain "provided I am in health." Public meetings were postponed when ailing officials failed to attend, or forced to new locations when contagious distempers raged. Plaintiffs and defendants pleaded illness as the cause of their missed court dates; tax collectors complained that sickness (both their own and that of those who failed to pay) had interfered with their collections; and those long absent from church claimed to be sick and abed. There was enough regularity in these claims to provoke investigations into malingering. But more often than not, the excuses and alterations occasioned by ill health stood as an accepted, if unfortunate, part of life.

I refer throughout this book to this sense of urgency and necessary allowance in confronting illness as the problem of *extremity*. There was a point in any given illness at which the desires and prerogatives of the workaday world were trumped by the force of extremity. Not every sickness, nor every sick person, exercised the same power, of course. Ailing soldiers were forced to forge rivers and sleep in the cold. Persons marked as inferior in law, such as enslaved and free blacks in Boston, were asked to undertake risks to their health that persons of higher station and clout were able to refuse. During the terrifying smallpox epidemic that beset the town in 1721, free blacks were made to clean up refuse strewn about the streets, this at a time in which it was unclear whether such materials harbored the dread disease. There was no absolute standard for extremity; like other aspects of early modern life, extremity was marked by power and privilege.

Yet even for those occupying the lowest rungs of the social hierarchy, extremity could confer power, demanding attention and accommodation. Sick soldiers could simply drop and bring the rhythms of expeditionary warfare to a halt. Blacks in a smallpox-ridden city could, like whites, become sick and require nursing, cleansing, and quarantine. Field hands could suffer injuries and illnesses that absented them from work. Elite gatherings could be thwarted by the indisposition of servants. One was said to be "held" in the grasp of a fever, "gripped" at the guts, made "helpless" by rheumatism. Illness would have its sway.

The problem of *locality* takes us to the concrete places where persons actually fell ill. If the body in a state of becoming helps us access a dimension of lived time in early America—the on-again, off-again rhythms of persons moving into and out of health—the question of where the sick fell ill directs our attention to the connections between space and authority in early American life. Although historians often treat this question on a grand scale, addressing the tensions of westward expansion and the creation of territorial boundaries, illness illuminates a more intimate and immediate aspect of the relation between space and authority, and territorial boundaries, in particular—the problems that ensued when persons with bodies in a state of becoming fell ill where they did not belong.[24]

Illness was ideally conceived as the proper charge of local society. Families, neighbors, and towns were asked to take care of their own in times of need. Problems arose when persons fell sick away from those local sites of care. Early modern society was a world in constant motion. Daily routines revolved around visiting and exchange; apprenticeships took youths from their houses and placed them with others; trade, commerce, and warfare called persons even further afield. In all of these instances and more, persons could fall ill far from those properly charged with their care, which led to two problems. On the one hand, the local institutions responsible for care might have to stretch well beyond their daily borders. Families were obliged to retrieve members working in other households, to fetch ailing sons from the theater of war, or to rush to the scene in the aftermath of a daughter's difficult pregnancy or illness. Towns received notices from places far afield claiming that one of their own had fallen sick and needed to be retrieved. Even provinces and states could insist that the ailing be returned to where they properly belonged. On the other hand, if the sick lay in extremity, care was an immediate necessity. Bills and obligations easily piled up before the final seat of responsibility could be determined.

New Englanders wanted to have it both ways. They depended on a continuous movement of people to sustain everything from local economies to the successful prosecution of imperial warfare. But they also insisted on local responsibility for affliction. The result inevitably fueled disagreement. Despite indentures that specified that masters were to care for their servants, poor laws that carefully defined criteria for local inhabitancy (and so rights to town coffers should one become impoverished or ill), and provisions for government to pay for diseases visited upon soldiers in war, when persons fell ill away from their proper localities, confusion and contest ensued.

Although the problems of extremity and locality associated with illness can be found throughout the Atlantic world, they had special resonance in New England because of its commitment to *protection*. Beginning with its origins as a refuge from the corruptions of the Old World and as a shining example of a godly society, New England had promoted the need for community to protect its own. In "A Model of Christian Charity," John Winthrop suggested that New England's "City Upon a Hill" would have to act as a "community of perils," requiring "extraordinary liberality" from its members. "There is a time," Winthrop explained, when "a Christian must sell all and give to the poor, as they did in the Apostles' times." And there were other moments, as in ancient Macedonia, in which Christians would have to "give beyond their ability," although not all that they had. The community envisioned by Winthrop, in which persons of different stations were knit together in brotherly affection, required an exquisite "sensibleness and sympathy of each other's conditions," a "desire and endeavor to strengthen, defend, preserve and comfort the other." By the eighteenth century, Winthrop's sense of the immediate possibility of failure, of the peril of the utopian undertaking itself, had waned. But the sense of New England's special role as a place where the vulnerable would be protected continued. In the claims during the imperial crisis that English society had lost its moral footing, in the claims after the Revolution that the nation should be as New England writ large, the region promoted its special virtues in attending to local need. And like Winthrop, who made it clear that there were times and seasons for different kinds of giving, the abiding question remained just how much was required of the suffering and their protectors alike.[25]

The idea that neighbors should be their brother's keepers and that government was finally responsible for protecting the people became a link between society and politics in the colonial period that was especially evident in times of affliction. From the outset of settlement, New England's "town state," as Barry Levy has dubbed it, was remarkably active in its conception of social welfare. Towns became central governing bodies, carrying forward and amplifying cutting-edge reforms prompted by the traumas of Elizabethan and early Stuart England, most especially widespread poverty and plague and the social dislocations that emanated from the two. Public health measures, and quarantine efforts in particular, were promoted with a vigor in New England that flagged elsewhere. Drawing on Elizabethan Poor Laws, New England's "warning out" system, which demanded that those without legal settlement in a town post bond (or have it posted for them) and stand ready to be removed, not only ensured ready employment of town residents through its careful control of local labor markets, but also offered financial security in the event that outsiders fell ill. The imperative of protection fueled an activist local government in New England that became deeply implicated in social relations.[26]

And yet, the pervasive presence of sickness was not so readily accommodated. The quarantine measures meant to protect the public's health achieved a success that was finally ironic: the advent of large pockets of the population left unexposed to contagious diseases, such as smallpox, became fodder for epidemics that burned through the region. The warning-out system, so elegant in its assignment of responsibility for misfortune to the localities in which a person had legal settlement or to those who sponsored outsiders in town, could not keep pace with the swift descent of maladies. Strangers who had been "warned" but remained in town (a not uncommon occurrence) fell ill and their condition demanded attention in its extremity, leaving caregivers and others to petition their towns for relief and towns to engage in protracted court battles with one another over rightful settlement. The steady integration of New England within empire only amplified the difficulties: commerce and Atlantic travel increased the possibilities for contagion, as did the four wars for empire fought between 1689 and 1763.

In the end, the pressures placed upon the sick and those implicated in their afflictions radiated outward in eighteenth-century life, from family, to neighborhood, to town, to provincial and later state government. Approaching their governors with their heads down and hands out, the people asked for relief. In this sense, the political culture of the colonial period was one in which governance was enacted not just by law, but by numerous exceptions and allowances accorded the afflicted in their time of need.[27]

The commitment to protection, within towns and communities and in the interaction of subjects and citizens with the General Court, highlights a key element of monarchical political culture that was forceful enough to carry into the early republic. When Congress first convened, it heard from hundreds of petitioners asking for consideration of their particular circumstances. Faced with the prospect of becoming the ultimate source of protection for all of the people in all of the states in the nation, federal officials worked to limit the kinds of claims they would consider. Congress continued to hear stories of distress from ordinary citizens, but it also made it clear that affliction was best addressed at the level of local society and governance. That shift in political culture, which we see most clearly in the case of sick and disabled soldiers asking for relief in the 1790s, represents the beginning of a major rethinking of the role of government in the lives of the people.[28]

Finally, I refer to the accumulated weight of the problems that inhered in extremity, locality, and protection as leading to *social suffering*. To an astonishing degree, suffering in New England was a social affair. The sickness of a single individual implicated many others, something revealed continuously in the diaries, correspondence, and government records from the period. Illness was visible because its costs—social, economic, political—were manifest to all. Each sickness created its own society. And when that society was pushed beyond its means, sufferers and their supporters turned to government—town, province, state—for aid. There was, finally, the possibility of a political answer to social suffering.

⁓

The Province of Affliction explores the personal, familial, and governmental struggles over who would be finally responsible for sickness and debility in early New England. In the end, the book reveals how affliction tended to overwhelm the individuals, families, households, and towns that knew the sufferers best. The latent power of illness steadily threatened to exceed the capacities of different levels of society. Families, households, and communities cared for their own, backed by the possibility of town support, until they were overwhelmed by disruption and distress. Towns, province, and state did the same, and the logic of illness pushed toward a larger role for higher levels of government.

The enduring theme throughout the eighteenth century was that the province of affliction continuously threatened to overrun the metropole of health, and as it did so, the building blocks of society and government were defined, tested, and maintained. At the turn of the nineteenth century, with an incipient bureaucracy tasked with accommodating social suffering, cost-conscious measures were introduced to limit the state and federal government's responsibility for mitigating the effects of illness. But the new medical charities that developed in the breach—such as the Dispensary, Female Societies for the Sick, and the Massachusetts General Hospital—also found themselves overwhelmed. A new era in accommodating affliction had begun, but the old problems endured.

The continuing relevance of these tensions today has drawn me to this material and influenced my sense of its urgency—an attraction, but also something of a liability, in writing the history of illness. My hope for this book is that it will provide historical depth to our present discussions without succumbing to "presentism."[29]

There is surely enough that is familiar in the story of New Englanders and their confrontations with illness to suggest ready and even necessary comparisons with our time. The social and political costs of their struggles are everywhere manifest in records of daily life. Their heavy labors and the considerable strain in designating responsibility for the ill counter our temptation to see in the past the warm glow of communities taking care of their own. As Darrett Rutman has written, the little communities of early America rested on "a congeries of interacting neighbors—more, of *good* neighbors—but only because it had to be that way."[30] They did what they felt compelled to do, following the Golden Rule and a social logic that called for interdependency. But they also spoke freely of their frustrations and worries in doing so. And in a world of dangers, where illness was considered both inevitable and costly, they looked upward and outward for assistance. To a striking degree, early American governance was bound up in social welfare. There was no positive and encompassing "right" to health care in early America. None of the state constitutions (or the federal constitution) provide such a right, beyond the stipulation that government was meant to protect the welfare of the people.[31] But in their efforts to seek relief from the costs of affliction, eighteenth-century New Englanders exercised their prerogative to ask government for protection, for allowance, and for exceptions to the rules. Recent scholarship has reminded us just how long the history of entitlements has been in America, reaching back at least to the early national period. In ending where those stories begin, I hope to show even earlier continuities in social provision, as well as what was lost as programs were created that singled out particular groups of citizens for benefits.[32]

But for all of its familiarity and contemporary resonance, there is enough that is odd and even jarring in these pages to remind us not just that this is the world from which we have emerged, but also that, for better or worse, much of it has been left behind. The book will have in some small measure succeeded if it can add people stricken by illness and all those implicated in their afflictions to our imagining of the past. Let us watch them take center stage in the province of affliction.

OVERVIEWS

CHAPTER ONE

A Tour of the Province: October 18, 1769

One does not have to venture far in the sources of early modern life to encounter affliction. The swift descent of epidemics of smallpox, measles, and assorted fevers; the lingering presence of cancers, ulcers, swellings, and sores; and the accounts of the indisposed and unwell: these were vital commonplaces inscribed in everything from journals and letters to the proceedings of courts and legislatures.

While subsequent chapters will consider illness systematically in family and household, town and province, and state and national government, this chapter takes a different approach, choosing a day on which a cluster of sources reveals how the routines of everyday life were forced to accommodate and absorb the demands created by illness. On an October day in 1769, we can see rural, intimate settings in which friends and good neighbors gathered around the afflicted, but also the measures taken by Boston selectmen trying to contain an outbreak of smallpox, and even the ways in which illness was implicated in the most pressing political matter of the day—an escalating imperial crisis. Our tour of the province of affliction begins in central Massachusetts.

I. OCTOBER 18, 1769: HOPKINTON, MASSACHUSETTS—NIGHT AND MORNING

The Reverend Ebenezer Parkman awoke that Wednesday morning and recalled that his friend and fellow minister, Samuel Barrett, had "several turns of Bleeding" through the night. Since their time as classmates at Harvard (AB 1721) and their call to pulpits a half-day ride from each other, Barrett and Parkman had seen each other frequently over the years, especially for "ministers' meetings" in which the two men and other clergy in central Massachusetts gathered together to discuss matters of doctrine, theology, church discipline, and controversies that regularly arose. A meeting was supposed to have taken place at Barrett's parsonage in Hopkinton on Tuesday, October 17. But after Parkman was the only minister to arrive, and hastily sent reminders to their colleagues had no effect, the two men resigned themselves to failure. They dined together, and Parkman agreed to spend the night. Parkman was well accustomed to adapting to such disappointments. Even though the intellectual arena was filled with minds sharpened by voracious reading habits and committed to preserving an orderly society, the social arena was anything but precise— missed messages, lame horses, harsh weather, and, of course, illness itself disrupted well-laid plans. For Parkman, this occasion, like many others, was at once a source of frustration and an opportunity to practice patience. "Probably the unusual cold, Windy, rough Weather might hinder the aged and infirm," Parkman surmised, "but what may be the reason of the delinquency of Others, I can't conjecture."[1]

That night, as the two men lay in Barrett's house, the sixty-eight-year-old Barrett had his "turns" of bleeding, the ordeal leaving him "faint and dizzy" in the morning. Parkman said little else about the incident. It was, like much else in his diary, an event recorded as noteworthy without further explication of its significance. But we can imagine several contexts that attracted Parkman's attention and imbued Barrett's bleeding with meaning. The therapeutic use of bleeding and the culture of self-diagnosis and cure within the medical marketplace, the spiritual significance of the bleeding and suffering body, and the social implications of accommodating one who had lost blood—all of these contexts help us better understand what Parkman saw and understood that night and morning.

It is possible that the "turns" were intentional. Bleeding, or the opening of a vein to release blood, was a common therapeutic device in eighteenth-century New England. Whether drawing on an earlier "humoral" conception of the body as composed of liquids (blood, phlegm, yellow and black bile) or more recent "solidistic" understandings of the body as machine, bleeding was thought a potent method of restoring the body to the perfect balance that was health. The letting of blood might rid the body of its excesses, brace it in the face of debilitation, prevent blockages, and open new pathways for vital energy.[2]

Barrett would have been well-acquainted with bleeding, though by 1769 he may have been out of practice. Barrett was one of the few remaining "preacher-physicians" in New England, a line of divines reaching back to the seventeenth century who had coupled their ministerial practice with that of healer. Such men were common through the colonial period in New England, a testament to the limited numbers of physicians in the early days of settlement, the need for ministers to find by-employments to supplement their meager salaries, and the broader cultural authority of men who could command the Word. In addition to being a minister, Barrett had been a sometime surgeon, a tooth puller, and a general physician. He had treated many, including Parkman himself some thirty years earlier, when he was stricken with a severe bout of rheumatic fever, the effects of which—periods of fever, numbness, and even partial paralysis— would continue throughout Parkman's life.[3]

But by 1769 preacher-physicians were on the wane, replaced by others in an increasingly competitive medical marketplace, not least by the steady growth of "doctors" (a term that might apply to one who undertook the practices, either singly or in combination, of a physician, surgeon, or apothecary), nearly five hundred of whom were in practice in Massachusetts in 1770. Trained through apprenticeship and, less commonly, through formal education in Europe, doctors increased at a faster rate than the population at large in Massachusetts, sometimes needing to resettle several times before finding an area not already saturated with practitioners. In 1758 Parkman and his family were regularly seeing three doctors whose circuit included Parkman's home town of Westborough, and the minister had discouraged a prospective physician from settling there; apparently, there would not be enough work. If Barrett had wanted to be bled in 1769, he would likely have had to call a doctor or his assistant. Midwives do not appear to have engaged in bloodletting, and while knowledgeable neighbors might bleed a sick animal, phlebotomy was left to trained male practitioners.[4]

But interest in blood, and in healing more generally, extended well beyond doctors. Even if Barrett's "turns of bleeding" were simply the loss of blood through the night, perhaps the most likely scenario, it is not surprising that Parkman took note. Body fluids were subject to public scrutiny and discussion in eighteenth-century life. Diuretics, cathartics, purges, and emetics were meant to expel sweat, urine, feces, and vomit from the body, and it was important to note the frequency of such emissions, their color and texture, and their smell. In a similar fashion, blood was analyzed for what it said about the body's health. When blood emerged from the inners on its own accord (as an "involuntary discharge"), it attracted attention, not least in efforts to properly regulate or stem its flow. Bleeding itself, whether from the nose, ears, eyes, mouth, and bowels—in "spitting blood," "vomiting blood," "bleeding and blind piles" (hemorrhoids), or "bloody flux" (dysentery)—was a common enough occurrence to be treated in some detail in popular healing guides of the time; these included *Every Man his own Doctor* (1734), John Wesley's *Primitive Physick* (1747), and William Buchan's influential *Domestic Medicine* (1769), all reprinted many times in America through the late eighteenth and nineteenth centuries.[5]

Because the well lived in close quarters with the ailing, they could not easily avoid the material products of sickness like blood. Many eighteenth-century folks seem, in fact, to have been drawn to comment on the condition of the ill. It was commonly believed that the exterior of the body might be read for signs of interior states; countenance, complexion, and disposition provided clues about the extent to which he or she was veering into illness. Even as the sick themselves noted how the peculiarities of their constitution interacted with the environment to produce illness or health, commonplace references by the unafflicted to the ailments of family members, neighbors, townsfolk, and the like suggest an abiding interest in the health of others. Parkman had a keen eye for bodily woes, which he noted in his regular accounts of visits to his parishioners and others. He had made just these sorts of notes on his friend Samuel Barrett and his wife for many years. He knew when Mrs. Barrett suffered from the "gravel" (kidney stones) and when the minister labored under a "very low and wasting state," which Parkman attributed to Barrett's service twenty-four years earlier as a surgeon during the Siege of Louisbourg. Now he could add bleeding to the tally.[6]

Beyond therapeutic bleeding and lay understandings of blood, Parkman may also have considered the spiritual aspects of his friend's "turns" through the night. Well into the eighteenth century, many thought illness presented a challenge to faith, a special "trial" in which the sick might examine the state of their soul, ask for forgiveness, and, with God's grace, be restored. Seventeenth-century writers such as Anne Bradstreet considered her afflictions to be the "corrections" of a generous God who gave her the means to bring Him forward and leave the ensnarements of the temporal world behind. Afflictions offered a means of improvement; her "greatest getting" came in moments of malaise. In Cotton Mather's *Angel of Bethesda* (1724), he wrote that afflictions might be considered "love-tokens" of a long-suffering God. Conceived of as a "Family-Physician," a practical guide for families in treating bodily maladies and preserving health, Mather's manuscript offered remedies for everything from gout to worms to asthma, but no cure could be effected unless the soul was cleansed. Each cough was a chance to pray; confession was the most

powerful emetic; and renewal came only through the heightened aware-
ness of the sacrifice of Christ. Illness was man's just punishment for original sin and his daily iniquities, but it was also an opportunity for self-
reflection, humiliation, repentance, and renewal.[7]

There were elements of this seventeenth-century world that Parkman
had left behind. Ralph Josselin (1616–1683), vicar of Earls Colne, England,
saw the black and "corrupt" matter festering in an infected navel as so
much sin oozing from his corrupt body. Mather thought it possible to
"cough up" sin. Parkman's view of sin, however, was not as palpably material as that of those living in the seventeenth-century Atlantic, nor as
tightly knit to the body as it was in what Robert St. George has called the
"densely metaphoric" landscape of colonial New England. While Parkman
was humbled by evidences of God's awesome wonders—the great storms
and natural disasters that wracked the eighteenth-century world—he was
less concerned with working out the little evidences of God's direct handi-
work in his life. While Parkman certainly saw connections between the
microcosm and the macrocosm, they were less specific and direct than
those noted by his seventeenth-century predecessors.[8]

But Parkman did subscribe, and profoundly so, to the idea that sickness was a call to turn inward and consider matters of the soul. Born in
1703, he had been instructed in the "school of affliction," as some called
it, and actively inquired into the personal meanings of suffering. In 1729
he sat down to record "the more remarkable Mercies of God to Me in the
Course of His Providence" since a "memorable dangerous Sickness" that
he had survived as a young schoolboy. Parkman returned again and again
to the many trials presented by his afflictions, to the dance of body and
spirit in which the decline of the body inspired fear, doubt, confusion, repentance, and finally new seasons of God's grace. As an evangelizing minister, Parkman encouraged his flock to view illness in this fashion. Some
bridled at the effort, resenting his intrusions and insistence that they turn
inward to consider their assurances of salvation as death approached. But
many in Parkman's church took his message to heart. Public testimonies
written by the laity or dictated to the minister and read before his congregation as evidence of God's saving grace often centered on affliction as key
moments of trauma and transformation.[9]

When Parkman witnessed Barrett's bleeding, it would have been perfectly natural for him to move from the concerns of the body to the larger
drama of the salvation of the soul. The failures of the human body were
evidence of man's fall and the suffering that was his fate to accommodate
and endure. One could only hope to be forgiven and cleansed through the

sacrifice of Jesus, itself marked vividly with the savior's blood. "O that God would pardon my numberless Defects," Parkman pleaded in his diary in 1770, "and wash me in the Blood of the Lamb!"[10]

Alongside the medical and religious aspects of bleeding, there was, finally, a social dimension, a balance to be struck between expectations placed on the sick and the accommodations that one who lay prostrate and weak could command. Without any record of their conversations about the arrangement, we can only surmise that both men had questions to ask of themselves and obligations to fulfill after Barrett's night of bleeding. In a ritual repeated with endless variations throughout the eighteenth century, the sick would be asked to continue as much as possible with workaday affairs; and those around them would be asked to accommodate as much as possible the inevitable delays and absences that attended affliction.

Before he left Barrett that afternoon, Parkman borrowed his friend's copy of Cotton Mather's *Magnalia Christi Americana* (1702), an enormously ambitious history of New England that chronicled the peculiar trials faced by God's chosen people in their errand into the wilderness, including numerous portraits of seventeenth-century divines and their special grace in suffering. Parkman could only hope to emulate their example. For his part, Barrett was prepared to follow suit. Having bled through the night and endured a woozy morning, he headed out with Parkman that afternoon to attend Wednesday lecture. Strong enough to journey to the meetinghouse but still too weak to preach, Barrett would sit with the others in his congregation. Parkman would be obliged to fill in. Such was the mixture of perseverance and forbearance that made up the province of affliction.

☙

We know about everyday events such as "turns of bleeding" because eighteenth-century New Englanders deemed them worthy of written record and comment. Blood could be "read" in many ways, a few of which we have highlighted here. But above all, linking its medical, religious, and social contexts, blood figured in contemporary efforts to record fluidity and motion in daily affairs. Turns of bleeding throughout the night remind us that the early modern body was "always in a state of becoming—and thus always in jeopardy."[11]

It was that movement of the person's body into and out of health, its rapid oscillations, that opened a field for thought and action. Bleeding meant change, and change invited comment—from lay healers and others who interpreted the material essence of blood; from the pious who would see in it another reminder that the temporal world was a fleeting thing and that one could rest with God alone; and from those who found their friends and neighbors in health one day and bleeding and weak the next.

It was one thing to notice sickness, to comment on a world in which sudden change was common and inflected in many ways. But sickness called for action as well. In addition to therapeutic and spiritual interventions, there were the questions of social expectation and political allowance: How much could be asked of the sick, of their caregivers, and of the public at large?

These questions arose in the Connecticut River Valley, where two young women were summoned during the night to the bedside of a widow lying in "extremity." Here, John Winthrop's fervent hope that New Englanders might act as if living in a "community of perils," sharing in each other's infirmity and misfortune, was very much alive.

II. OCTOBER 18, 1769: HADLEY, MASSACHUSETTS— AFTERNOON AND NIGHT

"Wednesday at several places of errands," Elizabeth Porter wrote with her usual brevity in logging daily affairs. "[D]rank tea at Moses Keloggs—at night I went and Silence Bartlett and I watched with old Mrs. Smith." At age twenty-one, Porter was two generations removed from Parkman and Barrett. Her home in Hadley, Massachusetts, in the fertile Connecticut River Valley, offered opportunities for large-scale agriculture that was as close as New England came to rivaling the booming production of tobacco, wheat, and other grains that sustained the Mid-Atlantic and Chesapeake. Porter came from a leading family, one of the so-called "River Gods," an elite class that, despite living deep in the hinterland of Massachusetts, was able to achieve a level of refinement and comfort more often enjoyed by the metropolitan elite (if not the grand style of the plantation South). "Forty Acres," the Porters' estate of some 640 acres, lay a few miles outside of town. Named in the fashion of English country manors, its Georgian architecture modeled from English pattern books and its public facades adorned with clapboards carved to look like stone, Forty Acres sat atop provincial society.[12]

In all of these ways, Porter's world was distanced from the more modest surroundings of Parkman and Barrett. But her active participation in the social economy of affliction would have been utterly familiar. If the graciousness of "tea at Moses Keloggs" set Porter apart from many others in town and beyond, "watching" through the night with the sick and dying was practiced everywhere, particularly by unmarried women, those past childbearing years, or those with daughters or servants old enough to manage the household in their absence.

Before Elizabeth Porter and Silence Bartlett watched together with the widow Smith that night, their days had likely been shaped differently by the imperatives and prerogatives of class. At age eighteen, Bartlett worked regularly as a tailor at Forty Acres. Her father, Caleb, owned an estate assessed at £52 in 1770, the median for Hadley (though a mere one-fifth of that of Charles Phelps Jr., Elizabeth Porter's future husband), and added to his income by sweeping Hadley's meetinghouse floors. Silence had begun to visit Forty Acres in 1768 with her mother, eventually tailoring for Daniel Worthington, who had for several years managed the Porters' farm, and spending a night or two at the estate as she completed her work. Even in Porter's terse diary entries, it is possible to detect a friendship between the women. A few years apart in age and unmarried (Porter would marry a year later), they shared the social world built around women's textile work, which had the potential to bring women together across class lines; in July 1769 Porter recorded "going up to help Silence Bartlett quilt" and staying the night when a thunderstorm roared in. And a half year after Bartlett started work at Forty Acres, we find Porter and two cousins taking her off for a late summer's day of "whortleberrying."[13]

But Bartlett was not at tea with Porter that afternoon on October 18, nor does it appear that she ever had tea with her. These were times reserved for Porter's "dear friends" and "ladies," as were the singing classes she also attended, in which one learned, practiced, and displayed the habits of the refined. Moses Kelogg, whose household hosted the tea that day, belonged to a leading family in town. Two Keloggs were among the largest landholders in Hadley, and while Moses possessed a more moderate estate, his family stood out in a town of some seven hundred persons. He had acquired a fine sleigh in 1769, the likes of which were owned by just a handful of families in town and, like carriages that brought the elite to other occasions (including community events such as quiltings), a mark of wealth and refinement.[14]

In the evening, Elizabeth Porter and Silence Bartlett arrived at the widow Smith's and watched through the night. The widow Smith had been ill for several months. She was in a low enough condition to warrant the church's prayers in late August, when Porter's mother had gone to visit her. Now, as she worsened, watchers were summoned. Watchers like Porter and Bartlett were expected to administer to the afflicted, who might request tea, simple conversation, a damp cloth to mute a fever, or consoling words from the Bible or devotional tracts. These were modest requests in comparison with the power commanded by the sick that one can find at other times and places. Jesuits in seventeenth-century New France, for example, recorded entire Indian villages engaging in feasts, games, and dances to fulfill the dream-inspired wishes of the sick. But as guardians of the afflicted, charged with the care and comfort of those who lay close to death, watchers in New England were engaged in a serious undertaking, and their labors were celebrated even by critics of the colonial world writing later in the nineteenth century. Even though many in the early modern Atlantic awoke at night for extended periods of reflection, writing, work, and intimacy, an entire night spent watching was onerous. Beyond their efforts on behalf of the sick, watchers had to confront the fear, cold, and damp that lay beyond the candle and fireplace. It was common for watchers to arrive in pairs, as Porter and Bartlett had, which afforded company, the ability to share the work, and the chance to talk together about critical changes in the sick person's condition before waking others in the house.[15]

Elizabeth Porter and Silence Bartlett had shared an intense experience, but we may imagine that the aftermath of the night revealed differences between the women. Porter did not record anything in her diary about the following day; perhaps it was a blur after the night spent watching. We do not know what happened to Bartlett, who like the vast majority of early Americans did not have the leisure time to keep a diary. But given that her wages were critical for her family's middling subsistence, she would not have had much time to recover. Although both women faced the moral imperative to be good neighbors in community, Porter had greater means to do so.[16]

By Friday, Elizabeth Porter was back at Forty Acres, hosting a deacon who lodged at the house. When Silence Bartlett returned to Forty Acres in early November to spend a week tailoring, perhaps the friends talked about the latest developments in the province of affliction—that the minister's wife had been "taken poorly" and several young women had gone to the parsonage to help, that the minister had been so weakened by rheumatism that another had preached in his place, and that the widow Smith, after several months of severe illness, had finally died.[17]

∞

"Watching" through the night represents one of the most enduring examples we have of the sacrifices that might be required of those living in a "community of peril." More than a century after John Winthrop had articulated his vision of a community that would be knit together through love and an exquisite "sensibleness and sympathy of each other's conditions," watchers like Elizabeth Porter and Silence Bartlett fulfilled the obligation to "strengthen, defend, preserve and comfort the other."

Winthrop's community of peril cast a long shadow. In the late nineteenth century, the physician, reformer, and antiquarian Edward Jarvis looked back on the rituals of community life that drew from the past—the corn huskings, barn raisings, quiltings, and the like—and found that many of them had been usefully replaced. While there was much to admire in this earlier spirit of "cooperation," the people of his hometown of Concord, Massachusetts, had developed more economical, efficient, and self-directed means of accomplishing what had formerly been done through collective efforts. Although Jarvis made it clear to his readers that his contemporaries were now more "happy," "prosperous," and refined in their manners, he also insisted that his fellow townsmen had not forgotten the best that the earlier world had to offer. Residents of his Concord were still "loving, generous and ready to aid in distress, poverty and sickness, whenever they shall present themselves in any family or neighborhood." Despite the changes in society, culture, and politics wrought in the nineteenth century, sickness and distress continued to create community, an observation borne out in recent scholarship that has emphasized the ongoing "social" realm of mutuality, reciprocity, and local allegiances that flourished in antebellum New England and beyond.[18]

In the twenty-first century, when "watching" and other community efforts surrounding affliction have waned, one needs to avoid the temptation to romanticize such practices. If watching was a source of community connection, it also was implicated in social inequality and exclusion. Watching placed unequal burdens on community members—women watched more frequently than men, single women more than married women, and young women more than old. In the nineteenth century, when women working for pay faced a conflict between the imperative to care for sick relatives and the benefits of wages for the worker and her family, it is easier to detect the social and financial stakes involved in nursing the sick. In the eighteenth century, although the sacrifices women made in the name of watching and in longer stints of nursing are not raised as explicitly in the historical record, they may be glimpsed in diaries of single women charged with caring for family and in the occasional murmurings of matriarchs that found their way onto the written page.[19]

Moreover, not every illness evoked the same community response. It mattered not just that someone in the community was sick, but who that someone was. Finally, there were limits to what communities would do for the ill, no matter what their station. We will return to these topics at some length in the following chapter.

For now, let us move from Hadley to Boston, where we can see the ways in which the extreme conditions of sickness first absorbed by family and neighbors could bubble up into the civic sphere and become a central focus of governance.

III. OCTOBER 18, 1769: BOSTON, MASSACHUSETTS— THE ROUTINES OF SMALLPOX

As Ebenezer Parkman was filling in for his weary fellow minister and Elizabeth Porter was preparing to spend a night watching, four of Boston's selectmen met to discuss ongoing efforts to contain an outbreak of smallpox. The immediate order of business was to decide whether a young family—one Isaac Tuckerman, his wife, Mary, their infant son, and two nurses who had been assigned to them—was fit to return to town after being quarantined at Rainsford Island in Boston Harbor. The significance of that moment derives not from any immediate fear registered in the selectmen's records, but rather in the routine measures employed to contain the potential for a lethal epidemic.[20]

The fact that Bostonians faced epidemics of smallpox was, ironically, a sign of the city's stringent and successful public health measures. Whereas cities such as Philadelphia suffered from endemic disease, an outgrowth of lesser precautions and sluggish enforcement, Boston had been at the vanguard of public health measures in the Atlantic world. The pioneering quarantine efforts in the late seventeenth century, aimed at isolating ships infected with smallpox and other infectious diseases and imposing quarantines on those suspected of contagious sickness, met resistance initially from the Lords of Trade and finally from the Privy Council, which deemed the measures capricious and subject to abuse. But the General Court persevered, and Boston's success in isolating infected goods and persons meant that exposure that would confer immunity to such diseases as smallpox was limited, leaving large portions of the population vulnerable to the disease at any given time.[21]

By the 1760s, although Boston had been surpassed by New York and Philadelphia in both population and commercial fortunes, it still lay at the center of trade and commercial exchange in New England. With a population of around fifteen thousand after several decades of slow decline, the town was ten times bigger than most other towns in the region. While Boston was not a primary site for immigration, many sailors, soldiers, and other "strangers" passed through the town or were confined to its almshouse or workhouse when they found themselves down on their luck. Still a key site for trade along the Atlantic coast with the West Indies and with regions in British North America and the wider Atlantic, Boston saw its share of "contagious distempers," including smallpox.[22]

The pox had been working its way through the town since June 1769. Compared to the terrors visited upon Boston in 1721—when, after a twenty-year absence, the pox had claimed 842 lives, infected nearly five thousand more, and led to near riots over the newly introduced practice of inoculation—the events of the last several months were tame. This time about forty people had been infected over several months, a regular enough occurrence in Boston to warrant a staid reception. By 1769 Boston had a well-known series of measures that the selectmen implemented at the first sign of infestation. Their response to the Tuckermans, and their handling of the outbreak as a whole, shows how potentially very dangerous situations were folded into daily affairs.[23]

The Tuckermans' case before the selectmen on October 18 was more complicated than others, though by no means unique. Mary Tuckerman had been stricken in early September. An initial inquiry revealed that she had recently delivered a child and in her lying-in could not be removed safely from the house. Under ordinary circumstances, she and her family might have been taken immediately to the province "hospital" on the west side of town (a "pesthouse" in which the sick might be placed); or else the family might have been sent to Rainsford Island in Boston Harbor, the primary site since 1737 for incoming ships to be quarantined when smallpox or other virulent distempers were detected on board. But given the weakened condition of mother and child, the selectmen arranged for local quarantine. This was not uncommon, but it involved considerable effort on the part of the town and disruption for those who lived near the infected. In this case, like many others, special accommodations had to be made for the severely ill.[24]

The selectmen ordered that a red flag be placed outside the Tuckermans' house, fences hastily built around it, and a guard appointed (Mary Tuckerman's brother William) to block all traffic to and from the house except for those given special permission. They also appointed a nurse to minister to Mary Tuckerman and her child; if no one could be found to serve voluntarily, the selectmen had the power to impress nurses and others in a time of potential crisis. As a last precaution, the selectmen asked that those especially vulnerable, such as children who had not already been exposed to the infection, leave the area. In all of these ways, the selectmen required that Bostonians accommodate an extreme situation.

While the Tuckermans were permitted to remain in their house, they, too, were obliged to follow strict orders; nothing could happen without the permission of the selectmen. For nearly a month, the stricken family was made to wait inside the house and let smallpox take its course. When the selectmen began to allow members of the household to leave, they did so cautiously, making a judgment in each case as to the suitability of release. A nurse placed in charge of the baby (likely a wet nurse who suckled the infant) was the first to be allowed to leave on September 27 and was promptly sent to Rainsford Island for cleansing. Next the Tuckermans were removed from the house and sent to the hospital in west Boston for a week before being carried to Rainsford Island to await permission to return to town.

Finally, on October 18 (the day of our tour) the selectmen decided that the family might come back to town, though all of their things "liable to Infection" would need to be sent to the island and cleansed.

⌀

The routine handling of smallpox outbreaks offers a vivid example of how extreme conditions were incorporated into daily life. Throughout the colonial period, periodic outbreaks and epidemics of measles, influenza, whooping cough, and mumps, as well as generic agues and fevers, struck New England. In the seventeenth century, the relative isolation of towns in the region had made it more difficult for contagious disease to thrive among the European settlers (the same cannot be said of the natives, who suffered nothing less than a demographic catastrophe: a lethal combination of new diseases and the devastating social consequences that followed in their wake). By the eighteenth century, epidemics increased in frequency and intensity in New England, promoted by increases in population and mobility. The terrible wave of "throat distemper" (now believed to be diphtheria or scarlet fever) that coursed through New England in the late 1730s and early 1740s proved especially devastating, killing large numbers of children and provoking a larger debate about whether the disease was contagious.[25]

Bostonians and other coastal residents were especially familiar with managing regular outbreaks of smallpox and other "contagious distempers." Boston had been vigorous and inventive in devising aggressive responses to smallpox and other diseases deemed infectious; it had faced major smallpox epidemics in 1701, 1721, 1730, 1752, and 1764. Between these larger epidemics were smaller outbreaks, particularly of smallpox, that threatened to develop into something much more severe, and therefore called for a robust public health response. These outbreaks were more common in the ports and along major trade routes than in less-traveled inland areas. Thirty miles west of Boston, residents of Ebenezer Parkman's Westborough could remain untroubled by Boston's woes in 1769; the same was true of Elizabeth Porter's Hadley, where connections along the Connecticut River to Hartford and New London were stronger than ties to Boston in any case. Neither Parkman nor Porter even mention the outbreak in Boston in their diaries for that year. For inland towns, it would take a more spectacular epidemic elsewhere or a more direct brush with the pox to register in local affairs. Coastal ports like Marblehead, Massachusetts, however, set up guards at town entrances in 1769 to keep out or quarantine all who had been to Boston, just as they had five years earlier during a much more severe outbreak in the city. In the meantime, Boston's townsfolk and selectmen had to deal with the threat of smallpox as a more routine affair.[26]

In comparison to developments in the United States later in the nineteenth century, eighteenth-century responses to public health threats can seem weak and fleeting. There were neither permanent boards of health staffed by medical men nor robust police forces capable of enforcing regulations. There was no fully realized vision of the importance of promoting health as a public good or as a means of increasing the country's productive capacities. In the long history of public health in America, the eighteenth century is most often contrasted with a much more powerful public health regime and a broader conception of public health that developed later.[27]

But during the outbreaks themselves, town fathers in eighteenth-century Boston and elsewhere in Massachusetts could exercise considerable power in the name of protecting the public, something that set the city apart from other ports in British North America. As we have seen, the selectmen could quarantine and evict the sick, impress nurses to care for them, and enforce a regimen of cleansing. Their powers also included substantial control over commerce, including the ability to admit or deny entrance to ships carrying persons or goods into town. All reports of potential cases, all directions to those tending the ill, and all public notices concerning the outbreaks had to go through the selectmen. Although the response to any individual case could proceed in an ad hoc fashion—for example, the necessity of quarantine could be made initially by a local physician—the selectmen enjoyed final authority and did their best to exercise it.

We might expect resistance in the late eighteenth century to the extent of the selectmen's powers in public health, particularly their ability to seize property and determine the placement of household members, including the head of the household. The legal authority of patriarchs to control their own property and the property and labor of their dependents— their wives, children, and servants—grew steadily through the eighteenth century and into the antebellum period.[28] The persons ordered about by the selectmen in an epidemic were not only the impoverished, but also freemen, whose household control was made to bend to the will of the town fathers. By 1769 in Boston and elsewhere, a larger public discussion was taking place about the nature of public authority, the consensual basis of governance, and the fear that property taken without consent, by taxation or otherwise, was tantamount to slavery. The Boston selectmen's intrusion in household affairs through the seizure of property, and the added insult that those stricken would be made to pay for such seizures and the attendant cleansing, must have rankled.

Yet there is little evidence of overt or extensive challenges in the 1769 outbreak to the selectmen's authority or of principled objections to their interventions. The absence of such resistance speaks to the deep and long-standing moral justification for the selectmen's action—that they took measures for the public's safety and protection. In the seventeenth century, the notion that the "fathers of the town" acted in the name of the public good might justify any number of interventions in household affairs. The ideal family was to function as a "little commonwealth" in which the patriarch protected his dependents in exchange for their allegiance and submission, mirroring the relations between the governors and the people at large. When family government seemed to break down, it was not uncommon for the town fathers to intervene. The selectmen's powers in regard to smallpox related to this broader authority of the orderly community to exercise oversight and discipline over its members. Over the course of the eighteenth century, the practice of intruding into family affairs appears to have declined, and the legal powers granted to household heads increased. But the notion that the people's governors were obligated to protect the public, and that public health regulations were a critical means of protection, endured. When laws concerning the "people's welfare"—for example, regarding quarantine and the regulation of noxious trades—were elaborated in the antebellum era, they were drawing on a well-established precedent from the colonial period.[29]

The selectmen thus had the legal and cultural authority during a time of potential crisis to exercise power. Outwardly, the selectmen presented the calm face of order, issuing stern warnings about the crime of willful "concealment" of the pox and announcing all of the latest news on the outbreak in the local papers while emphasizing the limited scope of infections and their successful efforts at containment.[30]

But if the public presentation of their response to the outbreak demonstrated control and composure, the meeting minutes of the selectmen reveal the anxiety that attended their duties. Even with a routine in place and relatively few persons sick, the selectmen met frequently, sometimes several times a week, to determine what should be done to avoid a crisis. They worried that some of the infected were not coming forward, particularly the British soldiers (and their wives and children) who had been brought to Boston a year earlier to quell what Parliament considered riotous behavior. They were concerned as well that some were intentionally infecting themselves with the pox through self-inoculation, a practice that would protect the inoculee but had the potential to spread the distemper further through town. They puzzled over different sources of the outbreak, which seemed to be emanating not just from the soldiers and their families and elsewhere in town, but also from ships and sailors.

The selectmen also worried about the aftermath of the smallpox outbreak. How deeply would the town's economy be hurt? In order to attract traders to the town, the selectmen needed to assure any potential arrivals that the threat of the pox was contained. But if the selectmen were too strict in their enforcement, the town might acquire a reputation as a place inhospitable to commerce. Certainly, merchants and ship captains had interests in a less strict quarantine, a brief stopover at Rainsford Island, and then on to trading in the town before profits vanished as ships sat in the harbor. At what point would traders move elsewhere, avoiding Boston altogether? While in times of crisis—after Boston's disastrous fire in 1760, for example—other towns in the region might come to its aid with charitable gifts, there was also a darker side to misfortune. For towns trying to rival Boston's commercial success, like Salem, even a small outbreak of the pox might be an opportunity; Boston's misfortune could be their gain.[31]

Finally, the selectmen might be obliged to consider personal stories of the sufferers and their families in the wake of the pox. What of the Tuckermans, for example? Isaac Tuckerman, Mary's husband, has left enough of a record for us to follow his fate. Born in 1727, Isaac married Mary Sutton in Boston in 1753, one year after the city had undergone a major smallpox epidemic. A few years later, at the age of thirty, Isaac became a member of one of Boston's nine fire companies, a means that young men had of entering civic life and cutting a figure in urban society and politics. In 1761 and 1762, Isaac Tuckerman followed another route to improvement (and much-needed cash in a money-scarce economy) by serving in the Seven Years' War as a lieutenant in at least two expeditions, against Halifax and Louisbourg. He was able to buy property in Boston a year later from Mary Lawson, a spinster living on the corner of Water and Congress Streets. By this time, Tuckerman had taken work as a "hatter," a respectable trade and one that placed him far above other day laborers who scrambled for work in the depressed town. By 1769, then, when Isaac and Mary were taken with smallpox near the Horse-Shoe Tavern, near Boston Common, he had built for himself a modest competency.[32]

The pox could have taken all of that away. There was always the possibility of death, of course; at its most lethal, smallpox claimed fully one-third of its victims. But even in survival, there were potential difficulties to confront. Isaac Tuckerman would have been kept from his practice as a hatter for four weeks and, given that the pox was thought to hide in soft clothing, his business as a whole may have suffered even after he had recovered and was allowed to resume his work. On top of possible lost business, Tuckerman would have been obliged to pay for the cleansing of his house and belongings, unless he could prove his poverty. As it turns out, Tuckerman seems to have weathered the crisis in fine form. When he deeded the property on Water and Congress Streets in 1780 to his brother-in-law William, a trader, he was listed as an "esquire." Within a few years, he was licensed to sell drink as a retailer on Tremont Street. And when he died, at the age of seventy-five, Tuckerman was an innkeeper on Common Street, an employment that he had evidently enjoyed for many years.[33]

Isaac Tuckerman had been fortunate; others would not be so lucky. Shortly after Mary Tuckerman was struck with smallpox, the newspapers announced that Mr. John Fillebrown, distiller, had died, leaving "a sorrowful Widow and seven young Children." For the selectmen, these would be the final stories to attend to, persons whose lives had been devastated by the pox and who might well need public relief.[34]

Looking back on the selectmen and their efforts during the outbreak, we can see the ambiguous situations that they had to confront and adjudicate in a swift and workmanlike manner. As fathers of the town, Boston's selectmen were charged with protecting the public. But smallpox made it difficult to know who that public was and what protection might mean.

The need to respect the extreme condition of the stricken, as in the case of Mary Tuckerman, might mean asking neighbors to sacrifice; the need to enforce quarantine might mean disrupting commerce; the need to have the sick pay for their own care might lead to hardship and impoverishment. There was a balance to be struck in all of these instances, a continual series of decisions to be made during a time of crisis, made easier only through the unfortunate necessity of being well-versed in the ways of misfortune. Such was life in the province of affliction.

If the selectmen could have finished their business in a timely fashion on the afternoon of October 18, we might imagine them making their way to Faneuil Hall, where a town meeting had been scheduled—not to address smallpox, but to consider other matters infecting politics.

IV. OCTOBER 18, 1769: BOSTON TOWN MEETING—VIRULENT POLITICS

Boston's town meeting assembled at four o'clock that afternoon to discuss the "virulent Endeavors" of the former governor of Massachusetts, Francis Bernard. It was the second meeting of the day, and one of numerous assemblies that had taken place since the annual town meeting in March. Governor Bernard had been recalled to England in August, eager to escape what he considered the crazed actions of Bostonians. His departure had many causes, but the immediate precipitant was the publication in April of his private correspondence with the secretary of state, Lord Hillsborough, written the prior year. Bernard had painted a portrait in that correspondence of near-insurrection in the town and recommended the replacement of the colony's assembly-elected council with royal appointees. And while he had not directly requested royal troops to restore order, the lawlessness he had described had been so great that Hillsborough had felt compelled to send two regiments to the town in October 1768. A year later, seething with each new discovery of perceived treachery and slander, Bostonians wanted to clear their good name.[35]

Bernard's unhappy tenure in Boston had coincided with a larger imperial crisis that had evolved and gathered in intensity in the town since the riots protesting the Stamp Act in 1765. Over the decade, Boston had not lacked for violence and intimidation. An effigy of Andrew Oliver, appointed as stamp collector, was hung from the liberty tree, beheaded, and burned with boards from a building that the crowd dubbed his stamp office; merchants who violated non-importation efforts in response to the Townshend Duties a few years later had their windows smashed and their houses smeared with "Hillsborough paint" (a mixture of urine and feces); and there was much else besides. Thomas Hutchinson, whose mansion had been nearly destroyed during the 1765 riot, had reluctantly taken over the governorship from Bernard in 1769. He was convinced that what he saw in Boston bespoke nothing short of a conspiracy to destroy Crown rule in America. Crowds were one thing. But it was the concerted effort of a small number of men leading the people, whose tirades against royal authority and the unconstitutional actions of Parliament had been widely covered in the press and disseminated through committees of correspondence, that Hutchinson found especially ominous.[36]

From the perspective of agitated Bostonians, there was good cause for protest. They had been subjected to repeated insults and injuries, from the quartering of troops in town to the unlawful levying of taxes, and their legitimate pleadings had not brought redress or relief. Formal petitions to the Crown and efforts to influence public affairs through the channels of sympathetic patrons in England had been to no avail. What also rankled was the slander that the town had been subjected to not only by Bernard, but also by other ministers and servants of the Crown in Boston. In the afternoon meeting of October 18, the town reviewed newly obtained copies of a letter by General Thomas Gage suggesting that there was "very little Government in Boston," along with other "severe" complaints. In considering all of these writings together, many Bostonians saw a plot to sully their reputation. The town formally resolved that "false scandalous and infamous Libels upon the Inhabitants" were "of the most virulent and Malicious, as well a dangerous and pernicious tendency," and that the "wicked Authors of these incendiary Libels" should be punished according to law.[37]

When one reads the records of the town meeting and those of the selectmen alongside one another, it can initially be difficult to see what the world of smallpox and the world of the imperial crisis had to do with each other. But two connections between politics and illness emerge, one directly related to the smallpox outbreak, the other less direct but more far-reaching in its consequences.

Most directly, the selectmen were concerned about British soldiers stricken with the distemper. Early in the outbreak, in June, the selectmen were given information that the pox had "broke out in the Regimental Hospital at the bottom of the Common," and they went to investigate. When they could "get no satisfaction as to the truth" of the report, they approached General Mackey "to acquaint him, with a Law of the Province relative to concealing Infectious Distempers." That law, enacted in

1732, had required heads of household to notify the selectmen when any within their house had been stricken. For the selectmen, the demand for compliance was not merely a matter of protecting the public health but also spoke to the larger issue of sovereignty at the center of the imperial crisis. Local law, created by legislators who represented the people and exercised power with their consent, would need to be obeyed. For his part, General Mackey was willing to defer to local authority. Within two days, he had made inquiries, found that one of his men was sick with the pox at the Regimental Hospital, and "readily consented" when the selectmen requested that the soldier be quarantined at the hospital in the west end. As other soldiers and their family members fell ill in the coming weeks, they, too, were sent off to be quarantined. In the realm of public health, local sovereignty would prevail.[38]

A second, more subtle connection between sickness and governance emerged at this time that would be of profound importance in the years to come. It concerned not smallpox but rather the ongoing and often vexing question of how to accommodate the poor. Faced with assaults on their reputation, Bostonians not only publicly protested their virtue and loyalty, but also undertook their own internal housekeeping as if to make good on the promise. They turned inward, as they had many times in the past, in an effort to purify local society. In the process, a spotlight was shone on the poor, a development that had particular implications for the sick among them.

Beginning with the annual town meeting in March 1769 and continuing into April, the town considered a proposal to promote the "Reformation of Manners." There would be no more drunkenness, profanity, Sabbath breaking, or other public disruptions. Above all, "idleness," long considered "the parent of all Vices," would have to be addressed. Some "effectual method to employ the many poor who are now Objects of Charity" would be the "most likely means to prevent the further spread of Vice and Immorality," and the best means of promoting "the Reformation of Manners so Justly desired." As it had over a decade earlier, the town turned to a plan to put idle children and youths to work in "spinning schools," to have the yarn spun by master weavers. The plan promised to transform idleness into productivity and sin into virtue, and in the process to vitalize the town's depressed economy.[39]

The plan was, in part, a direct response to the impact of the nonimportation movement on the town's economic fortunes, a solution to the problem of "employing the Poor of the Town, whose Numbers and distresses are dayly increasing by the loss of its Trade & Commerce." The overseers of the poor reported to the town meeting that there were some 230 souls at the almshouse, an alarming number. In addition to these recipients of "indoor" public relief, many were being provided for "out of doors," not in the almshouse or workhouse, but in their own or others' homes with the aid of money from the town coffers. Outdoor relief alone had cost £600 in 1767 and £620 in 1768. In order to cut costs and put the idle to work, the overseers suggested that spinning schools might absorb the labors of as many as "two hundred of the Poor of the Town who are now ready, and are desirous of being employed in Spinning and Carding and that their Numbers are dayly increasing."[40]

In this sympathetic rendering of the plight of the poor, they were idle because of the failure in the town's economy and eager to get back to work. But the report also suggested another way of interpreting the relationship between idleness and poverty in its conclusion that by training the poor in the ways of industry through spinning work, it might "annually lesson the number of those who are esteemed proper Subjects of the Almshouse." Spinning would "habituate the People to Industry" and, in doing so, remove the primary source of their misery. The basis for the "workhouse movement" in England, well under way by the early eighteenth century (most large English towns had a workhouse by 1723), was the idea that many of the poor could, if given the incentive, labor steadily and productively. That idea had been the impetus for the first workhouse in Massachusetts, which opened its doors in Boston in 1739. The darker implication was that persons receiving public relief had been brought into poverty not through misfortunes beyond their control but rather through their own vicious habits.[41]

If we look at the residents of the almshouse in 1769, however, it is difficult to imagine who among the poor the overseers and others had in mind for reform. The records for the almshouse reveal just how bleak a scene it was. One hundred nine persons were admitted in 1769. Forty persons died during the course of the year, 17% of all the residents in the house. Among the ten who died in October were the widow Zerviah Smith and her child. Smith had come originally to New England from Cape May in New Jersey, eventually settling in Marblehead, Massachusetts. When she arrived in Boston in January she was in the final stage of a pregnancy. Being "near laying in & not having wherewithall to support herself," the selectmen provided for her removal to the Almshouse, where she was admitted on January 30. When she passed away some nine months later on October 6, Smith was just thirty-seven; her child, age seven months, followed her to the grave a week later. Was Zerviah Smith to have taken hold of the spinning wheel in a weakened state and worked her way into a new, improved, industrious self?[42]

Zerviah Smith's case betrayed the disjuncture between the theory and practices of poor relief in early New England and beyond. The theory held that the poor could be neatly separated into the worthy and the unworthy. The worthy were the "impotent" poor, persons who had through age, infirmity, sickness, or misfortune been reduced to poverty. The unworthy were able of body, but unwilling to labor for their upkeep—the so-called "sturdy beggar," the vagrant, or the malingerer, who might be made to labor in the workhouse or denied aid altogether. A second critical component of poor relief—again, an elegant idea in theory, if not in practice—was that each person was the proper responsibility of other persons or places to whom they legally belonged. Families were responsible for their members, masters for servants, towns for their legal inhabitants, and so on. In practice, however, the response to persons whose extreme conditions called for accommodation involved numerous complications. Questions of worthiness or unworthiness, belonging or estrangement, were secondary to the imperative to tend quickly to persons in distress.

The extremity of Zerviah Smith's physical condition landed her in the almshouse, even if she did not properly belong there. When Smith was admitted, she was placed on the "province account," which meant that she had no legal residency in any town in the colony and the money for her keep would be drawn from the province treasury. In theory, after expending enough energy and effort to locate someone responsible for the care of Smith and child, the overseers would have been within their rights to send Smith away, back to the last place she had come from, perhaps back to another colony. The selectmen might have "warned out" Smith upon her arrival, serving her legal notice that Boston would not be responsible for her care, and laying the legal basis for physical removal should the town desire it.

But such actions would be time-consuming and costly, and Smith's case was pressing. She was quite late in her pregnancy and likely showing it. The extremity of her condition trumped other concerns. As in similar cases, the overseers were willing to make exceptions, allowing even those who were clearly not from Boston to be admitted into the almshouse. In addition to Zerviah Smith, there were some thirty-six other persons admitted to the almshouse on the province account in 1769, a third of the total admissions.[43] This sort of poor law provision for strangers had been an innovation in New England, and accommodations in Massachusetts were especially capacious. Beginning in the dislocations of King Philip's War, which had left many in the colony homeless, the "province poor" accounts had swollen by the eve of the Revolution. In 1769–70, Boston's selectmen were awarded £677 to care for the province poor in the almshouse. Two-thirds of the overall allotments for the province poor went to Boston in that year, and in other years before the Revolution around 10% of province appropriations, save for servicing the debt, went into the province poor accounts.[44]

Brief notes by the selectmen, who gave special permission to the keeper of the almshouse to admit these province poor, suggest the desperate circumstances that occasioned relief. At a minimum, the selectmen justified each decision by noting that the person in question was a "stranger" (not belonging to any town in the province) and "not having the wherewithall to support" themselves. In some cases, the selectmen explicitly, if briefly, noted why the pauper needed help. When John Collfar was admitted in September, the selectmen explained that he was "a sick person . . . not having wherewithall to subsist himself" after arriving from the West Indies. Collfar would remain in the almshouse for six months. That the population of province poor were in feeble health can also be gleaned from what physicians billed the town for their care. In March Dr. Joseph Gardner had his bill of £124 7s. 4d. (likely for the year 1768) accepted by the town, and he submitted again in May for £174 13s. 4d.—substantial sums at a time in which Boston was trying to cut costs.[45]

Because the selectmen required special permission for support of the province poor, their care left a clearer mark in the public records than that of the town poor, but it is reasonable to assume that Zerviah Smith and John Collfar were not exceptional. Both province and town poor died in high numbers. And even as the overseers suggested that many poor in Boston might be made to work, thereby cutting public outlays, they acknowledged that the town was already overwhelmed by persons in legitimate need of relief. Reporting on the overall state of the poor in April, the overseers noted that some forty persons had been placed in the workhouse because there was simply no room to place these "worthy" poor in the almshouse where they belonged. This had been a chronic problem for Boston. Since the 1750s, some of the "distracted" persons, unable to care for themselves because of their mental condition, had been placed in the workhouse, and special compensation offered those who tended them. In 1769 Joseph Lasenby was offered £27 12s. for keeping the "sick and distracted" at the workhouse; he had for many years received similar compensation.[46]

Even as they proposed to create a spinning school that might inculcate the habits of industry in the idle poor, the overseers must have known what they were up against. The 1769 plan would fail, just as similar plans had failed in the past and would fail again in the future. They were expensive and relied on volunteers who were not readily forthcoming. But at a more elemental level, the schemes betrayed an almost willful blindness to a problem all too visible in Boston and elsewhere: that poverty often was intimately related to the debility of the body. Industry might be the way to redemption, but it lay outside the capacity of many on Boston's poor rolls. Thus, faced with individual cases of poverty and physical and mental distress, the overseers were moved, as gentlemen, to offer assistance and protection.[47]

Over the next half century, the idea that idleness was the cause of poverty would slowly eat away at such practices. Individual accommodations for the problems of debility and distress would be supplanted by policies and institutions that judged whether people fit specified criteria for relief or did not. In the meantime, in 1769 the ideal of improving the poor would sit alongside the practical realities of accommodating persons whose distressed lives blurred the boundaries of worthiness and unworthiness, local belonging and estrangement. These were the everyday ambiguities faced by those living in the province of affliction.

V. OCTOBER 18, 1769: A DAY AMONG DAYS, WEEKS, MONTHS, AND YEARS

We could extend our tour further by venturing to other places or other days. George Washington, who would six years later assume control of the newly assembled Continental army at Cambridge, spent October 18, 1769, fox hunting at Mount Vernon in the company of gentlemen, including Robert Fairfax, younger brother to the sixth Baron Fairfax of Cameron, and happily reported killing a fox. The ship rigger Ashley Bowen of Marblehead, Massachusetts (whom, along with Ebenezer Parkman and Elizabeth Porter Phelps, we will meet again), spent a day that New Englanders would have considered more industrious: he finished a mainstay and hired a hand to help him complete some shrouds. Neither man says a thing about illness that day, a reminder that illness punctuated daily life but did not fill it.

Yet one does not have to travel far to find affliction. Just a few days earlier, on October 14, Washington had written to the Reverend Jonathan Boucher to congratulate him upon his "easy passage over the Sickly months"; Washington noted, "We have had a much more troublesome time of it in this family," and his family had only now "tolerably well recovered" from the prevailing local disorders. Ashley Bowen, too, would find his wife ill enough on the prior Sunday to keep him home from church, and her ongoing troubles that year (likely tied to a pregnancy), coupled with a serious illness facing his eight-year-old son in August, made for "much sickness in my family" despite his being "well employed" at his business. New Englanders did not have a grim "sickly season" in the manner of those in the malarial South, though they tended to suffer from more respiratory ailments in the late spring and intestinal disorders throughout the summer. But without too much prodding, we can find the ready presence of illness in their daily lives.[48]

Eighteenth-century New Englanders saw sickness and reported on it. What should *we* see? Perhaps not any one thing, but rather a dynamic process at work, one that would in significant ways hold firm through the eighteenth century and, indeed, well into the nineteenth century. Many aspects of the early modern world were "circular" in motion, based on the recurrent rhythms of days and weeks and seasons. Illness within the province of affliction can be thought of this way. Illness created a circular motion in daily life. Part of the motion was caused by a world in a state of "becoming," which we have seen. To complete the circle, we need to add the act of "reckoning."[49]

Early New Englanders were comfortable with a world of becoming. Children were born and raised; land was broken, planted, and harvested; seasons turned. Nothing was permanent in the temporal world; everything changed. At particular moments, individuals and society brought this world of becoming to a stop. They "reckoned." The godly assessed the growth or decay of grace in their lives; accounts were taken of ongoing relationships of credit and debt within the barter economy; death brought the final settlement of legacies. For a moment, at least, becoming was stilled by reckoning.

Sickness added another layer of complexity to this world. The sick person's body commanded attention in its movements: it needed to be cared for, watched, and excused. The dynamic force of illness created many moments of reckoning: for some, it was a matter of determining the relation between body and soul; for others, a question of locating the body somewhere along the vast expanse between perfect health and death. And in the end, there would be a final reckoning, social and financial costs to be assessed. What adjustments had been made? What work left undone? What social favors granted? What accounts outstanding? Minor illness may have been absorbed into daily life without a thought. But more serious bouts of sickness as well as chronic conditions warranted sustained consideration.

Every illness posed the challenge of a body in a state of becoming, yet that fluidity could be reckoned in contrary ways. The following chapter explores the very different social and financial practices that attended the illnesses of the well-connected, on the one hand, and the poor, on the other.

Illness in the "Social Credit" and "Money" Economies of Eighteenth-Century New England

It is curious to see how completely social ethics and relations have changed since olden days. Aid in our families in times of stress and need is not given to us now by kindly neighbors as of yore; we have well-arranged systems by which we can buy all that assistance, and pay for it, not with affectionate regard, but with current coin.

The writer is Alice Morse Earle, whose *Home Life in Colonial Days* (1898) is both a rigorous treatment of domestic life in early America and tinged with the nostalgia of the colonial revival. There was, Earle confessed, "one curious and contradictory aspect of this neighborliness, this kindliness, this thought for mutual welfare, and that was its narrowness," especially in New England. For the poor and vulnerable removed from town to town and denied a place in community life, the colonial world could be cruel. But Earle considered this a "restraint of vision," an incidental blot on a grander way of seeing one's fellow beings. Somewhere between the colonial period and the late nineteenth century, something precious was lost when "current coin" supplanted "affectionate regard" as the means to address misfortune.[1]

Histories of the "market revolution" in America have found such observations attractive. The change Earle describes seems discrete and profound: from an economy of goodwill to an economy of money; from informal institutions of care in families and neighborhoods to "well-arranged systems" of care mediated by cash. But discovering when, where, and why these changes occurred has proven to be extraordinarily complex. There is no agreement about the timing, tenor, and final meaning of the changes wrought by the market. Even the notion of "revolution" has been called into question. As Richard Bushman has argued, the idea of a market revolution in farm society is built on an artificial "two-part typology" of "household" and "market" producers, in which the latter replaced the former. But the scheme fails to account for evidence of intensive production for distant markets in the seventeenth and eighteenth centuries as well as the persistence of local barter, exchange, and limited trade in surplus well into the nineteenth century. At best, Bushman suggests, we might shift our focus from the temporal dimensions of the revolution to the spatial: ports and inland towns all over early America undergoing transformations at different times, speeds, intensities.[2]

Historians of medicine in early America face similar challenges. In an effort to show historical change, one may draw too sharp a distinction between the world "before" and "after" the intrusion of the market. Paul Starr's influential *The Social Transformation of American Medicine* may stand in for many. Starr's primary concern is the slow, contested growth in professional medical authority in the nineteenth century and the rise of the medical industry in the twentieth, developments that he argues are inseparable from the growth of the market. With the growth of towns and cities, the care for the sick "increasingly shifted from the family and lay community to paid practitioners, druggists, hospitals, and other commercial and professional sources selling their services competitively on the market." Starr acknowledges that "the family continues even today to play an important role in health care," but he argues that "its role has become . . . secondary. The transition from the household to the market as the dominant institution in the care of the sick—that is, the conversion of health care into a commodity—has been one of the underlying movements in the transformation of medicine." By the time he is finished, it is difficult to see anything but withered remnants of the pre-market past in the commercialized present.[3]

For historians of early America, there are two major problems with this account. First, the commercialization narrative downplays the degree to which family and domestic medicine continued into the modern period. Histories of informal care in the modern period suggest that even as the cultural authority of medical professionals increased in the decades before World War II, women continued to shoulder the burden of caregiving in their families—and tensions abounded. Women were obliged to pick between directives by professionals that seemed reasonable and those that seemed harsh and too difficult to carry out. Chronic illness raised particularly troubling questions. Poor white women and women of color had to choose between the paid employment crucial for their family's financial well-being and the unpaid domestic caregiving crucial for its physical well-being.[4] Such dilemmas suggest that, rather than thinking of domestic care as being supplanted by professional medicine, we might fruitfully explore the ongoing negotiations between the domestic and the professional.

Moreover, by focusing on the shift from the familial to the professional and institutional, one risks minimizing how medical services could become part of family care. Works on the "mixed economy" of healing in early modern Europe demonstrate that institutional care, including care of the sick poor, was often an extension of family care. Rather than seeing informal and institutional care as opposites, it may be more accurate to think of them as overlapping and often complementary.[5] While the social history of medicine in early America is still in its early stages, it is clear that in addition to the informal care afforded by family members and neighbors, medical treatment could be sought from an enormous range of lay and learned practitioners in the eighteenth century. Although much is still to be learned about the roles of practitioners in any given area, domestic medicine in eighteenth-century New England had a commercial context that suggests important continuities with the nineteenth.[6] Rather than repeating a narrative of money replacing neighborly goodwill, we might more profitably consider the ways in which money and goodwill had a long and interconnected, if not always tranquil, history in American life.

This chapter examines the relation between familial and commercial "medical marketplaces" in eighteenth-century Massachusetts. It draws upon diaries and town, court, and provincial records to explore the spectrum of ways in which assistance for the sick was provided. At one end was neighborly support, with family members, neighbors, and the community rallying around their own in times of illness, as we saw in Hadley. At the other end lay the harsher realities of charitable and civic provision experienced by the sick poor, as we observed in Boston. Traveling along this spectrum, we understand how health care and sickness could operate in both a "social credit" economy, where care for the afflicted was part of a system of social credits and debts, and in a "money" economy, where explicit sums were attached to care for the sick. The tensions between these two methods of provision raised pressing questions about individual and communal responsibility in the face of incapacity.

I. ON SOCIAL CREDIT, MONEY, AND NEW ENGLAND

An examination of the "social credit" economy of early New England helps us move beyond thinking of altruism—or kindliness—as the driving force behind the extraordinary labor and allowance that could be accorded the sick. As studies on the intersection of sociability and communal labor in early America have shown, interdependence was the norm in farm society; scarcities in labor and material resources meant that only through relations of exchange could the needs of any farm be met. The favors granted the sick further illuminate the breadth, depth, and limitations of those networks. While the exchanges surrounding illness were rarely recorded in formal accounts, diaries and correspondence may be read as ledgers of "special kindnesses" offered and received. A tally of those records allows us to explore the degrees to which any individual or family could command a social response to their incapacities, as well as the extent to which illnesses could push the limits of goodwill.[7]

By contrast, the "money economy" refers to those exchanges in which debts had to be discharged with cash or coin. However, we should not make too neat a division between "social credit" and "money." As Craig Muldrew's work on the "credit economy" of early modern England has shown, many transactions were registered in coin in account books, but in fact were discharged through instruments of credit; money was a measure of value, not the favored medium of exchange in an economy in which coin was scarce. The "value" of exchange turned on questions of trust, reputation, and other considerations that informed one's ability to access credit. In the British colonies, imperial regulations kept coin limited and insured that what coins there were flowed back across the Atlantic. The "complex barter" system of New England—in which debts could be reckoned in monetary terms but paid in labor exchange, exchange in kind, and exchange in commodities such as lumber or fish—was an artifact of money scarcity. Any simple and universal division between credit and money is untenable.[8]

Nevertheless, colonists were required to discharge some debts in cash or coin: taxes, fees, and land sales, as well as long-distance transactions and those with strangers. Poverty and poor relief also became intertwined with questions of money. Persons called on to help the poor could expect money from public coffers; those helping the poor needed to be paid in cash by authorities because the poor often lacked the wherewithal to pay them in kind (although the labor of the poor might be used to pay at least some of their costs of care). For those at the margins who were selected by towns to care for the poor, poor relief itself was a way to procure limited cash. But entering the money economy could also be a significant cause of impoverishment. The poor themselves, particularly if they were transient, were limited in the credit they could draw, and so were asked to pay debts in money, further increasing their poverty.[9] While some scholars of the medical marketplace have emphasized its liberating potential, the connection between money and impoverishment should give us pause.[10] The fact that social relations of poverty, including care for the sick poor, were infused with questions of money goes a long way to explaining the politics of poor relief.

New England is an interesting—and somewhat unusual—site to investigate social credit and money as they figured into the medical marketplace. The founding ideals of New England, its relative social homogeneity (compared to the ethnic diversity of the middle colonies and slave societies of the South), and its unusual political economy set the region apart in mainland British North America.

Scarcities in labor and a basic want of material resources (plows, draft animals, tools) intensified mutual dependence among New England households over the century.[11] And the political economy of the towns in the region ensured special protections for town residents: free education for children, a carefully regulated labor force that favored locals, and social insurance via the town's poor law provision. Such developments allowed New England to grow economically without significant immigration or a large enslaved population. But it was a costly endeavor, and provisions for residents could be made only by keeping careful watch on outsiders. Strangers—whether poor or middling, able-bodied or suffering—were "warned" on their arrival in towns with a legal notice that would allow them to be removed should they become impoverished or otherwise draw on town coffers.[12]

Town concerns about cash outlays for the poor relate to larger debates about the great shortage of hard currency in the region, a problem that was exceptionally divisive in New England, where the lack of a stable medium of exchange could make ventures into the money economy confusing and dangerous.[13]

We turn now to a family's experience of illness in an eighteenth-century town, an experience embedded in the economy of social credit but also touching the money economy.

II. SICKNESS AND SOCIAL CREDIT:
WESTBOROUGH, MASSACHUSETTS, 1739

A diary that details the vicissitudes of the ailing body and the social response to it can tell us much about social networks of care. One particularly rich source comes from the pen of Ebenezer Parkman, whom we met in the previous chapter as he visited his fellow minister Samuel Barrett in

1769. From 1723 until his death in 1782, Parkman vigilantly recorded matters pertaining to his household and family life, his farm, and his pastoral duties in Westborough, Massachusetts, a town some thirty miles west of Boston. Sickness appears throughout. As a minister, Parkman saw illness as a crucial opportunity to apply himself to the afflicted and inquire into the state of their souls. As a farmer and the head of a household, Parkman knew well the disruption that illness occasioned. Minor ailments required special attention and changes in social schedule. More serious afflictions consumed family life.[14]

Parkman's diary vividly illustrates how sickness became enmeshed in an economy of social credit. The year 1739 was particularly trying for the minister and Hannah (Breck) Parkman, his second wife. Ebenezer Parkman was in his mid-thirties, a respected figure. Hannah Parkman turned twenty-three that year. A relative newcomer to Westborough, having married the minister two years earlier, she, too, was embedded in community relationships, despite overseeing a household that included children from Parkman's previous marriage. Ebenezer's and Hannah's serious illnesses during the year reveal the strength and limitations of a town's capacity to care for its own.

The year began with the death of the Parkmans' infant daughter, Elizabeth (January 14, 1739). Hannah's condition and that of the child had been severe enough to warrant a steady stream of watchers for the two weeks before the infant died. Watchers came again a week later when Hannah's pains increased and it was feared that she would follow her child to the grave. Hannah recovered slowly, being "exceedingly pained under her Breasts" (December 30, 1738) and later having "pain from her Hip to her Toe" brought on by swelling in her legs (February 6, 1739). Not until mid-February did Hannah feel "somewhat better," allowing the Parkmans to send the afternurse home after a seven-week stay (February 14 & 17, 1739). In September and October, Hannah was unwell enough (perhaps in relation to another pregnancy) that Ebenezer pleaded that his house was in "great Trouble" (September 28, October 15, 1739). A final blow came at the end of November, when Hannah fell from her horse (November 26, 1739). The accident was perhaps responsible for the year ending in much the same way it had begun: "About 12 (although she had gone but about 5 Months) She was deliver'd of a tender, lifeles, Male Child, The Measure of which was 13 ½ Inches long" (December 25, 1739).[15]

Ebenezer Parkman became seriously ill at the end of October, which posed significant problems for the family because his wife was also unwell at the time. The diary narrates his dramatic decline over four days, as Ebenezer slipped from being a fully functioning man to being a help-less dependent: "Not well at Wards" (October 26, 1739); "Not well, but yet in my Study" preparing for Sabbath (October 27, 1739); "Grew worse. Not able to go to Meeting. A.M.–P.M. preached on Rev. 2.21 but with much Difficulty, being very ill and feeble" (October 28, 1739); "At Eve my pains exceedingly increas'd. Neighbor How came and got my bed down into the lower room, and lifted me on to it" (October 29, 1739); "I grew More help-less" (October 30, 1739). Neighbors and friends had come to visit and no doubt to help the Parkmans during this time, but when the Parkmans' family physician (who was also Ebenezer's brother-in-law) arrived at the parsonage and judged the minister to be afflicted with "high Inflam-matory Rhumatism," a more formal response from the community was needed (November 1, 1739). For the next two and a half weeks, the fam-ily secured watchers who sat up with Ebenezer singly and in pairs during the night. At the end of three weeks of severe illness, the long recovery process began. Not until the end of December did Ebenezer return to the pulpit, two months after he had become bedridden.

The Parkmans relied heavily on their neighbors, friends, and relatives to help them through this especially trying year. Ebenezer recorded their help in spare, unsentimental entries, such as "Rebecca Hicks watch'd" or "Nathan Maynard was sent for Doctor" or "Nei[gh]bours on the South side came and got wood." The diary was a record of social action, a register of "special kindnesses" that were undoubtedly performed in the spirit of friendship and Christian charity. But by noting them in the diary, Ebene-zer ensured that good deeds would not be forgotten. With the exception of the doctor or midwife, most of those whose names were registered in the diary would not be reimbursed with money or the exchange of goods. They could expect to be repaid instead with like action when they found them-selves in desperate circumstances.

Ebenezer was particularly attentive to who watched through the night, a gesture that involved considerable sacrifice given the rigors of daily work. Circumstances at the Parkman house were dire enough that year to require watchers on forty-one separate occasions. Some thirty-five dif-ferent persons watched, most only once. Hannah Parkman's circle was smaller than her husband's and exclusively female. In the two weeks following her daughter's birth, eleven women took turns watching her. Four—her afternurse, a young woman hired to help run the household, and two neighbors—watched twice. During his fever, Ebenezer was watched by twenty-two people, fourteen of whom were men. Only one—again, a neighbor—watched more than once. Only three people—all women, two neighbors and a hired "girl"—watched both Ebenezer and Hannah Parkman. Because Ebenezer recorded very little other than the name of the watcher and the date on which he or she watched, one is left with more questions than answers. How was the care organized? Who decided who would watch? What stresses did watching place on watchers and their families? Although the records do not answer these questions explicitly, three themes emerge.

First, care was distributed throughout the community. The principle of dispersal explains why there was less overlap than one might expect between the healers who helped Hannah deliver her child and the women who tended her in the weeks thereafter. With the exception of the midwife, of the seven women who assembled initially to help with what turned out to be a false alarm, only two, both neighbors, served as watchers in the following two weeks; one of these had been called out by Hannah's false alarm and did not assist in the birth a few days later. One suspects that it was understood that these women had already performed an exhausting service, and there was no reason for them to watch while others could do so. In particular, older, experienced women might have needed to save their energies to help with future childbirths. Within the families that sent watchers to the Parkmans, the task was also dispersed. The adult sons and daughters in these families most commonly watched; presumably it was less taxing to send energetic youths.

Secondly, certain families played critical roles in care, as the Hicks family did for the Parkmans. Ebenezer Parkman was related to Rebecca (Champney) Hicks through his first marriage. Sometime before 1736, Rebecca and her husband, John, moved to Westborough, where they became neighbors to the Parkmans. In the years that followed, the families saw each other regularly. Ebenezer helped "brother Hicks" get settled in town, and John Hicks reciprocated, helping with special projects and field work on Parkman's farm and watching with the minister during his illness. "Sister Hicks" and Hannah Parkman appear to have been especially close. In 1738 and 1739, they attended each other in childbirth and sat up together as those children lay dying. Two of the Hicks girls were caregivers as well, watching with both Ebenezer and Hannah. In all, the Hicks family watched for the Parkmans ten nights.

A final theme concerns social power. Although few of those who tended the Parkmans were as close to them as the Hicks family, the Parkmans were able to draw many watchers into their home. As a minister, Ebenezer had healed divisions in the town; his advice was sought in many non-ecclesiastical matters as well. His public position may well have drawn a deacon and other leading men in the community to serve as watchers. Moreover, Ebenezer may have commanded a greater response to his illness than other prominent men of the town could have expected for themselves. As minister, he tended to the sick and dying; in the past few years, he had visited many of the families of persons who watched for him in 1739. When Ebenezer became ill, he drew on these informal social debts.

Because Ebenezer did not regularly record his wife's visiting, one cannot know her connections with all those who eventually came to the parsonage to help. Her circle of female watchers was smaller and perhaps more intensely connected than her husband's. It is clear, however, that Hannah's sickness constructed a network of neighborly exchange. Rebecca Hicks and her daughters and the neighboring Maynard families tended to Hannah more often than others. Yet Hannah's connections were not limited to local visiting. Her husband's diary makes it clear that she went beyond her immediate neighborhood to show fellowship with those who were afflicted. Not infrequently Hannah accompanied her husband to private meetings in the houses of the seriously afflicted and to funerals. As the parson's wife, she had a special stature in the community of suffering.

In all of these ways, the Parkmans were unusually capable of drawing watchers into their home. Through connections and calling came ready access to the social credit economy. And yet, even for the Parkmans, social credit was not enough to sustain them during their trials. On two occasions in the year, the length and severity of their illnesses forced the family to enter the money economy.

Two and a half weeks into Ebenezer Parkman's confinement, the orderly system that had brought watchers into his house appeared to be unraveling. The bulk of the watching in the first week had been undertaken by the Hicks family and close neighbors; by the second week, Ebenezer had to assemble a more eclectic group, dipping deeper into his social reserve and finding a deacon and a leading citizen from the far side of town to watch. But in the middle of the week, things began to go awry. Two watchers in succession failed to show, leaving Hannah to sit up with her husband. The matter was more than an inconvenience for the minister and his wife. Hannah was four months pregnant and had not felt well for some time. Ebenezer was acutely aware of the dangers in exposing an ill wife to night watching; his first wife, Mary, had died three and a half years earlier under similar circumstances. This time the minister made plans to hire a maid from Boston. During 1739 the Parkmans had summoned young women from neighboring households to help Hannah with heavy work for a few days at a time. The decision to call for a maid from Boston was different, more like hiring an afternurse in the wake of childbirth or hiring farm workers from April through September. It meant that, in all likelihood, Ebenezer would be contracted to pay wages—something he did not do lightly.[16] But sick and facing the prospect of a long recovery, his wife pregnant, ill, and caring for five children, and having already called repeatedly on friends and neighbors, Ebenezer may have deemed it prudent to hire long-term help. The economy of social credit had effectively provided for the Parkmans for periods of a few weeks, but it could not continue indefinitely.

Perhaps Ebenezer had these costs in mind when he had his second encounter with the money economy. In December the town met to grant more money for a minister who had substituted for Ebenezer while he lay ill. That night Ebenezer wrote, "Sundry Neighbours here. N.B. Mr. Tainters advice to offer the Town to bear Some part of the Charge of preaching, he not duly Considering the great and extraordinary Charges which I was brought into by my Sickness." One can imagine the conversation from Ebenezer's perspective. Although his salary comprised a hefty chunk of the town's budget, it had never been enough to support himself and family—for that he had to add the labors of a farmer to his calling as a minister. Now, at his most vulnerable, he was being asked to pay beyond even the "extraordinary charges" of his sickness. Because Ebenezer's account books and almanacs from this period no longer exist, it is impossible to know what these "charges" were. Certainly the doctor, afternurse, and maid would be paid in money, goods, or notes. The watchers and visitors would be acknowledged in an informal tally of social credits and debts. But how much of the labor of neighbor David Maynard's son Jotham, who performed various tasks on the minister's farm while Parkman was sick, would appear as debts to be paid? Would the neighbor who brought victuals or drink think to add this to his account? Or did Ebenezer have in mind all of the extra firewood that burned through the night while he lay ill, or the cost of entertaining the concerned persons who came to the house? However these would be tallied, it was clear that despite all of the "social work" done for the minister and his family at no cost, Ebenezer still felt the connection between sickness and extraordinary charge.

If the Parkmans, with all of their social credits, on the one hand, and the minister's salary, on the other, felt the severe financial burden placed upon them in sickness, what kinds of additional pressures were faced by those who were sick and impoverished, who found themselves without social connections in the towns in which they lived or strangers in towns they were merely passing through? We turn now to the stories of the sick poor and the politics of providing them with care in the money economy.

III. THE SICK POOR AND THE MONEY ECONOMY

In October 1738, John Jackson, a stranger "providentially passing through" Attleboro, Massachusetts, fell sick and died under the watch of Thomas Slack, innholder. We know little more about Jackson. Evidently he had no place of legal settlement in the Massachusetts Bay Colony. When pressed about his residence, Jackson declared that he belonged to Great Britain.

Jackson's life simply left a long bill. After Jackson's death, Slack drew up an account of his expenses in caring for the sick stranger and attached it to a petition to the Massachusetts General Court. It detailed a mug and a half of buttered flip; hiring a man and a horse to fetch the doctor and subsequent charges for his visit; and charges for those who nursed and watched with Jackson. There were charges for the interment, funeral, and liquor that flowed after it. Lest anyone forget more mundane expenses, Slack added to all of this "The Trouble and Charge in the House not above Expence as Fire, Wood, Candles, and Washing & four days Trouble." All of this amounted to £9 19s. 9d. Slack subtracted every possible ounce of worth left to Jackson: the six shillings he had in cash, two oxenbridge shirts ("part worn"), a pair of shoes and stockings ("almost worn Out"), an old hat and two old jackets ("of small value"), all of which amounted to £1 6s.[17] The town selectmen pronounced the charges "just and reasonable." Attleboro's representative to the General Court drew up the petition on Slack's behalf and was given permission by the innholder to receive any money granted. As an outsider who belonged to no town in Massachusetts, Jackson was considered one of the province poor, for whose care the General Court was obliged to field individual bills and authorize the provincial treasurer to pay.[18]

With no ties to family, neighborhood, or town, every element of care for Jackson was reduced to a monetary price. From a financial perspective, Slack had been fortunate that Jackson had died quickly. In just a few days, the cost of his sickness had well surpassed Jackson's ability to pay. Had he lingered, Slack would have likely suffered a loss. While the General Court was responsible for strangers like Jackson, large bills received especially strict scrutiny. But with the backing of the town selectmen who verified his charges and the help of the town's representative to the General Court, the financial burdens presented by a humble stranger worked their way to the highest levels of government. Innholder, selectmen, and representative alike must have been relieved when the initial committee review of the account subtracted only 20s. from the request.

In theory, public relief for the sick poor should have been an untroubled affair. In contrast to the "sturdy beggar," whose poverty was thought to be a product of idleness and vicious habits, the impoverishment of the sick, infirm, and impotent was understood to warrant compensation. But in many cases, as scholarship on early modern England has suggested, the sick and those caring for them could not expect immediate public relief and had to devise strategies to tap into public coffers.[19] In eighteenth-century New England, both the indeterminacy of illness and questions arising from the local provision of care led to confusion and contest. Given the continuum between perfect health and death, any sickness raised the question of the degree to which accommodation was warranted. How extreme was the condition and what public allowance should it be granted? Following the precedent of the Elizabethan Poor Laws, families and towns were obligated to care for those determined by law to belong to them. But when the sick fell ill away from their family and place of legal inhabitancy, bills piled up well in advance of determining who was responsible for them.

Beneath the complaints about the care of the sick poor lay a fundamental disjuncture between the biological and the political: sickness and compensation operated according to two vastly different schedules. While the sick person's condition called for immediate measures to ease the pain of infirmity or to address the urgencies of acute illness, the political arrangements were slow and uncertain, as the sick, their families, and towns tried to sort out the tangled lines of responsibility for the costs of care.

The poor were the responsibility of the town in which they had a legal settlement, most often due to birth, marriage, parentage, or continuous residence. The most common type of assistance in rural towns came in the form of outdoor relief, where submissions for nursing the sick who were legal inhabitants were added to the cost of their board, clothing, and other sundry charges. Physicians in rural areas made a variety of arrangements to accommodate the poor and near poor, accepting payments in goods and labor, forgiving portions of their charges, and running accounts directly with towns. In urban areas like Boston and Salem, indoor relief assumed greater importance over the eighteenth century, and physicians contracted with almshouses for annual salaries and fee schedules for visits. Finally, for those impoverished by epidemics and wartime illness, and for strangers like John Jackson, the sick and their caregivers could turn to the provincial government for relief.[20]

While poor law provision could be confusing and contested, it is worth underscoring just how capacious that provision was in the early modern world. As in England, local residents had a lifelong entitlement to relief in their legal place of settlement. In Massachusetts, the province poor accounts went further still, offering care for those with no legal settlement in the province (and after independence, the state). In towns across New England, the poor were provided with medicine, nursing, food, and shelter. That such provision might be spare was a function of just how stretched residents could be in a cash-poor economy where schools, roads, and the local minister also required support. But we should not diminish the poor laws' elegant solution, in theory, to the problem of responsibility for the impoverished, including the sick poor: either someone had a town of legal residence that was responsible for care, or the province poor accounts could be tapped.[21]

Nevertheless, in practice, provisions for the sick poor were not automatic—and could be fraught. Towns met yearly to "look into the circumstances" of the poor and decide on what method and extent of aid they "thought most proper"; contested cases reveal the pressures facing the sick and those tasked with their care. Consider the case of Thomas Stockbridge, of Scituate, Massachusetts, who urged the court of general sessions at Plymouth to intervene with town authorities on his behalf. Stockbridge had asked his selectmen for an abatement of his poll tax, an assessment on all male householders over age sixteen and a measure of the productive capacities of the household. Although Stockbridge had a ratable estate—he was not destitute—he argued that, at age seventy-nine, he was so disabled that he should be excused from his poll, something the town had refused to allow from 1778 to 1781. He had "for above nine years [been] so lame as not to be able to do one Day's work in a Day since, by reason of Rheumatick Disorders setting in both his knees; and for 3 or 4 years so blind and deaf as not to be capable to act or carry on Business, but that he has been obliged to leave it to his sons to manage his affairs. . . ." Others pleaded in a related vein: "lameness," "bodily indisposition," and the decay of old age had incapacitated them from the labor that was taxed. Some, like Stockbridge, were awarded their back taxes; others were not. Regardless of outcome, the cases suggest the moral pressures faced by those asking for exemption. Towns might tell men who had worked their entire lives that ill health did not excuse them from the public's claim to their labor or its cash equivalent.[22]

Stockbridge petitioned on his own behalf, but he made it clear that he was dependent on his sons. Before public relief could be issued to the aged infirm, families were legally bound to offer assistance, an obligation that could occasion anxiety and resistance. While extended family may have felt morally bound to care for their kin, the law defined family responsibility quite narrowly: grandparents, parents, and children were responsible for one another. Towns regularly helped poor families care for their own with food, fuel, and clothing, or with limited cash outlays. But that relief was a fraction of what might be required, especially when the poor were sick or infirm. The case of the Plymouth shipwright Samuel Kempton is instructive. When Kempton petitioned the court of general sessions in 1739, he pleaded that he had supported his aged mother-in-law, Bathshua Donham, who was "much impaired in her health and Senses," with just £4 allowed by her town selectmen. Despite repeated entreaties to other sons and daughters-in-law, no one would help. When the court found in Kempton's favor, it demanded that the children and grandchildren pay him £36 a year, fully eight times his allotment by the town. It is little wonder that persons like Kempton feared that the "Necessitous Circumstances" of the aged indigent could become their own.[23]

Nor is it surprising, given the costs, that some families neglected their legal responsibilities. Many petitions state that family members had been applied to and refused to contribute: brothers, sisters, and grandchildren left a few of their hapless relations to shoulder the burden of care for those who could no longer support themselves. When these cases reached the courts, the aggrieved were prepared to argue that others were able but simply unwilling to help. This may have been true, but the court's solution—dividing financial responsibility among those legally responsible for care—also suggests that refusal to provide for kin may have reflected the potentially overwhelming burden of tending the aged indigent. When the court divided care into sixteen portions, as it did when it assigned the son of the aged and infirm Ruth Drew five-eighths responsibility for her care and her six grandchildren one-sixteenth each, it was not only implementing "family" obligation but also recognizing the need to disperse the burdens of care.[24]

When families could not be made to care for the aged infirm, the burden fell to the towns of their legal inhabitancy. Small farming towns like Wenham, where cash and coin were scarce, gave especially close attention to finding ways of limiting outlays. The provisions for Sarah Batcheller, widow, who was boarded out to Lieutenant Josiah Herrick in 1770, were typical. Herrick was to take her into his family for the year, to provide her with food, drink, washing, and lodging, and to return her clothes and bedding in the same condition in which they arrived. The town promised him nine dollars, granted the "Labour the sd widow can do, being Constantly Emply'd as she is able during sd Term," and offered to pay the "Necessary Charges of Doctors & Nursing" in case of sickness. Even as it acknowledged that the poor widow might face sickness during the year, the town traded on the cash value of her future labor; her prospective employment, however limited, became part of the negotiation. For her part, the widow could hope that the expectation that she labor "constantly" would be eased in her indisposition, and that the "necessary" charges for her care would not be done on the cheap.[25]

When we turn to the town's provision for strangers, transients, and others not entitled to relief, we find different sets of negotiations over costs and responsibility for illness. Towns protected their coffers by "warning" outsiders, serving them legal notice that they would not be relieved should they become ill or impoverished. When non-residents came to town, the law demanded that they or their hosts announce their presence to officials and post bond for future care. In theory, such measures allowed people to visit and labor without rendering the town vulnerable, but complications arose in practice. Officials and residents learned to recognize persons posing future liabilities, such as pregnant women, and have them summarily removed. But illness was not always manifest; one could enter a town healthy and fall ill soon after. Moreover, the illness that made sick strangers costly also made it quite difficult to remove them; it was not proper to expel a dangerously sick person laboring under extremity. In the meantime, care was provided without clarity about the ultimate responsibility for payment.

The case of Nicholas Shaw, a yeoman of Abington, Massachusetts, speaks to this ambiguity. Shaw complained at the Plymouth Court of General Sessions in 1766 that Sarah Richards, a single woman who had lived in town for several years in "poor and necessitous" circumstances, had come to his house and "fell sick there and became burthensome to Petitioner for her support, though [he] is not nor ever was under any legal obligation to maintain her. . . ." We don't know why Shaw allowed Richards in his house in the first place; perhaps it was an act of charity or an effort to secure household help. Whatever the case, Richards was soon confined to bed, and Shaw had to pay for her board, lodging, washing, nursing, watching, doctor's visits, and medicines. Shaw argued that the town should pay him for his "great expence," but the Abington selectmen and overseers of the poor refused, a common strategy when an indigent's residency was in question (and one less aggressive than suing the townsman who harbored a stranger without properly notifying officials, a measure that towns also pursued). The court found in Shaw's favor and ordered Abington to pay Shaw £25 6s. for forty-five weeks of care and an additional £4 8s. for the expenses of her final seven weeks, including digging a grave and the funeral. It was certainly a victory for Shaw, but his need to provide immediate care for Sarah Richards put him in considerable debt for a year, no doubt causing difficulties in his other transactions.[26]

In like fashion, the sick transient figured in debates between towns. Because warnings did not necessarily mean removal, when outsiders became sick, costs mounted as towns tried to sort out legal responsibility. Plymouth selectmen, acting on the behest of the town of Plympton, had warned out Deborah Drew as early as 1757. When in 1762 the selectmen found that she was "sick and so poor she can't support herself" in Plympton, they applied to nearby Halifax, which they claimed was her legal residence. But the Halifax selectmen refused to pay for Drew. It was five weeks before the aggrieved selectmen presented their case to the court of general sessions and were awarded costs. They had been fortunate. In many other cases, the dispute over which town was responsible for the poor continued without resolution. Ambiguous settlement histories, failure to warn out in a timely fashion, improperly served notices, and a host of other difficulties meant that although bills for care were immediate and pressing, the political solution could drag on.[27]

Finally, the difficulties posed by the sick stranger rose to the General Court, where they were heard in petitions and accounts from individuals and towns asking for relief. Some involved transients with no legal settlement in Massachusetts whose "stroll" through the countryside and ports was interrupted by severe illness. Cases like John Jackson's, with which we began, dot the provincial records. In Boston, New England's cultural capital and commercial center, selectmen placed a range of sick and ailing strangers on province rolls, including travelers and sailors from countries throughout the Atlantic, wanderers from neighboring colonies, and free blacks and Indians from the province who had no access to legal settlement.[28] Other petitions and accounts for the province poor arose from the surges in violence and dislocation that punctuated colonial life. Starting with King Philip's War (1675–76), Massachusetts made special allowance for those wandering unfortunates who were "forced from their habitations" and found themselves in towns to which they had no legal claim to assistance. The Acadian exiles deported to Massachusetts—a massive infusion of over two thousand impoverished refugees whose homes and farms had been destroyed by the British—provide the most extreme example of colonial dislocation, and their circumstances became deeply enmeshed in provincial government. Starting with the initial deportation in 1755 and continuing for a decade, dozens of towns from every corner of the province submitted accounts for the support and medical attention given to "French Neutrals," the geographic range of claimants widening as the exiles were relocated in response to towns' pleas about the overwhelming financial burden of providing care.[29]

IV. CONCLUSION

Any given sickness in eighteenth-century New England called forth a different arrangement of individuals; each sickness created its own society. At one end of the spectrum lay a family like the Parkmans. Deeply rooted in community and enmeshed in the social credit economy, the Parkmans could draw on a vast network of helpers during the family's time of need. Such help would not be forgotten; it would be recorded as a social debt to be paid at a later date, a major strand of interdependence in community life. At the other end of the spectrum, the sick poor lay wholly at the public charge. Government commissioned society to care for those deemed incapable of providing for themselves, and almost every conceivable cost associated with care was assigned a monetary value. Individuals, families, and towns then struggled to sort out responsibility for care and payment.

Between these two extremes lay a realm that has only been hinted at here, dominated by a cruel logic in which either isolation or severe illness could lead toward dependency. One path was traveled by those isolated from the community of social credit: the fewer social connections one had, the more likely it was that in times of sickness one would have to enter the money economy and become indebted. The other path was traveled by those whose illnesses were severe: even for those as well-connected as Ebenezer Parkman, the more severe one's sickness, the more likely it was that the economy of social credit would not suffice, and one would need to enter the money economy for additional support in times of need. In either case, one would acquire more and more debt through the very conditions—isolation, weakness, incapacity—that would make it all the more difficult to repay these obligations. The medical marketplace in early New England may have afforded those privileged with access to money and credit the ability to seek medical attention and household support. But for the marginal and seriously afflicted, the forced confrontation with the market could fuel a dynamic of dependency, leading the sick and their caregivers to turn to the town, province, and state for relief. Governing officials would place a price on their suffering.

The overall picture of social provision for the sick poor is a mixed one. On the one hand, poor law provision in early modern New England was unusually generous, extending developments in social welfare that had their origins in Elizabethan England to include provision for the sick stranger with no legal place of settlement. And towns regularly accommodated, as best as they could, the illnesses and other debilities of their members. The individual and social consequences of illness were everywhere on display—visible in a way that is immediately striking to the modern reader—and registered in town, province, and state records as stories not only of individual suffering, but of all of those who were brought into the orbit of the sick.

On the other hand, in practice, poor law provision for the sick could be riddled with difficulties. The extremity of the sick could generate considerable bills, but the payment schedule was often slow and plodding, as families, towns, and province tried to work out lines of responsibility. Capacious but also vexing—this was the world of poor law provision for the sick and their caregivers.

COMPETENCY

CHAPTER THREE

Family Competency: Scenes from the Life Course of Illness

Family was a potent word in early America. The orderly family served as foundation, model, and metaphor for a stable society and godly life. It was also a primary site in which sickness was accommodated and absorbed. This chapter explores the ways in which illness shaped social relations within family life in eighteenth-century New England. What were the cumulative costs—social, financial, cultural—of a family's afflictions? These questions help us to probe the boundary between those who could support themselves and those who could not—the great gulf that separated the competent from the dependent.

The term "competency" has helped scholars of early America move from the well-documented world of behavior to the elusive world of motivation and desire. Simply put, we know much more about what early Americans did than about what they sought to achieve in even the most elemental of endeavors, such as daily work. Competency fills this void. As Daniel Vickers has suggested, in early New England competency was an ideal: one worked to achieve "a degree of comfortable independence." In the seventeenth century, one possessed a competency if one had property sufficient "to absorb the labors of a given family" and protect family members from having to depend on outside employment. By the nineteenth century, competency no longer meant property but rather suggested one's skill at work. While the change in the term, as Richard Bushman has argued, reflected a profound (if gradual and often imperceptible) transformation in economic life, the goal remained much the same in the nineteenth century as earlier. "The capacity to provide for oneself in all circumstances, including illness and old age," inspired labor strategies ranging from farm to factory work.[1]

Although broad and necessarily imprecise, competency is neverthe-less useful in illuminating the strains that sickness placed on achieving and maintaining a "degree of comfortable independence." New England-ers were, for the most part, able to find ways to negotiate the burdens of illness. But their difficulties in doing so suggest that we might profitably turn Bushman's formulation on its head: rather than thinking of a com-petency as a means to protect families against life's calamities, we might think of family competency as surviving intact because of successful efforts to manage those calamities. In addition to care for the afflicted, illness raised challenges—rearranging social schedules, delaying tasks, drawing on social credits and neighborly exchange, hiring help—that needed to be integrated into work that historians have traditionally seen as securing a competency: land purchase and management, the sale of sur-plus goods on local and distant markets, the search for by-employments in rural areas and factory work in towns. The consideration of the fam-ily's management of illness incorporates the collective efforts of all fam-ily members and extends the concept of family or household competency beyond the labor of fathers and sons. Finally, the study of illness sheds light not only on actions to mitigate the effects of affliction but also on the social and economic importance of incapacity itself. Family competency waxed and waned with the health of family members.

To illuminate the connection between illness and competency in fam-ily life, this chapter will trace the strains that afflictions placed on fami-lies during different stages of their development, examining most closely the impact of sickness on the evolving relations between parents and chil-dren.[2] For the sake of continuity and depth of analysis, we will again fo-cus on the Parkmans of Westborough, Massachusetts. The Parkmans were atypical in several respects. The family was large—two marriages yielded sixteen children, of which fourteen survived into their twenties, unusual in an era of high infant mortality. As the years passed, however, the bal-ance changed. By the time Ebenezer Parkman died in 1782, seven of his children had preceded him, several after long illnesses.[3]

The central problematic here is the tension between family being at once the source of and solution to the presence of affliction in daily life. A significant part of family labor for the Parkmans entailed address-ing the needs of its ailing members and filling in for tasks that the sick were unable to perform. The broad ideal of competency, for them and for others, could only be achieved if the incapacities of the ill could be accommodated.

I. EARLY CHILDHOOD

Although historians have investigated the cultural construction of childhood and the place of children within a family's economic strategies for several decades, they have tended to focus more on childhood mortality than on childhood sicknesses. Early New England childhood mortality rates were quite high by modern standards, though estimates are fragmentary and necessarily speculative because of the spotty record. Laurel Ulrich has calculated that Martha Ballard, a midwife in late eighteenth-century Hallowell, Maine, saw one infant death per twenty-four births, with 40% of these deaths stillborn and the remainder dying within a day. Christopher Jedrey has proposed that "perhaps as many as one child in three died before the age of twenty" in Chebacco Parish (Ipswich, Massachusetts). And Daniel Scott Smith and J. David Hacker have estimated that half of all deaths in colonial New England would have been children under the age of eleven. New Englanders regularly lived into their sixties and beyond (two of the Parkmans' children lived until their sixties, two to their seventies, three to their eighties, and one to his nineties), but they had to survive childhood sicknesses (and other traumas) in order to do so.[4]

Childhood mortality was a real presence. It may well have animated fears that any illness could lead to death—a theme we will return to shortly. But the majority of illnesses did not end in death. If one-third of New England's children died before age twenty, two-thirds survived, and those who eventually succumbed had most likely labored under many afflictions before a final illness. What, then, were the social implications of living in a world in which many children, threatened by numerous ills, lived through them? The following two sections sketch some of the broad outlines of the problem.

The major diseases afflicting children in colonial America are well known, thanks to durable work on the social history of medicine tracking outbreaks of contagious disease in the seventeenth and eighteenth centuries. These epidemics cut swaths through towns: throat distemper, canker, quinsy (diphtheria), measles, chin cough (whooping cough), bloody flux (dysentery), smallpox, influenza, and mumps, to name some of the more prominent. In addition to these diseases were afflictions that defy retrospective diagnosis—fevers, agues, indispositions, and assorted pains—not to mention poisonings, falls, scaldings, burns, and other accidents. In short, children faced ailments that ran the gamut of ailments from the lethal to the relatively innocuous.[5]

TABLE 1. Ebenezer Parkman Family Genealogy
Ebenezer Parkman (1703–1782)
Marries Mary Champney (1699–1736) on July 7, 1724
Marries Hannah Breck (1716–1801) on September 1, 1737
The Parkman children:

Name	Birth	Marriage	Death	Age at death
Mary	September 14, 1725	August 6, 1752	January 16, 1776	50
Ebenezer	August 20, 1727	September 21, 1752	July 5, 1811	83
Thomas	July 3, 1729	—	October 23, 1759	30
Lydia	September 20, 1731	—	June 21, 1733	20 months
Lucy	September 23, 1734	April 28, 1757 November 13, 1793	March 13, 1804	69
Elizabeth	December 28, 1738	—	January 14, 1739	17 days
William	February 19, 1741	September 9, 1766	February 5, 1832	90
Sarah	March 20, 1743	September 28, 1769	March 12, 1825	81
Susannah	March 13, 1745	October 13, 1768	November 30, 1772	27
Alexander	February 17, 1747	December 12, 1768	April 1, 1828	81
Breck	January 27, 1749	January 9, 1777	February 3, 1825	76
Samuel	August 22, 1751	February 11, 1773	June 11, 1824	72
John	July 21, 1753	—	September 10, 1775	22
Anna Sophia	October 18, 1755	September 21, 1780	November 26, 1783	28
Hannah	February 9, 1758	—	October 14, 1777	19
Elias	January 6, 1761	December 25, 1785 March 13, 1794	September 30, 1828	67

Note: Genealogical material adapted from Ross W. Beales Jr., "The Reverend Ebenezer Parkman's Farm Workers, Westborough, Massachusetts, 1726–82," *Proceedings of the American Antiquarian Society* 99 (1989): 141. Additional data from the Ebenezer Parkman Project (http://diary.ebenezerparkman.org/diary-themes-people/#Children), which contains substantial genealogical material on each child, as well as American Ancestors (https://www.americanancestors.org/index.aspx) and ancestry.com. The table uses January 1 as the start of the new year.

In his long-running diary, the Reverend Ebenezer Parkman had ample opportunity to note diseases that we might recognize—the "meazles" swept through his house on more than one occasion—and others that seem to be clusters of generic symptoms. What is of greatest interest is the intensity and repetition of Parkman's accounts of his children's health. Parkman watches closely as his children become ill, grow worse, continue in their condition, or recover; he listens to their coughs and scrutinizes their swellings and ulcers; he calls healers of all sorts (midwives, doctors, knowledgeable neighbors); and he procures (or, more often, has others procure) physic and notes treatments (vomits, purges, blisters, bleedings). In a diary that records action, a major part of what his young children "do" is to engage in endless cycles of illness and recovery (and, in the process, worry the minister and disturb his work).

The illness of Parkman's children played out in three ways: sicknesses that commanded urgent response, consuming the minister's attention and energies as did the final weeks of his wife's pregnancies; overlapping sicknesses, when more than one child was ill at once; and, finally, serial sicknesses that continued, one after another, for weeks, even months at a time. All three of these patterns appear in 1736, which, like other severe years the Parkman family endured, was particularly trying.[6]

All four of Parkman's surviving children—Molly (age eleven), Ebenezer (age nine), Thomas (age seven), and baby Lucy—became ill during 1736. Young Ebenezer was the first, with acute symptoms that were of immediate concern to his father. Ebenezer had been to the Sunday afternoon service, but "At Eve he was somewhat aguish" (January 11, 1736). On Monday, Ebenezer was worse, "indisposed with a Fever and Cough," and his father cut pastoral visits short to return home to his sick son. By Wednesday, Parkman had called on a doctor who was unable to come to the parsonage, and the minister tended his son through the night. On Thursday, Parkman sent a field hand to another doctor who was also not able to come but sent "some Remedys," which toward night made Ebenezer "Easier and better," though his condition was of enough concern that Parkman's maid sat up with the boy. While the fever abated on Friday, the cough continued, and Parkman's sister-in-law watched with Ebenezer. The physic he took the following day "worked kindly" but made him "Weak and faint," and Ebenezer required two watchers that night. Finally, on Sunday, Ebenezer showed signs of improvement. It had been a week of worry, but the episode had come to a close.

Perhaps because of the knowledge that young children often died from them, illnesses such as young Ebenezer's were taken seriously. Parkman had watched twice with his son during the week, traveled for a doctor, drawn on the help of his sister-in-law and the labor of hired workers (a field hand and maid), and facilitated arrangements for care. Had Parkman detailed his wife's labors during the crisis, which were likely significant (as we will see below), the overall burdens of care would appear greater still. The power of the illness to shape routines and command attention was considerable.

Yet the ultimate impact of this incident lay in its ubiquity. All across New England, families coped with children in dire circumstances. Some would die; many others, like young Ebenezer, would live. Taken alone, a week or two was manageable. But a house full of children often meant that families endured more than one illness at a time as the Parkmans did in 1736. The following narrative of those illnesses will include only a momentary pause for the dramatic focus of the year, the death of Ebenezer Parkman's first wife, Mary, eight days after contracting a fever at the end of January shortly after her older son's recovery. Her death deserves treatment beyond the bounds of the present discussion: it was a defining moment in Parkman's life (and undoubtedly in his children's lives as well).[7] But for our purposes here, Mary's illness might be considered one in a long line of illnesses in the family.

On Monday, January 19, Parkman wrote in praise of his son Ebenezer's apparent recovery: "the Glory be to God our Healer!" Yet even at the time, he noted, "Almost all the Family indisposed," especially his infant daughter, Lucy (age fifteen months), who was so ill that Parkman "got up several Times in the night" (January 19, 1736). The following day, Parkman included among his rounds a visit to a doctor in neighboring Marlborough "on Account of little Lucy," but met with little success; the doctor was not home, and at evening Parkman found Lucy "very ill" and his wife "much indisposed." By Wednesday, things had worsened: "A sick House— *Lucy very* bad and my Wife taken very ill of a fever" (January 21, 1736). In the following week, the situation intensified. Help was hastily assembled. Neighboring women were fetched while others arrived on their own accord and offered to watch; Mary's sister was retrieved from Cambridge; a doctor visited and consulted with the family several times; a maid was brought in to tend Lucy, whom the Parkmans tried to wean to avoid any more unnecessary "exposure" of the mother. As hopes of recovery faded on January 28, the minister asked his wife to pray "For me and the Children *with this dying Breath*." She begged Jesus to come quickly, and Parkman recalled later, "Some of the last Things I heard her Say I think were—*My Dear!—My Dear Lucy!*"[8]

Even as the house sunk under the weight of the death, the family for whom Mary prayed continued to labor under affliction. In the first half of February, Parkman's eldest daughter suffered from "Ague in her face, her Teeth and Ear" and "broke out" from her treatment, a blister applied to her face (February 8 and 18, 1736). She was evidently troubled well into March: "Molly very grievously exercised still, with her Hands breaking out and remaining exceeding Sore" (March 24, 1736). Young Ebenezer became sick at the end of February and into mid-March with a fever and faintness, though the child's condition was clearly of less concern than his fever and severe cough a few months earlier. The immediate family had been ill from January through March.

The year closed with the Parkman children falling ill again. On October 17, young Ebenezer had a bout of fever and vomiting and, more ominously, two days later a "Canker rose very visibly" on the inside of his throat (though Parkman was relieved that the swelling was minimal and did not seem to overly trouble young Ebenezer); Thomas followed suit on October 29. By 1736, the deadly "throat distemper" was working its way through New England, causing particular concern.[9] Both Parkman's maid (along with her sister) and his hired farmhand watched with Ebenezer. But the minister had less help the following week with Thomas; he had hoped his maid would watch, but she left to visit her mother and failed to return to the parsonage until four days later.[10] A week after Thomas's illness, Parkman lamented, "My little *Lucy* taken ill of a Fever in the Eve" (November 7, 1736). Although Lucy recovered two days later, the minister may have decided that, after a troubling year, he could not manage a house (or oversee its management by a housekeeper and assorted kin) with an infant. On November 15, Parkman carried little Lucy to his sister-in-law's in Cambridge, where she would remain for two years. During the visit, Parkman stopped at his brother Elias's in Boston, where his daughter Molly had been staying for the previous three weeks. Finding Elias "indisposed," Parkman brought Molly back to Westborough with him. Parkman wrote, "through Divine Goodness she bore the Journey very well" (November 19, 1736). And with that, the family's experiences with illness for the year 1736 came to a close. In total, Parkman's family had been ill for nearly four months; if one adds the afflictions of Parkman's hired help in the middle of the year, there was hardly a month at the parsonage in which someone was not sick or lame.

From our perspective, it is not difficult to imagine why illnesses overlapped and persisted. Children without immunities to any number of diseases contracted them and passed them on to their siblings. The larger the household, the greater the probability of sickness at any given time. Each family would have to go through its own periods of "seasoning." But why does this pattern matter? What does it illuminate in eighteenth-century life?

For Ebenezer Parkman, the death of his wife forced the minister to find a way to discharge responsibilities formerly shouldered by Mary. He did his best to patch things together with household help, but for any number of reasons, that was not always reliable. Writing in the middle of the year after his housekeeper Deborah was slowed by her indispositions, Parkman lamented in his diary that the house was out of control: "My House very much like a Boat adrift—by means of my sore Bereavement and the Circumstances of my Friends and Relations *below*, which keep them at a Distance from me; and by means of Deborahs indispositions and heartlessnes" (June 21, 1736). In truth, Parkman had received a good deal of assistance from friends and extended family—neighbors, brothers and sisters, and in-laws—not to mention the significant contributions of his hired help. But without a wife, or someone to assume the control of domestic cares, Parkman's household had lost its moorings. Although he remained devoted to the memory of his first wife, it was not long before the minister began to search for another partner. In September 1736, Parkman prayed that God might recognize "the broken State of My family" and grant him success in finding a "Fellow-Helper" who could "make my Life Comfortable again So as I may again attend to my Ministerial Duty with some freeness and Delight" (September 13, 1736). Marriage and comfort folded together in a kind of "social competency"; the minister sought a measure of independence in the labors of a wife. Without her, he was lost in a sea of dependencies.

The sicknesses of young children added significant work to the already taxing obligations of child rearing. Illness played into a dynamic that made young couples vulnerable to the forces of dependency at work in daily life. More of a drain than an asset on family farms, young children had to be fed and maintained for several years before they could contribute significantly to the family economy. Childhood illness added to this burden, asking the family (including hired help) to provide care, to take time away from other tasks, and, in serious circumstances, to call on midwives, doctors, and other healers. Parkman became responsible (or more responsible than he would have liked) for all of these things and more in the absence of a "fellow helper." A wife would afford him time, order, and the freedom from the constant worries that attended child rearing. Perhaps Hannah Breck had these heavy burdens in mind when she refused the minister's proposals in 1736 (she would marry him the following year), citing his house full of children as one of the primary reasons that the marriage was unsuitable.[11]

As children grew, they continued to endure illnesses, but they also began to contribute economically to the household in substantial ways, and so the loss of their labor while they were unwell registered keenly in the diary. The sicknesses of older youths, then, assumed a different importance and were construed in different ways than the afflictions of young children.

II. YOUTHS AND YOUNG ADULTS

If one of the primary things that young children "do" in Ebenezer Parkman's diary is fall ill and recover, youths have a more extensive repertoire. While his children were not often the central focus of any entry, on the margins of Parkman's notations one watches his growing children extend their range of movement, take on new tasks, and build connections outside the house.[12]

One development crucial for the purposes here is that Parkman's growing children began to become active participants in the economy of affliction and its urgent requirements. Starting at around age ten, Parkman's boys began to ride on their own and were able to fetch doctors, midwives, neighbors, and medicines, as well as visit a healer by themselves. In August 1738, young Ebenezer was within a few weeks of his eleventh birthday when he took himself off to a doctor in neighboring Marlborough to seek advice for a "bad swelling" in his neck (August 10, 1738). In December of that year, Ebenezer rode to Marlborough again, this time to fetch the doctor for his stepmother, whose pains and swellings in the final month of her pregnancy had caused alarm (December 16, 1738). The night after the delivery, Ebenezer brought home the midwife (December 29, 1738). As Ebenezer's seven younger brothers came of age, this pattern would become quite familiar.

Parkman's sons and daughters also helped with some of the more onerous tasks of tending the sick, such as watching through the night. The minister's eldest daughter, Molly, was only fourteen when she sat up with a nurse to watch over her newborn sister, whose "Ghastly pale" visage and difficulty breathing presaged her death a week later (January 9, 1739). When they were older, Parkman's sons and daughters would watch on their own. Thomas was twenty-seven when he watched with Mr. Rogers, bringing back word that the man was "but just alive" (October 9, 1756); two years

later, after watching with Deacon Tainter's boy, Thomas was given a gift
of white gloves, perhaps "mourning gloves" for the funeral (December 1,
1758).[13] In most cases, if there was only one person to be tended, persons
of the same sex watched over each other. But twenty-five-year-old Billy
Parkman was considered responsible enough to watch Elizabeth Whipple
in 1766, a woman who suffered numerous fits after an apparent prank by
"sundry foolish vain young fellows" who threw snow down the chimney
of her loom shop (January 24 & 27, 1766). And Parkman's daughter Anna-
Sophia ("Sophy"), age fourteen, was called to watch over an entire house of
sick folk (several members of the family and their maid); perhaps the fact
that the ill in the house were "growing better" helps to explain why young
Sophy was given such a tall order (December 21, 1769).

The point is clear. As the Parkman children entered their teens, they
watched not only family members, but participated in a larger economy of
affliction. Their efforts sometimes resulted in gifts, but more often were
placed in the realm of neighborly exchange and social credit. Although
Parkman's boys were important in the process, his girls were likely even
more so. As each of his six daughters who survived childhood made it into
their teens, they changed the character of the parsonage, which now was
filled with the comings and goings of "young women." Save for some explicit references to quiltings or the minister's catechetical exercises with
groups of young women, the details of their rides, visits, and conversations are beyond the purview of the diary. Nevertheless, Parkman took
seriously the extremely important place that young women played in the
economy of affliction, and not just because his wife relied heavily on her
grown daughters for help (a topic we will return to momentarily). While
they may have lacked the healing wisdom of their mothers, young women
had an energy and flexibility that enabled them to smooth the regular disturbances that arose in daily life. They could be called on in an instant to
attend to very serious business. As Parkman put it in 1756 when yet another family on the southeast side of town had been stricken by lethal illness, death brought its own sorrows, but the death of young women made
the blow that much more severe: "N. B. Betty Bellows dyed about 10 a.m.,
Aetatis 18. Extremely Sorrowful in that House and Neighborhood, there
being no other Daughter in that family; and but one or two more Young
women in that Corner of Town" (March 17, 1756).

As Parkman's family moved through the life cycle, his family was
better able to absorb the burdens of affliction. Yet at the same time, the
illnesses of Parkman's older daughters and sons generated fresh problems
that had to be addressed. First, when Parkman's children left his house

and fell ill, he still maintained ultimate responsibility for their well-being. The bonds of family would have to be resilient enough to stretch beyond the household. Second, when his older children were unable to work due to illness, the value of that labor became apparent. Illness of adult children exposed the costs of their absence while sick.

Parkman's son Thomas repeatedly fell ill away from home. The failure of two apprenticeships, and almost a third, were tied to the young man's health. One month after Parkman had sent the fourteen-year-old to a Boston goldsmith, Parkman heard the bad news that his son was "much out of Health" and that his master was "discourag'd about him and would have me send for him home" (May 19, 1744). On June 1, Parkman collected his son, noting somberly in his diary that his "hopes [were] all blasted" for his son's training, as the goldsmith had given up on the boy (June 1, 1744). The following year brought more of the same. Just before he was to start an apprenticeship with a weaver in neighboring Grafton, Thomas fell ill, deferring his starting date by several days (April 12, 1745). One month after he began, Thomas "came home ill" from Grafton. Parkman sent the youth off to a doctor in Marlborough the following day and again two weeks later "that he might get suitable Directions and Druggs of him" (June 1, 1745). Thomas resumed his apprenticeship the following week, but returned to Westborough for good one week later, "being in such Pain and under So great Discouragement that his master sends all his Things home with him" (June 15, 1745). An agreement reached in the fall of 1749 with a saddler in Concord ultimately proved successful, though the master had to overlook several weeks in February when Thomas returned home to recover his health. Thomas ultimately finished his indenture three weeks later than planned; though there was no explicit discussion between Parkman and the saddler, it may be that Thomas simply added time to his indenture to work off days missed due to illness.[14]

What are we to make of Thomas's repeated illnesses: Would some modern diagnosis explain his case? Was the boy homesick or malingering? According to the diary, no one seems to have questioned the validity of his afflictions. Indeed, his case fits a much larger pattern in which youths (and, indeed, adults as well) fell ill away from home. Society encouraged youths to widen their orbit and expected them to leave the house as they grew older (although ideas about the acceptable range and manner of travel were gendered, and the means, opportunity, and necessity of travel were sensitive to family fortunes).[15] That some became ill is not surprising. Contemporary medical understanding suggested that a change in environment could be dangerous; present-day biomedicine might frame the problem as an encounter with a new set of microbes. Whatever the explanation, there were consequences. When the young left home and became ill, both their families and society at large had to make accommodations.

Ebenezer Jr. was eleven when he took a trip to Boston with his parents, the first since he was a babe. The boy found the "Evil Smells" of the city objectionable, perhaps even sickening; a day into the trip, Parkman wrote that his son was "under great Infirmitys—weak and Sick and a bad cough" (May 31, 1738). Parkman took Ebenezer to a doctor the following day. But when Ebenezer showed no signs of recovery, Parkman left him in Boston and traveled home. It was Friday, and the minister had Sabbath preparations and services over which to preside. Beyond these personal concerns, leaving young Ebenezer may have seemed only prudent; it was considered dangerous to journey while in a precarious state. Two weeks later Parkman's cousin brought Ebenezer back from Cambridge, where in-laws from his father's first marriage, the Champneys, had apparently taken him in.

In 1742 illness thwarted several attempts made by Parkman over the course of a month to retrieve his seventeen-year-old Molly from Boston, where she was attending school. On each occasion, after troubling to secure someone to bring his horse into town for Molly to ride home, Parkman received news that Molly was too ill to travel. Finally, Parkman rode into town in the company of a Mr. Smith (likely the Reverend Aaron Smith of Marlborough), who brought along his chaise. A few days later, Parkman began the journey home on Smith's horse with Molly riding in the chaise. But when Molly worsened on the ride, Parkman left her at Smith's house in Marlborough to recover. Not until two weeks later was Molly able to return home to Westborough with Ebenezer Jr., who had come to Marlborough to fetch a doctor for his father.[16]

In most cases, we don't know if compensation was made for these stays. Controversy surrounded young Ebenezer's care in Cambridge, but it did not involve money or other restitution—it was about female authority and respect. When Parkman's cousin returned the boy, he relayed a message from the minister's in-laws, mother Champney and her daughter Lydia—apparently special cautions to be taken for his son's welfare. Parkman let it be known that he thought this too "strict a Charge," and the women became quite "disquieted" when they heard about it some weeks later (July 4, 1738). Reliance on the goodwill of relatives might mean minding their advice, particularly the healing authority of the women who cared for the boy. During Molly's stay with Parkman's sister Betty, the teen may have lessened her burden by making herself useful. When Parkman retrieved his daughter, he noted that though she "had long been laid up with a Severe ague," Molly "Still kept house" (November 30, 1742).[17]

Only on rare occasions does one find explicit financial arrangements made between Parkman and the family members or friends who took in his children when they fell ill away from home. When twenty-two-year-old Susanna ("Suse") Parkman fell ill while visiting at the house of Reverend Ebenezer Morse in June 1767, it was several weeks before she was able to return to the parsonage (July 20, 1767). There is no hint in the diary leading up to that point that she was ill during the time. But in December of that year, Reverend Morse made a visit from his home in neighboring Shrewsbury to the Parkmans, and among his purposes was to reckon with the minister for "Boarding and Doctering Suse" (December 8, 1767). Morse seemed almost sheepish in asking, saying, "3 Dollars will suffice." Perhaps if Parkman's surviving account book was complete, these sorts of transactions would appear more often.[18] It is equally likely, however, that such transactions would not appear; they are buried within the unwritten intricacies of the barter economy, part of a calculus of goodwill and practical limitations that we cannot access.

⁐

If the first major problem of youth and their sicknesses lay in negotiating afflictions away from home, the second problem cut in the opposite direction. As young persons of the family became valuable members of the family economy, their inability to labor due to sickness was keenly felt. Parkman's diary makes clear the ways in which illness is linked with performance. Not every illness or ailment was recorded. Certain contexts prompted Parkman to make note of affliction. Consider the following comments on Parkman's ten-year-old son Billy. On November 29, 1751: "Billy has been not well for some time. Pain in his Neck and Face." We have no way of knowing how long Billy had been unwell (he is last mentioned a month earlier hauling a side of beef), nor why his condition was worthy of comment at this point. But subsequent entries provide a clue. A week later Parkman gave his son a once-over and noted, "Billy not well, but is better" (December 5, 1751). The matter was then dropped. And in the following weeks, Billy returned to the diary as a boy of action—writing, tending the cattle, taking corn to a mill in nearby Southborough, helping his older brother sled wood. What mattered to Parkman in the space of the diary was not to note every pain he perceived Billy to have during this time. As long as the boy was "better" (perhaps "not well," but not getting worse either) and could perform the tasks expected of him, there was no need to write of his pains. Parkman would continue to record alarming conditions, new ailments, and changes that threatened to become worse. But increasingly, as his children grew, these reflections would be inseparable from his worries about the labor that they could not undertake as they lay ill. Sickness highlighted the costs of non-performance in a world dependent on active employment.

From their early teens into their twenties, the minister's sons were relied on to do farm work. Parkman did not have anywhere near the amount of land to promise them a future in farming, nor was husbandry the calling that he hoped they would pursue. But he did need their labor at certain times. Breaking and plowing the land; planting, hoeing, weeding, and harvesting corn, rye, and wheat; mowing, raking, gathering, and carting hay; watching, feeding, and butchering livestock—these were some of the tasks that needed attention. Although Parkman would draw on the services of many persons at different times of the year, from the late spring through the early fall he counted on having at least two reliable laborers, usually a young boy in his early teens and a young man in his late teens or early twenties who could do heavier work. At various points, his sons might fill either role. When they could not, Parkman secured workers elsewhere.[19]

By 1755 both Billy and Thomas Parkman had acquired ample farm experience. Thomas had worked on the farm between apprenticeships; beginning in the early 1750s, he set up a saddling shop on his father's property, where he practiced his craft and worked on the farm. Over the past several summers, Billy had increased the range of his activities on the farm. In the spring and summer of 1755, Parkman expected Thomas and Billy, who turned twenty-six and fourteen that year, respectively, to be his principal laborers. As fate would have it, both sons became ill during the summer, and Parkman scrambled to make up for their absence.

Thomas fell sick in early June. After observing his son "drooping for Several Days," Parkman made the diagnosis: "My Son Thomas has Fever and Ague" (June 5 & 6, 1755). The condition could be immediately threatening, but more often it was something that lingered. Parkman accordingly arranged for others to labor in his son's place. By Tuesday the minister had Rody Smith hoeing corn with Billy (June 10, 1755). When Thomas was still indisposed at the end of the week, Parkman hired a father-and-son duo to help Billy (June 13, 1755). Then Billy fell ill on June 20, though the "drooping" lad did his best to resume work the following week (June 25, 1755). By early July, both of Parkman's sons were having intermittent fits, and while there would be occasional signs of improvement, not until the beginning of August could Parkman write that "Thomas and William are Somewhat better and Stronger" (August 9, 1755).

In the meantime, Parkman tried to get help and welcomed acts of kindness. Some fellow townsfolk recruited labor; others offered their teams for plowing; still others, like Parkman's neighbor Mr. Rogers, brought over his team to cart away rye that had been gathered and bound—a chore that the grateful minister noted was "done gratis" (August 5, 1755). Many others would be paid by the task. But in the height of the summer, it was difficult to find anyone, paid or unpaid, who could come consistently. Equally frustrating were those like Jonas Twitchell who promised to work in lieu of paying his ministerial rates, but later refused the minister's requests.[20] Toward the end of July, Parkman was turning away members of the church seeking counsel so that he could focus on the "urgent" business of the farm: "There was no Hand could be hir'd, and both my sons, Thomas and Billy incapable of any Labour at all" (July 23, 1755). Parkman managed to get though the season, but only by cobbling together a variety of laborers—a few men paid by the task; two "young men" who worked at miscellaneous chores for nine days in August; sundry labors performed by Ebenezer Jr. (who was living in Parkman's first house and had his own farming and family concerns) and son Breck (age six); and the occasional labor of the minister himself. Parkman would have to pay out wages. He would also make sure that some "Friends" who had helped were given two hindquarters of veal, a "token of Gratitude to them both" (August 25, 1755). Cash outlays, expended favors, and the confusion and strain of assembling a labor force—these were the costs of his sons' summer illnesses.[21]

We know much less about the place of Parkman's young daughters within the family's domestic economy. A fragment from a diary kept by Parkman's daughter Sophy in 1777 affords a brief view. The diary records twenty-two-year-old Sophy sewing, knitting, spinning and carding wool, washing and ironing, and doing "sundries in the Kitchen" and "a variety of things." A comment that "Crosby cleans the Garretts" suggests that certain types of work may have been reserved for others. "Crosby" was almost certainly the widow Mrs. Mary Crosby, who served as a maid for the Parkmans from 1775 to 1777. Some types of dirty work were perhaps beneath the station of young Sophy, who, in addition to her chores, drank tea, engaged in conversation, wrote letters, and attended singing school—all part of preparing for and participating in polite society. If Sophy was typical, Hannah Parkman received substantial, if not complete, help from her daughters.[22]

It comes as no surprise, then, that the illness of her grown daughters could be especially trying for Hannah Parkman. From the late 1750s through their marriages in the late 1760s, Suse and Sarah Parkman were the eldest daughters remaining at the parsonage. Two years older than Suse and perhaps responsible for more of the housework, Sarah had repeated illnesses during these years that put pressures on her younger sister and mother alike. When Sarah fell ill in 1759, a year in which the entire family was afflicted by various maladies, Ebenezer Parkman wrote nervously, "Sarah indeed seems to be worse. The Care and Labour of the Family very heavy upon my poor Wife, Suse having gone to Marlborough yesterday with her Cousen Maynard" (October 10, 1759). In 1766 Parkman sounded a similar theme, though the burdens of affliction succeeded merely in dampening a celebration and possibly embarrassing the minister in front of his guests. On July 24, 1766: "Publick Thanksgiving for Repeal of the Stamp Act. . . . N. B. Sarah so poorly, and Suse at Boston, Mrs. P____ makes no great Provision." Later that year, as Sarah was slowly recovering from a period in which she suffered headaches and pains in her breast, Parkman noted with relief that while "Sarah [was] but weak and poorly," Suse "is in Family Business again" (August 28, 1766). The smoothly operating "business" of family relied on the healthy bodies of its female members.

For both Ebenezer Parkman's sons and daughters, reaching maturity meant greater responsibilities in the economies of production and affliction. The disruptions caused when these young adults fell ill spoke to their growing importance in sustaining the family's competency.

III. NEW FAMILIES

Concluding his biographical sketch of Ebenezer Parkman with a list of the minister's progeny, Clifford Shipton muses that "any extended account of Parkman's sixteen children and the equally distinguished people whom they married would be a history of their century."[23] The remainder of this chapter contributes in a modest way to this ambitious project by considering the organization of illness in the Parkman family as the minister's children set up households of their own.

Two dimensions of New England's demographic history set the scene. First, over the course of the seventeenth and eighteenth centuries, new towns were established, populations grew and open land became scarce, and the young and marginal migrated to the peripheries in search of new land or, later in the eighteenth century, to opportunities in port towns and cities. This "hiving out" process was enacted repeatedly.[24] The settlement of Parkman's adult and married children offers a variation of the pattern, moving in all directions but different distances. Some stayed close. The minister's fifth son, Breck, lived nearby in Westborough and became a successful shopkeeper in town; Ebenezer Jr. began his married life in Westborough and ended his days living with his brother Breck; Parkman's youngest surviving daughter and her husband lived at the parsonage during the minister's final years. Others moved further afield, mostly to other towns in central Massachusetts. With few exceptions, however, Parkman's children stayed within a forty-mile radius of Westborough. The result was that almost every child lay within a ride of a day or two, making it possible for Parkman's family and those of his children to respond to each other's illnesses.

To this movement across space we need to add the movement of New England families through time. Thus far, illness in the family life cycle has been explored in the context of changing relations between parents and their children at various stages of maturity. When children married and created families of their own, the cycle was repeated: infants and young children presented numerous illnesses without being able to contribute to the family economy; and the disruptions caused by ailing youths and unmarried adults highlighted their increasing importance in economies of affliction and production. It would be a mistake, however, to think of these "new families" as moving through this process in isolation; in fact, the term "new family" should be applied not only to those starting out but to those left behind. Illness allows us to see some of the ways in which families at different stages of the life cycle intersected with and influenced each other.[25]

For purposes of analysis, we might distinguish four periods in the organization of illness in these intersecting families. The first period begins in the 1750s, as Parkman's eldest children created family households of their own. "Going to housekeeping" could involve a sharp break between parent families and their newly married children, but if married children stayed close by, there might well be considerable exchange between the households.[26] This was the case with Parkman's eldest son and his family. When the minister moved from the parsonage to live closer to the new meetinghouse, Ebenezer Jr. was allowed to remain at the original house and farm the land, a fortunate but not unheard-of occurrence for a young man in his early twenties, although he did not hold title to the house and would have to wait for his portion. Young Ebenezer married Elizabeth Harrington within a year, and the couple had a son eleven months later. By 1756 they were a family of five. Meanwhile, Hannah (Breck) Parkman's reproductive years were not over—her last child was born in 1761. On the same day that Ebenezer Jr. and Elizabeth had their first child, Hannah delivered her eighth. In short, older couples like Ebenezer and Hannah Parkman might well share part of the life cycle with their adult children: both couples had young children to tend to in their houses. The major difference between the families was that the older couple also had youths and unmarried adults in their brood.

The year 1756 reveals the intricate relations that had developed between the two families. Parkman's unmarried children moved frequently between the parsonage and "t'other" house, staying with their brother overnight for days, even weeks at a time. There was an element of reciprocity in such movements. Parkman's older boys helped Ebenezer Jr. with his farm work, especially after he fell behind in the early spring. Ebenezer Jr., in turn, worked on his father's land, harrowing fields, getting in the last of the oats, and carrying loads from the ministerial meadow. His wife, Elizabeth, may have helped by watching her husband's young brothers, Samuel and John (ages four and nearly three), who occasionally stayed at the new house (March 13, 1756). For their part, Hannah Parkman and her thirteen-year-old daughter Sarah were instrumental in helping at the new house. Sarah moved there in the middle of April, undoubtedly to aid her sister-in-law in the final weeks of a pregnancy. Hannah Parkman participated in the delivery the following month.

Instances of illness during that year reveal both the depth and the limitations of family reciprocity. Three weeks after the delivery, Ebenezer Parkman Sr. wrote, "My sons Wife So weak etc. we have not only Sent *Sarah* over to them but my Wife herself has gone over and changed Children," leaving their seven-month-old daughter Sophy and returning with his son's infant (June 8, 1756). The following evening Ebenezer Jr. brought Sophy back to the parsonage but did not retrieve his daughter. "[M]y wife has both of them to keep and Suckle over Night," Parkman worried. "We fear a tedious Task" (June 9, 1756). Hannah Parkman returned the child two days later and suckled her a final time the following week. Daughter-in-law Elizabeth was able to repay the favor, at least in part, in September. When Hannah Parkman wanted to visit Boston and little Sophy was unwell, arrangements were made to leave the child at the other house, where she would be suckled by Elizabeth and tended by Sarah (September 29, 1756).[27]

We might interpret these events in two ways. On the one hand, there is a remarkable sense of harmony and order here—a happy fit between two families at overlapping and yet distinct stages of their life cycle. A nursing exchange was made possible because Hannah Parkman and her daughter-in-law were both in their childbearing years; the Parkmans were able to spare the labors of their teenage sons and daughters because they had several adult children remaining at the parsonage; and the free-flowing exchange of people was possible because the two families lived close together. When all of these elements came together, family could be a significant source of aid with mundane cares and of support in times of crisis.

On the other hand, tensions lurked below the surface. Hannah Parkman had the difficult charge of nursing two children at once, a labor that the minister considered his sacrifice as well. As he put it: "we worry through the Night" and "we fear a tedious Task" (June 8–9, 1756). Nor was everything well with Ebenezer Jr. and his wife. Even with the nursing help and young Sarah Parkman's efforts around the new house, Ebenezer Jr. felt the limitations of his wife's incapacity. Several days after Hannah suckled her grandchild for the last time, Parkman wrote, "Ebenezers Wife Still weak—he in much trouble for a Maid" (June 18, 1756). Family aid could only go so far. It certainly could not guarantee comfort. It could lessen but not remove intense pressures.

In the end, the relations between the two families could not be fully reciprocal. Hannah and Ebenezer had greater depth in family resources—and greater responsibilities. Ebenezer Jr. and Elizabeth could offer the minister's children a place to stay and perhaps meals. But they could not (or would not) absorb the burdens of afflictions that were not properly their own. The fate of two younger members of the minister's family who became indisposed at the old house during the year illustrates the point. In late August, Ebenezer Jr. asked his father about the prospect of sending nine-year-old Alexander to live with Ebenezer Jr. until he turned fourteen (August 30, 1756). Yet when Alexander fell ill with the fever and ague in October and was not better within a week, Parkman wrote that the boy "returns to tarry at Home" (October 24, 1756).[28] It was much the same with seven-year-old Breck, who was "brought home from Ebenezer because he is Lame, having cut his right Legg with an Ax, before the former Sore on his left is healed" (December 22, 1756). We have no way of knowing who initiated the returns—the children, the minister, or Ebenezer Jr. But the diary makes it clear that these youngsters had a "home," and that it was not with their older brother's new family. Parkman and his wife would assume ultimate responsibility.

In the project of launching a family competency, Ebenezer Jr. and Elizabeth were net consumers of family capital; they absorbed more than they could possibly replenish. The minister, his wife, and children may have borne added responsibilities in keeping Ebenezer Jr.'s family afloat—the strains of fear and tedious worries—all in support of the competency of a young family.[29]

⁂

On November 16, 1758, Parkman made a simple notation in an entry otherwise filled with the business of town and church: "Thomas returned from Brookfield and brought Suse and Breck with him, and left Sarah in Suse's Stead." A mere two years after his children had shuffled back and forth between the new house and the old in Westborough, they were now doing much the same between Westborough and Brookfield, a town thirty miles to the west. Parkman's oldest child, Molly, had settled there in 1752 after marrying Eli Forbes, who became a minister in the town. Ebenezer Jr. and family followed suit in 1757 after they were forced to leave the old house (Parkman needed it rented or sold, in part to help his son buy a farm of his own). The most recent addition to Brookfield was Parkman's second eldest daughter, Lucy, who moved to town after her marriage to Lieutenant Jeduthan Baldwin in 1757. In the late 1750s and well into the 1760s, the minister's unmarried adult children were spending weeks, even months, at a time in Brookfield, helping with farming, infants, and young children, and perhaps thinking about settling there themselves.

This arrangement of family differed from the configuration a few years earlier in two significant ways, both with implications for the organization of illness. First, the Parkman children had developed in Brookfield a center of gravity apart from the parsonage. Even the most basic elements of that world are difficult to detect in a diary that has its home base in Westborough. But comments captured in the diary make it clear that, at a minimum, the families had an easy familiarity with the health of their members: "Mr. Forbes and Sarah from Brookfield. They inform that Lucy is often very poorly but that Neddy Parkman is better" (July 30, 1764). (Neddy was likely one-year-old Edward Parkman, Ebenezer Jr.'s sixth child.) Mr. Eli Forbes and Sarah Parkman knew that their sister Lucy was not only poorly, but often poorly, and that their nephew Neddy Parkman had been ill, for now he was "better." The Brookfield families were close enough to pick up on these kinds of details. One gets an occasional glimpse in the diary of how this world of affliction works, but more often than not, Parkman simply records that his children come and go to Brookfield, and we have to imagine what transpires while they are away.

The second development in this period concerns what might be thought of cautiously as the balance of social power between Westborough and Brookfield. There was no overt competition here; indeed, Parkman was deeply concerned that his children remain industrious, and may have been only too pleased to have them productively engaged with their siblings. Nevertheless, both those in Westborough and those in Brookfield had needs, leading to subtle strains in times of affliction.

The year 1759 provides a good example. When Hannah Parkman became severely ill with an intermittent fever during the month of April, the Parkmans received an astonishing amount of help from the community: their youngest, fourteen-month-old Hannah, was sent out to wean and was later boarded by another family; the widow Newton, following a night of watching, took three-and-a-half-year-old Sophy home with her; and an array of others, mostly daughters of families with whom the Parkmans had frequent contact, visited and watched. Sarah Parkman, now sixteen, assumed a central role in maintaining the household, not only watching several times with her mother but also working alongside the hired help to maintain the household. Despite these numerous efforts, the house suffered as one hired helper after another was either unwilling or unable to stay: Patty Dunlop, who had helped the family in the past, decided for some unknown reason to leave after five days of service (April 10, 1759); Persis Rice took over for a week until she became "so indisposed" that she went home (April 16, 1759); Jemima Maynard filled in to help with Sarah, but a week later Parkman was "Abroad after a Maid again" (April 23, 1759).[30] Finally, son Thomas was sent to Brookfield to fetch daughter Suse, who returned on April 28. Presumably Parkman's daughter was thought to be a more steady source of support than the hired help.

Hannah's sickness was not the only trouble that month for the minister and for the family at Brookfield. Billy fell ill with the measles immediately after returning to the parsonage from Brookfield. He thought "he took the Distemper at his Brother *Parkmans*, he having been there several Times while the Children were coughing and ill of it" (April 11, 1759). This added a burden to the minister, who slept poorly as he tended his son (April 12, 1759). Billy's illness also points to distress in Brookfield. Given that the measles lasted a week or more and that more than one of Ebenezer Jr.'s children had contracted the distemper, one suspects that his house, too, was in some trouble. Yet the minister had been obliged to ask Suse to return from Brookfield. One imagines that there was simply too much to be handled at the parsonage with her away. In the contest between the two centers, the parsonage had the stronger pull.[31]

By the 1770s, a third era in the organization of family illness had begun
with the emergence of several centers of family life. Now Parkman's children were scattered more widely, settling in Ashburnham, Concord, Boston, and Rochester—the latter sixty miles away from Westborough, the
rest within a forty-mile radius. Movement through time had produced
settlement across space.

This settlement pattern stretched family resources thinly, with several
implications for the management of illness. First, the minister more frequently registered the inconvenience caused by the absence of his wife and
children as they tended to his married children. Although Hannah Parkman was afflicted with recurring rheumatic pains through much of the
1760s, she was perhaps more mobile in the early 1770s than before. The
diary from that period finds her visiting frequently with friends and local
relatives as well as taking more "journeys" in part because of her new freedom: Hannah's last child had been born in 1761. By the 1770s her youngest
children no longer needed the vigilant care reserved for the steady stream
of infants that the minister and his wife had brought forth for over two
decades. Hannah not only had freedom to travel but also lures drawing her
away from Westborough. The first of her biological daughters gave birth
in 1771, and the majority of her biological grandchildren were born in the
1770s and 1780s. Nothing in Parkman's diary indicates that Hannah was
indifferent to the children born of his first wife, but she seems to have felt
a special draw to her own flesh and blood. Perhaps a mixture of ability and
desire inspired Hannah to take more journeys during this period.[32]

From the minister's standpoint, Hannah's journeys could be trying.
With his wife visiting her daughter Sarah (Parkman) Cushing in 1771, the
sixty-seven-year-old minister fretted, "I had but a poor night—pained in my
Mouth, Sweating, restless. . . . Am lonely also, my wife tarrying So long,
am full of Fears that all is not well among them" (August 16, 1771). Sarah
would deliver her first child the following day. Yet it was an excruciating
four days until news came that Sarah had gone "through a tedious Travail,"
but her mother had been with her and all was fine. Lonely and in pain, Parkman perhaps wanted some care himself. Visits could be equally troubling
when children lay sick at home with their mother gone: "Have been in
daily Expectation of Mrs. P____ from Brookfield," Parkman quipped, "but
She doth not come. Both Hannah and Elias not well" (August 26, 1773).[33]

If others had been there to tend to the obligations of the family, Parkman might have been more complacent. But by the 1770s, only two daughters lived at the house, and they, too, could be called on by others. This meant that Parkman had to assume more of the burdens of family affliction. Hannah Parkman had been ill for just over a week when the minister was invited to preach in nearby Grafton the following Sabbath. The minister had to decline, explaining in his diary that with "the Circumstances of my Family, at present (my Wife Sick and I have not one of my Children at home etc. etc.) I can't gratifie him" (August 20, 1778). Parkman felt the importance of his wife and children most keenly in their absence. With fewer people to take care of family affairs, he needed them present and healthy in order to tend to his own routines.

Another change occasioned by this period of family dispersal is the way in which illness prompted what might be called heroic visiting. Except for the few children who remained in Westborough, there were simply too many families spread out over too great an area to visit any of them regularly. Especially with their children who lived farthest away, visits were often prompted by dire circumstance. When Parkman got word on November 9, 1772, that his daughter Suse "was nigh Expiring last Evening" after having delivered a child a fortnight earlier, he and Hannah made immediate preparation to leave from Westborough. After a delay in finding suitable horses (none would work with the Parkmans' chaise), they left the next morning and arrived the following day. Suse was alive but her case "doubtful." The following week was filled with "various turns," signs of improvement and decline. Then, after Parkman had written to son Breck that he would be gone for another week, Suse gained in strength to such a degree that Ebenezer and Hannah journeyed home on November 20. Within a week they received news that Suse's cough and fever were back again. Suse died on November 30—her parents were given the somber news ten days later.

The ability to traverse space could not keep pace with rapid changes of the body. When one lived at a distance, illness moved faster than news of family members. An alternative was to come home. Twenty-two-year-old John Parkman returned from Lancaster, Massachusetts, in 1775 to recover his health. He spent several months among the family, and then, when his condition became dangerous, he was watched for the last three weeks of his life by his parents, three siblings, several neighbors, and the Parkmans' hired hand. As family scattered across Massachusetts, the parsonage became one of the few places where the remaining unmarried adults could receive both long-term and intensive care.

In the years after Ebenezer Parkman's death, his grandchildren continued to move out across the countryside. The children of the minister's most successful sons were able to stay closer. But a family genealogy points to a larger pattern of diffusion characteristic of late eighteenth- and early nineteenth-century New England. Grandchildren found their way into Connecticut, Rhode Island, New Hampshire, Maine, New York, and Ohio—one of Parkman's grandsons made it as far as Alabama. Parkman's fourth son, Alexander, and his family typify this trend for New Englanders. Alexander lived for many years in Leicester and Framingham, towns within roughly twenty miles to the west and east of Westborough. But in 1779 he moved his family to Marlboro, New Hampshire. Then in the late 1780s, they continued on into central New York. Alexander's son Robert Breck Parkman extended the movement. When he reached his majority, Robert Breck moved to Cayuga County, New York. Pushing still farther west, he became an agent for his uncle, a Boston merchant, who speculated in the vast lands of the western reserve. In 1804 Robert Breck and his family were among the first settlers of what became Parkman, Ohio.[34]

The travels of people like Alexander Parkman and his family raised the question of how far family ties could stretch. Connections to family back East would increasingly be made through letters or the rare visit, heroic or otherwise. Places like Parkman, Ohio, would become a new family center as generations dispersed across the countryside.

IV. CONCLUSION

Parkman's diary peppers the reader with so many accounts of illness and unease that one may become numbed by the assault. Nonetheless, some broad patterns emerge in and through the details. The frequent illnesses of young children drained family resources, adding to the burdens of young couples already in a vulnerable position. As children grew, they were better able to contribute to the economies of production and affliction. But maturity presented its own difficulties. When youths fell ill, it meant that crucial tasks around the house and farm were left undone. And as grown children moved further afield, the family would have to negotiate the problem of family members who fell ill away from the house. The entire cycle started again as married children commenced families of their own. As successive children moved away, the ties of family necessarily became more attenuated, and serious illness increasingly required family members separated by long distances to tend to their own.

When seen through the prism of family, affliction adds to our understanding of early New England life in three ways. First, studies of the family have emphasized the distinction between those living in the family household and those who live elsewhere, whether they are bound out, serving an apprenticeship, or in households of their own. According to one historian, children were moved from their family of origin with such frequency as to call into question the family of origin as the primary affiliation; on removal to a new household, a new unit of family labor, a child might well be considered a member of another family household. Families absorbed new laborers in their households, blurring the lines between servant and blood kin.[35]

Illness, however, points to the elasticity of family boundaries, the ways in which one's family of origin assumed new significance in times of distress. When minors and unmarried adults lived away, family might well be called on to retrieve them if they fell ill. When New England families fetched their young sons from the northern frontier in times of war (a topic we will return to in chapter 6), it was but an extreme example of what happened regularly in more mundane circumstances. Even when married couples set up households, their own illnesses or those of their children could construct and strengthen connections to their parent families. The organization of illness in family life suggests that we might place greater emphasis on the ties of family across space while recognizing how those spatial ties were attenuated over time as the family dispersed across the land.

Second, a consideration of illness in the family allows us to think of competency in new ways. A competency could allow families the wherewithal to manage during times of affliction but was itself dependent on family health; a family member's physical incapacity affected the ability of the family to maintain a middling subsistence. If the management of illness was an important part of sustaining a comfortable independence, then the women of the house must be considered central in supporting that ideal. Not only were women the primary caregivers in family life, but when the women of the house were sick, the daily immediacies of household maintenance required special and rapid accommodation.[36]

The Parkmans survived the numerous illnesses in their immediate family with their competency intact. They owed their success to industry and perseverance—but also to good fortune. The family had the collective resources to weather their afflictions that others might not: money from the minister's salary; items to barter; social credits earned in living for decades in the same town; the ability to hire maids, nurses, and farm workers who could be asked to help in a time of crisis; a prominence that commanded attention in times of need; and, significantly, family afflictions that, for all of their disturbance and alarm, resolved quickly in most cases. Others could face greater pressures and feel more acutely the force of illness pulling them toward dependency.

Finally, illness points to the ways in which interdependency upheld the ideal of independence. This family did not require town provision for the poor, but such provision remained a last resort for those in extremis and a remarkable achievement of towns that provided social welfare for their members, however spare. But the Parkmans could not have survived without a range of help originating outside of the family of origin. We have seen in-laws, neighbors, and town laborers (and those from further afield) aid the family in their time of need.

What was to be done, however, in the event that the laborers and others who worked alongside family became ill? We turn now to ways in which the sicknesses of household laborers figured into the larger project of competency.

CHAPTER FOUR

Household Competency:
Work, Responsibility, and Belonging

For much of the seventeenth and eighteenth centuries in New England, the rubric of family encompassed not only relations between parents and children but also those between masters and mistresses and the laborers who lived within the household, including slaves, servants, and long-term hired hands. In many ways, the problems that attended the illnesses of these laborers did not differ from those presented by other family members—the ailing needed care, and in their incapacity, someone had to take over their neglected tasks. Illness created burdens, the successful management of which helped to preserve a family's competency. Despite the similarities, however, the illnesses of servants, slaves, and hired hands were construed in ways that set them apart from family, calling into question the structure and meaning of "family" and the ideal of "family competency."

At issue was the instability of the worker's body, which highlighted the uneasy relationship between performance and belonging that integrated the laborer into family life. Workers earned a place in family in a variety of ways, not all of which were tied to their productive efforts. A servant might be taken in as a favor to neighbors or kin, one of the endless exchanges that constituted interdependent relations in early modern life. Workers might endear themselves to their masters through loyalty or ingenuity. But in the end, the ability to work steadily, industriously, and competently was fundamental. Afflictions like illness impeded work or stopped it in its tracks, prompting a series of troubling questions: At what point was the ailing worker's inability to labor at full capacity deemed unsatisfactory? When did a worker's incapacity dissolve the bonds of responsibility and benevolent oversight that held master to servant? Who should be made to pay for a worker's illnesses, understood as an aspect of living in the uncertain temporal world? Not easy questions to address, they arose repeatedly and presented New Englanders with the difficult and sometimes controversial task of finding solutions.

The chapter begins with a brief section on the sicknesses of enslaved persons, and then moves on to consider the afflictions of servants and hired workers. In each section, two dimensions of the problem are examined most closely. First is an investigation of efforts to anticipate the instability of the worker's body and to mitigate the effects of its failures. Here the sources consulted are indentures, contracts, and province and state provisions. Such efforts were necessarily fraught with ambiguity, and contests ensued over responsibility for a worker's illness and compensation for his or her absence. The second approach to the problem is less dramatic, but perhaps closer to the daily practices of coping with a worker's ailments. Here the chapter looks in detail at a few case studies of sick slaves, servants, and hired hands, which open onto more subtle questions of the relationship between responsibility, performance, and belonging.

I. SLAVES

Although one could find major concentrations of enslaved workers in Newport and Boston, in coastal towns, and along major riverways, in most parts of the region, slaves were not a central part of the labor force and never amounted to more than 3% of New England's population. Even as the number of African Americans in the region grew over the century, enslaved persons could be found in less than one-eighth of New England households by 1764. And while some households held as many as sixty slaves, most households that owned slaves possessed only one or two. With important exceptions such as Rhode Island's Narragansett region, New England never sustained anything resembling a slave society.[1]

The significance of slavery in New England arose chiefly from the critical role of the slave trade in the region's economy, fueling debates over the nature of liberty, property, authority, and coercion. Critics of the slave trade argued that one did not have to possess slaves to be implicated in slavery: human chattel was an integral part of the broader web of Atlantic exchanges that brought goods into and out of New England. At the same time, the capture, purchase, transport, and scattering of enslaved persons throughout ports and the hinterland raised practical problems. The rights and responsibilities of masters and slaves had to be established in law and adjudicated in courts. Central to the contests over the enslaved lay an inescapable contradiction, as true in New England as in the South: slaves possessed a doubled identity as property and human being, which raised perplexing questions in the event of sickness and disability.[2]

The central problem was this: If enslaved persons inhabited bodies they did not own, who was responsible for their illnesses? The master? The state that supervised the sale and maintenance of human chattel? The slave him- or herself? The worth of the slave was based on his or her ability to perform assigned tasks consistently and over time. But enslaved persons who were healthy and able to work at one point might well be ill and disabled at others. A slave in sickness could be physically present but no more able to work than a runaway. And, like escapees who might fashion an alternative identity, the enslaved might in some instances feign sickness in order to avoid sale or escape labor.[3] But sickness involved more subtle dynamics than those between master and runaway. Even if masters thought a slave to be malingering, the sick slave had broken no law. And in many cases, masters clearly believed slaves were truly sick. In the meantime, costs accumulated, care had to be provided, and labor was lost.

The complications wrought by enslaved persons' sicknesses began at sea. The terrible rigors of passage ensured that some of the human cargo aboard slave ships would become ill. The pursuit of profits dictated two very different courses of action. Some held that rather than providing for ailing slaves who would likely die, resources were better spent on those who would survive until sale. Anti-slavery advocates seized on the cruelties that flowed from such logic, notoriously illustrated by the *Zong*, a British slaver sailing from the coast of Africa to the West Indies in 1781. Faced with an epidemic on board that had already killed sixty slaves and seven of the crew, the *Zong*'s master ordered 133 ill slaves thrown overboard, apparently with the idea that while insurance would not pay for slaves who died a natural death, restitution was available in cases of drowning. While this incident was extraordinary in the number of slaves killed, there was strong suspicion at the time that similar practices regularly took place on a smaller scale.[4] Yet an alternative logic ensured that sick slaves would in fact be brought ashore. The press for profits dictated that slavers arrive at port with as many live slaves as possible, whether ill or not. Masters went to considerable lengths to save sick slaves, changing routes and hurrying to ports once illness broke out, and absorbing losses on shore, where the ailing might sell for a fraction of the price of the healthy.[5]

The difficulties surrounding sick enslaved persons continued after arrival in New England. Mortality rates for newly arrived slaves were high and, in some cases, on par with the Chesapeake, where as many as one-quarter of all enslaved persons died within their first year. How many of them were already sick upon entrance is impossible to know. But as William Pierson has written, slaves sold in New England were often considered the "refuse" of the Atlantic slave trade. Transported from the West Indies to the Lowcountry, the Chesapeake, and along to the Mid-Atlantic, those who were not wanted—the very young and aged, the obstreperous, the ailing—found markets in New England, where demands for slave labor were far more varied than in the plantation South. Massachusetts made provisions for the inevitable death toll, allowing drawbacks on the impost levied on slaves if they died within six weeks after their arrival in the province. Petitions to the General Court suggest that exceptions to the six-week limit were made as well, as importers scrambled to recoup their losses in the wake of an enslaved person's death.[6] Allowances were also made for slaves whose ailments, while not lethal, nevertheless made them less than fully productive members of the household. Massachusetts taxed slaves as personalty, valuing each "male negro above fourteen years of age and upwards" at £20 and each "female negro of fourteen years of age and above" at £15. But collectors were allowed to make exceptions for the limitations of "age or infirmity" and abate taxes accordingly.[7]

If legislation was devised to accommodate some of the losses that emerged from changes in the enslaved person's body—collapse in the face of a new and harsh environment, vulnerability to the assaults of age—contracts surrounding slave sales tried to do the opposite. These contracts generally promised that at the time of sale the slave was of "sound mind and limb," "Sound and in Good Health," "well and in Good Health," and "Free from Incumbrances."[8] Conflict arose when enslaved persons fell ill after sale. Josiah Stertevant's suit against Isaac Howland is a case in point. In the May 1731 session of the Plymouth County Court of Common Pleas, Stertevant complained that the defendant had in the winter of 1729 "Bargained and Sold and Delivered to the Pla[i]nt[iff]" for £95 "a Certain Negro Boy Named Primas and warranted and avouched that he was then Sound and in Good Health." Stertevant argued that, in fact, Primas was "Unsound and Disseased" with a "Swelling in his Throate" at the time of the sale, leading to his death three months later. Howland pleaded that he had been ignorant of the affliction. The jury found in the defendant's favor and dismissed Stertevant's charges that he had been defrauded and deceived. On appeal, however, the decision was reversed by verdict; Stertevant was awarded £95 and the costs of the litigation.[9]

Although no record remains of the reasoning behind either the jury's initial decision or the reversal, one may surmise the questions that had to be tackled. Had the slave's sickness or the seeds of it been present at the time of the sale, or had it developed later? Was the defendant Howland a scoundrel committing fraud in selling an ill slave, or an innocent? Did Stertevant deserve protection, or in buying living property did he assume the risk that the enslaved person would not survive? Things could become even more difficult when the agency of the enslaved came into play. In the December 1730 session of the Plymouth County Common Pleas, Nicholas Litchfield sued Israel Cowing because a slave promised in sale committed suicide before she could be delivered. In this case, the jury found for the plaintiff, and, again, the decision was reversed on appeal without record of deliberation. Was the slave clearly "Mad Distracted or Possesed of the Divil" at the time of sale, as the plaintiff argued? Or had she acted impulsively, perhaps upon hearing news of her sale? And, if she was deemed deranged, who would be responsible for such providential misfortune? The lack of clear answers in such cases left ample room, as the jury verdicts and reversals suggest, for opposing views. The personal history of the slave; the specific details of the contract; popular knowledge, perception, and interpretation of specific afflictions like swellings of the throat or derangement—such factors helped to determine the authenticity of the seller's assessment and representation of the enslaved person's health.[10]

When the enslaved sought out or received medical attention against the wishes of their masters, other issues emerged. Enslaved persons might have healers tend to ailments that they had not brought to the attention of their masters for reasons ranging from modesty to fear of sale. Slaves hired for outside work might be taken to doctors who charged more than a master desired. Matters were complicated by the urgency of some sicknesses, when care might be deemed vital for survival or necessary for public health. John Saffin, a Boston merchant and sometime jurist, petitioned the General Court in 1703 for immediate relief from many of the charges assessed on his slave Adam, including medical attention. In 1694 Saffin had agreed to give Adam his freedom in seven years provided that he serve faithfully. At the end of the term, Adam requested his freedom, but Saffin refused, maintaining that the slave had behaved poorly. Adam turned to the courts to uphold the agreement. In the meantime, with his status still uncertain, Adam contracted smallpox, and Saffin was held accountable for "all manner of Necessarys, as Cloaths, Bedding food and Physick, and attendance" that were bestowed upon Adam in his illness. Despite his plea that these costs and others generated by Adam had made Saffin "a meet Vassall to his slave," the court found against the merchant, holding him accountable for all charges.[11]

Incidents like these revealed the complications arising when persons dependent in law but, in significant ways, independent in body became ill and sought attention for their ailments. The charges that arose from the slave's affliction could easily mount without any certainty about who would pay: The master who owned the body of the slave? The healer who provided a service without consulting with the master first? The state that demanded in certain illnesses such as smallpox that a rigorous and costly protocol be followed?

Legal cases concerning sick slaves illuminate tensions that may have lain dormant in everyday life. But it would be a mistake to imagine that the conflicts that emerged in trials were routine. In fact, to the extent that New England's slave owners kept diaries and recorded their slaves' bouts of illness, they often noted the attention given the sick, sometimes involving extraordinary amounts of time and attention. We conclude this section, then, with a portrait of one family's efforts to care for a sick slave that proceeded without controversy.

Early in May 1783, Elizabeth Porter Phelps, whom we met in chapter 1 as a young woman watching at a sick neighbor's bedside, noted the passing of one of her slaves: "Wednesday about 2 in the after-noon our Little Negro Girl Phillis expired—she was a very prety Child, I hope she sleeps in Jesus, being washed in his Blood" (May 4, 1783).[12] Phelps rarely recorded the everyday work and activities of her slaves, but she did take special note of significant events in their lives, including births, sicknesses, marriages, and deaths. Phillis was of the third generation of slaves living at Forty Acres, the Phelpses' large estate in Hadley, Massachusetts, in the lush Connecticut River Valley. Born in 1775 and named for her young aunt who died the same week after a protracted illness, Phillis came to an early end at the age of eight. In sparse entries that mark changes in Phillis's health and efforts to treat her ailments, Phelps left a thin biography of her slave's affliction, if not a full portrait of her daily life.

Phillis appears to have been sickly even as a very young child, causing Elizabeth Porter Phelps and Phillis's mother, Rose, concern. "I made a visit at Mr. Dickinson's—Rose brought our Phillis there for Mrs. Dickinson to see—we fear she has the Rickets" (May 11, 1776). The disease was not uncommon in children, who were most frequently struck between the ages of nine months and two years. But the range of early symptoms—which included swellings in the face, flesh that was soft and flabby, and a distended belly—may have been harder to detect and assess than the advanced stages of the disease, marked by a misshapen back, legs, and breastbone. Did the two women take the thirteen-month-old child to Dickinson to confirm their suspicions? Did this healer attach a name to the child's cluster of symptoms and perhaps offer a course of relief, which might have included changes in diet, dress, and exercise to strengthen the weakened constitution? The diary is silent on these matters. What the diary does provide is an occasional record of those moments at which the child seemed to have taken a turn for the worse, with her condition listed as "poorly." The term was tangled in hope and resignation, an embrace of a life that in its weakness could easily be extinguished: "Satterday Phillis poorly—O Lord may she Live (if it may be thy will) for good" (January 19, 1777).[13]

It appears that by the time Phillis was nearly seven years old, both Phelps and her husband believed that the enslaved girl suffered from something beyond rickets. On February 3, 1782, Elizabeth wrote: "Husband and I up to Mr. Aram's at Muddy Brook, he a seventh son—we took Phillis with us—think she has a Kings evil." Both the diagnosis of the "King's Evil" and the healer visited here were somewhat exotic in late eighteenth-century America. So-called because it was thought to be curable by the healing touch of the king, the King's Evil was a particularly slippery disease with a wide range of possible symptoms, including swellings along the neck, ears, chin, armpit, breast, and groin, and ultimately ulcers on the hands, feet, and even the internal organs. Although Queen Anne was the last British monarch to use the royal touch, those who claimed special healing powers, such as the seventh son of a seventh son, still practiced their craft in early America, despite repeated attacks on these healers as quacks and their patients as dupes.[14] After the initial visit with Mr. Arams, Charles Phelps brought Phillis back to have her "stroked for her Kings evil" at the end of the month and retrieved her the following week. While Muddy River was not as far away as Boston or New Haven, towns that Phelps had occasion to travel to throughout the year, it was still some forty miles to the north; the journey, which involved crossing the Connecticut River, would have required some planning.

If Aram's healing touch provided Phillis with any relief, she was nevertheless "poorly" again the following December. Elizabeth Porter Phelps brought her to a doctor in Hadley, hoping that this "means might be blessed for her recovery." When recovery did not come, Phelps and husband set out at the end of January to take Phillis to yet another doctor. By April the situation was becoming far more serious, and Phelps recruited help to nurse the child at home: "Satterday our old Peg came back to stay to take care of poor Phillis she very poorly" (April 20, 1783). Peg was

Phillis's grandmother, a woman who had for many years been a free servant at Forty Acres before selling herself into slavery in order to join her husband. Charles Phelps had later purchased Peg from her new owners, and she was allowed to go free in June 1782. Now, the following April, Elizabeth Phelps asked Peg to return and help with Phillis. Although the diary makes no record of it, one assumes that Phillis's mother, Rose, had nursed the child during bouts of sickness in the past. But Rose herself had died after a lengthy illness some two years earlier. And while Phelps herself had noted a few occasions in which she tended Phillis—staying with the child to allow Rose to go to church and "tarrying at home" with her a few months after Rose had died—she was in no position to take on full-time nursing. Phelps had her own young children, a household to supervise, and neighbors and church members to watch. Two weeks after Peg returned, Phelps came home early from errands in town to find Phillis "very bad." The child died the next day.

The case of Phillis offers a quite different view than the contests over the care of enslaved persons that could rage in court. Without special comment or complaint, Phelps and her husband went to great lengths to care for the sick child, taking her to no fewer than three different healers in a little over a year and hiring a nurse in Phillis's final illness. And their approach to Phillis's illness was not exceptional; other ailing slaves at Forty Acres also received generous treatment. While the care of slaves varied from master to master, the Phelpses do not appear atypical in their efforts. Historians of slavery in both eighteenth-century New England and the South have noted that it was not unusual for slaveholders to make strenuous attempts to care for their slaves. Jared Hardesty has found that Dr. Elisha Story of Boston treated some twenty enslaved persons between 1766 and 1775, and in one instance Captain John Tyley had his slave Joseph seen ninety times in just five months. As Philip Morgan has argued in reference to the Chesapeake and Lowcountry, while sick slaves could be subjected to both experiment and abuse, "masters involved themselves too personally and with too much care in treating slave illnesses for their behavior to be dismissed as mere calculating regard for pieces of property."[15]

How are we to regard Phillis, then? Not merely property. But should she be seen as a member of the Phelps family? Phillis exists in Phelps's diary as a shadowy figure, appearing, like other enslaved persons, most visibly at points of greatest vulnerability and weakness. We see Phillis through her affliction; her life in health is not worthy of comment. In Phillis's illness, Phelps exerts her paternalistic control. She arranges care for the sick child and even does some of the nursing herself. But Phillis is not allowed the representational space in the diary accorded to others in Phelps's immediate family, nor even to those who visit the estate. She shines brightly only in her death, cleansed in the blood of Jesus, a "prety" child who reminds Phelps that she and others caring for dependents must "discharge our Duty faithfully" (May 4, 1783).

II. SERVANTS AND HIRED HELP

The controversy surrounding sick slaves most often festered at the borders of family life, before an enslaved person was incorporated into family, before the words of genteel ownership were applied to them—"our Phillis," "our Rose," "our Cesar," "our Peg," or "our people" as Elizabeth Porter Phelps had occasion to remark.[16] In the case of servants, the controversies over illness could extend well into a term of service. Their ties to family were far more tenuous than those of slaves, and when they fell ill, pressures were applied to make up for the failings of their bodies: their wages might be docked, their terms extended, or their employment abruptly terminated. The crucial importance of servants in the household pressed for such measures. But law, indenture, and contract could also hold masters responsible for the care of their servants, who were to be provided for under the cover of family protection. And so in the midst of a term of service, the ailments of a worker opened a field of confusion and negotiation, where the rights and responsibilities of workers and those charged with their care had to be apportioned.

Throughout the seventeenth- and early eighteenth-century Atlantic world, laws commonly held masters responsible for the illnesses of their servants during their term of service. Plymouth Colony held that masters were to provide for and maintain "diseased lame or impotent servants." Virginia not only demanded that masters care for their servants but also forbade them from dismissing sick and lame servants before their terms expired; the servant could not be "put away" to save costs under "the pretense of freedom." The same was true in the West Indies, where masters in Barbados, Jamaica, and Antigua could be severely fined for turning away servants who were ill. A financial motive underlay such laws: sick servants who were released by their masters could easily become a public charge. But the structure of social authority was also at stake. These statutes established and reinforced the power of the patriarch of the household and the responsibility that came with the title. As the town of New Haven put it, the sickness of strangers who belonged to no family would be borne by the public, but those of bound servants were the province of the family's "Governor." The master was expected to be a just and wise ruler who would preside over his servants in sickness and in health.[17]

Yet the illness of a servant presented complexities that could never be fully anticipated in law, something we have seen earlier in chapter 3. Consider William Buckley's suit in 1661 against the widow Thamar Quilter. As Goody Quilter related the events in her deposition, she had apprenticed her only son, Joseph, to Buckley of Ipswich, Massachusetts. When Joseph fell ill and became "unserviceable," the master called on Quilter to tend her son. After three weeks of nursing him at Buckley's house, Thamar Quilter herself became sick and returned home. Shortly thereafter, Buckley put the ailing Joseph in a tumbrel, carted him to Quilter's house, and dumped him there. Though Buckley had not asked for her permission and though she was "very ill," Quilter later recalled that she "had a mothers bowell yerneing toward my child, & did not turne him back." She had seen and heard enough about Buckley's "harsh" treatment of her son to fear for his life. Quilter nursed Joseph for the next ten weeks. Upon hearing that his servant was recovering, Buckley visited the house and demanded the return of the apprentice. Quilter refused, stating that Buckley had never come to see Joseph while he was sick, nor had he offered "anything in satisfeaction for the charge & paynes" she had incurred during the child's illness. Buckley sued, charging Quilter with "harboring and witholding his apprentice." Quilter shot back that Buckley had "broken his covenant" by not teaching Joseph a trade and "by returning him to her." In the end, the court found in favor of Buckley, and the boy was ordered to resume his apprenticeship with the master.[18]

Cases like these speak to the ill-defined boundaries of household and family life in early America.[19] Who was responsible for Joseph Quilter's sickness? Mother and master pointed to each other. Quilter's petition to the court portrays Buckley as an unfeeling master who has violated the trust placed in him to care for the dependents within his household. He cares only for those workers who are "serviceable." Buckley's indifference to her child places Quilter in a vulnerable position. If she refuses to help, her son may die. If she takes her son in, she risks further injuring her own health and may well be forced to absorb the costs of Joseph's illness. She wavers in her effort to balance physical and financial well-being with her "mothers bowell yerneing" for the child, nursing Joseph at Buckley's, leaving him there when she falls ill, and finally, reluctantly, tending Joseph at home. Given that we don't have Buckley's account of the incident, we have to imagine his motives. Did he think that Joseph's infirmities somehow absolved him as a master from his duty to care for the youth? Or did he think that by drawing on the services of the boy's mother he was, in fact, arranging for care? A deposition by another man who was at Buckley's house suggests that the master flirted with the idea of sending Joseph to Rowley, a town just north of Ipswich, but that Thamar Quilter had said that she would rather the boy go home with her. Perhaps Buckley thought himself a generous man who had been cheated by the cagey widow. In deference to Quilter, he had not sold Joseph's indenture and may have considered that she kept her son hostage by demanding the costs of nursing the boy before he could be returned.

We do not have an account of the court's reasoning in this case, but it raises interesting questions. Courts in early New England were accustomed to dealing with clear violations of the agreements between masters and servants. Masters who mercilessly beat servants were punished, as were servants who ran off or stole from their masters. The battle over Joseph Quilter presented no such clear-cut infractions. If Thamar Quilter was to be believed, Buckley had not been attentive to her son's distress— but had he been actively abusive? Quilter had kept her son at home after he had recovered—but had she stolen from Buckley, who owned the indenture and the rights to the boy's work? The case points to the potential difficulties in deciding the province of familial and household authority as the servant's afflicted body lay suspended between the two.

While indenture contracts differed in the details, the general provisions were similar. Servants most often were bound until their majority, age eighteen for girls and twenty-one for boys. They were to obey their master's commands, keep his secrets, protect his goods, and neither absent themselves nor marry without his permission. Masters were to provide servants with many things: reasonable food, washing, and lodging; perhaps lessons in reading and writing and instruction in a trade; and, often, two suits of clothing, one for everyday wear, the other for the Sabbath. Many indentures did not broach the issue of the servant's health. Those that did most commonly added "physic" to the list of things the master would supply, or else used stock phrases such as the stipulation that the master was to provide "necessaries in Sickness and in Health."[20] But these phrases were sufficiently vague that they could be interpreted in many ways. What type of medicine or other remedies would be called for? Who would do the nursing? And how long was care deemed necessary? Contracts could establish the general outlines of responsibility, but individual cases like that surrounding the ailing Joseph Quilter reveal the contingencies and conflicts that could arise.

What could be expected of the sick and ailing in early modern life? At what point did their incapacities void a contract? The extreme case was perhaps the easiest to address. The historian Helena Wall has found cases in the seventeenth and early eighteenth centuries in which a finding of total disability on the part of either the master or the apprentice would void a contract. Disability served as an instance in which either party might point to non-performance of essential duties as reason to terminate a contract.[21] And yet cases like that of Joseph Quilter illustrate how difficult it may have been to determine what constituted total disability, a category that, as Margaret Pelling has found to be the case in early modern England, was rarely applied to the young.[22] Young Quilter was incapable of work at some points and yet able to work at others—weeks and even months of incapacity did not signal total disability. Had he remained either healthy or totally incapacitated, there would have been less room for contest.

Some indentures addressed such issues squarely and allow us to imagine similar arrangements that never made their way into print. Parents were particularly concerned that their indentured children be protected against unnecessary assaults that would ruin their future health. In preparation for a sea journey in 1726, one Captain Storey bound his young son John to the Reverend Ebenezer Parkman, with whom we are familiar from earlier chapters, with an eye toward the lad's future health. Parkman recorded the terms set out by the captain in his diary: "Let him Serve you as he is able, impose not on him those heavy burthens that will either Cripple him or Spoil his Growth. But in all regards I am willing he should Serve you to his Utmost" (January 20, 1726). Parkman could expect faithful service. But he would have to decide what the young boy was "able" to do and assume the moral responsibility for tasks that might be beyond the boy's means; if the youth was "spoiled" or "crippled," it would come at the expense of Parkman's reputation (and perhaps his purse as well).[23]

Charles Phelps Jr. of Hadley provided an incentive for his indentured servant to maintain good health. While preserving his role as the upright guardian of his servants, Phelps's indentures gave him some protection against their infirmities. His agreement in 1783 with Elisha and Rachel Searl concerning their twelve-year-old son, David, stipulated that Phelps would provide "Drink washing and Lodging Phisick & Nursing in case of sickness," but David would also receive a £15 bonus at the end of the term if he proved "well and healthy as Boys in general are. . . ."[24] As he had in the case of his ailing slaves, Phelps provided for the boy in his affliction while establishing an indirect penalty for ill health. If gentlemen like Phelps assumed at least partial responsibility for the health of their servants, thereby adhering to the general tone of the law, there were others who lay the responsibility of sickness squarely at the feet of their servants. When J. Robert Jones of Providence, Rhode Island, was indentured in 1735, he agreed to the usual requirements that he serve his master faithfully and well but also acceded to the master's demand that "In Case tho said Apprentice shall loose any time by sickness or Lameness or put his afd. master to any Extriordinary Charge by Reson thereof all such Loss and Charge shall so [be] deducted out of the said Apprenticesses wages."[25] One wonders what an "extriordinary" charge would be; but it seems clear that the apprentice would shoulder the costs of any serious illness.

Laws and indentures tell us about the struggles to define and anticipate the burdens caused by a servant's illness, but we turn again to the diary of Ebenezer Parkman to see how these burdens played out in daily life. By affording a view of the ailing laborers—male and female, servants, apprentices, and free laborers—on his family farm, the diary provides an elaboration of our inquiry.

⁕

As the historian Ross Beales has illustrated in his extensive work with Ebenezer Parkman's diary, the minister's farm depended on two types of laborers: younger boys who did light tasks, such as tending livestock and cutting and hauling firewood, and young men who did heavier work, especially during planting and harvest.[26] In the years in which Parkman could not count on his own boys to do the lighter work, he might well take in "lads" like John Storey, who would be given room and board and some instruction but typically no wages. Such boys would usually stay from one to several years. Though they were never prominent in his diary, Parkman nevertheless kept brief records of their comings and goings, the special tasks they performed, and their moments of indisposition.

Benjamin Clark, who was eleven when he came to live with Parkman in 1773, was typical in many respects. One month after Benjamin arrived at the parsonage, Parkman sent him off in December to Miss Mary Bradish, who had recently opened a school at a neighbor's house (December 23, 1773). The following month he was back at the parsonage and helping one of Parkman's sons sled wood. The "Extream Cold" of January affected both boys, freezing John Parkman's heels and two of Benjamin's fingers (January 22, 1774). Benjamin's father, David, arrived a week later and spent the night, perhaps to check the injury or simply to visit his son, now absent from his family for over two months (February 2–3, 1774). By April, Benjamin was back in form, helping to drive Parkman's cattle to Boston for sale, though the boy got lost on his way back, perhaps due to youth or inexperience, and did not arrive at the parsonage until late at night (April 27, 1774). Mixed into work and school life was Benjamin's participation in the world of illness. During the family's very difficult year of 1775, the boy was sent on a few occasions to fetch the doctor for Parkman's ailing daughter Hannah when her condition became "more urgent" (January 27, 1775). Benjamin was sick himself during his summers with the Parkmans. On July 18, 1774, Parkman noted that the boy was "troubled with pain in his stomach and lies by from Day to Day," waiting to be restored before returning to work. And in August the following year, Parkman noted again, "Ben Clark not well" (August 29, 1775). Short bouts of illness or the lameness that resulted from accidents and injuries were expected in taking on a servant "lad," and Parkman seems to have been quite satisfied with Benjamin's performance. One month after his service was up and Benjamin had returned home, Parkman asked David Clark if the boy could return to the parsonage to help, but he found the father was not inclined to send him. Perhaps the young teenager was now too valuable an asset on the family farm to relinquish (March 27, 1776).

In other instances, the afflictions that youths suffered were so severe that Parkman had to send them home. This was the case with William Winchester, the son of one of Parkman's cousins, who lived with the family during the winter and spring of 1779/80. Parkman agreed to do what he could "conveniently and reasonably in teaching and influencing" the boy in reading, writing, and ciphering; Winchester would care for Parkman's cattle and cut wood for the parson. Work and learning would proceed as "Capacity should admit it" (December 27, 1779). However, within a few months, Winchester's capacity was called into question. At the end of March, Parkman was concerned enough about the boy's state to begin to write down what he had evidently been observing for some time. On March 27, 1780, Parkman noted, "William Winchester remains much unwell." The following day he continued, "William Winchester still complains of much Indisposition," but then added, "yet has been to the barn." Did the minister suspect the boy of malingering? Or did Parkman in this case, as in so many others, judge a household member's state of health as much by what he or she could *do* as by what he or she *said*? Within a day it was clear that William appeared "worse," and a doctor who had called to see the minister gave the boy some physic. The following day, the physician returned to offer the boy a vomit, which Parkman observed "works well," but William nevertheless was still "sick and exercised with Pain, in both Head and Stomach" (March 31, 1780). Winchester remained "poorly" the following week, with pains in his hip and his head. And so it went for another month, with the boy occasionally making progress, working "at times in the Garden," but most often laying by in his sickness and able to "do very little." Finally, on May 8, 1780, William left the parsonage and returned home to his mother.

From the perspective of farm work, William's illness was an inconvenience at best. With the boy indisposed, Parkman had to find help to fill in for chores left undone. Cattle had to be tended and the garden worked. The absence of someone to mind the garden proved an especially vexing problem during the spring, as the swine of one neighbor and the sheep of another broke through the minister's fence and freely partook of his unwatched vegetables. To compound matters, the parson was failing in his search for seasonal hired help, a search made all the more difficult because young men from New England were being called off to join the military service during the Revolutionary War (a topic we will return to in chapter 6). Although a neighbor and one of Parkman's sons who owned a business as a shopkeeper in Westborough was occasionally able to help, Parkman needed more steady support to keep the farm running properly.

In mid-April, several weeks into William Winchester's illness, Parkman wrote in frustration, "Having no man yet and young Winchester lame and infirm, my business is behind" (April 14, 1780). By early May, Parkman was forced to make some compromises to salvage what he could from the growing season. He relinquished control of one of his fields and hired it out at halves. To do so meant lesser profits, but it undoubtedly pleased Nathan Kenny, who had earlier been hired for a day to fix Parkman's fence and had agreed to the deal in the event the minister could not find a term laborer (April 14, 20, 28, 1780). Parkman also abandoned the search for a hired hand who would contract through the fall, instead settling on a day laborer. "While much embarrassed and pritty lame, Stephen Batherick came within Reach, and was very much at Leisure. I hired him for 15/ per day . . ." (May 4, 1780). With an infirm lad of his own and no one reliable to work the farm, Parkman found *himself* "embarrassed" and "lame," forced to accept the services of Stephen Batherick, and perhaps to overlook the undesirable features of a man who was "very much at Leisure" in a tight labor market. At times like these, the household head confronted an unpleasant truth: the vulnerabilities and limitations of his workers became his own.

Despite the inconvenience of William Winchester's illness, Parkman waited for five weeks before releasing the boy back to his mother. Perhaps Parkman hoped the boy would recover. After all, William's bouts of indisposition were punctuated by moments in which he could work. Perhaps Parkman wanted to delay until he had secured the services of another long-term worker. The boy went home just three days after Parkman had finally hired Batherick. Especially in the spring and summer months, one could not be careless in dismissing workers, even youths like Winchester who were never responsible for heavy work. But beyond any expediency in having William remain on the farm, Parkman tried to honor his moral commitment to instruct and provide for the boy. While the minister had clear reasons for returning Winchester home early, dismissal meant that Parkman had in some measure failed at his charge. Parkman let him go on a humble note. "William Winchester left us to go to Ashburnham. . . . I gave him 10 Dollars, Mr. Barnard's Sermons to young people and on the Earthquake, and furnished him with various Things to accommodate him for his Journey. May God grant him Health and Grace!" (May 8, 1780). At least the lad would carry home with him the rudiments of what he might have received had he been able to remain at the parsonage.

Along with lads like Benjamin Clark and William Winchester, Parkman relied heavily on hired seasonal help, young men in their late teens and early twenties who typically agreed to work six-month stints from April through October. Like the boys on the farm, these workers also fell ill or became otherwise indisposed during their tenure. But Parkman seems to have conceived of their afflictions in a different manner. The conditions under which lads came to the parsonage derived from an older system of labor relations in which a master was held accountable for the care and well-being of his servants, but the growth of a free labor market in eighteenth-century New England ushered in new conceptions of employers' responsibility for the health of workers. While Parkman was certainly not indifferent to the plight of his hired workers, he often held them responsible for the failings of their bodies, whatever the cause.

Parkman rarely made explicit provisions concerning his hired workers' health; such arrangements were evidently assumed. The agreement he reached with twenty-one-year-old Ebenezer Maynard Jr. in 1769 was exceptional in this respect, though quite typical in its basic provisions. Parkman noted in February of that year that he hired Maynard to "live with me Six Months from the first of April to the First of October. He is to fill up the Week Days, and make allowance if he be not well and able to work. He is also to find an Ax; I am to find other Tools—Diet, Washing, etc., and give him 10 £ Lawfull money" (February 27, 1769). For hired workers, the term of service, suitable wage, conditions of room and board, and other lesser matters were negotiated on a case-by-case basis. A worker who could get his washing done elsewhere or who brought his own tools might ask for more money. Another who wanted exemptions, perhaps extra time off to visit relatives or time to attend Thursday lecture, might ask for less. Why Parkman decided to add a provision about Maynard's health in this agreement when he failed to do so elsewhere is uncertain. But the requirement that Maynard "fill up" his time on the farm and "make allowance" if he was unable to labor was something Parkman asked of all his workers. The minister worried about a worker's idle time, whatever the cause. Parkman's diary is filled with the frustration of "time lost" on the farm— weather that leads workers to quit early, draft animals that are not brought when they are supposed to be, or emergencies that take hands away from their daily tasks. Parkman understood that such inconveniences were part of living in the temporal world, but he also knew they were costly. And where possible he appears to have demanded that his hired hands find a way to work or make up for their absence.

Accidents and illnesses were the chief afflictions leading farm workers to become "not well." Some workers fell ill for weeks at a time, others for just a few days. In the latter case, Parkman would scrape by. Longer bouts of illness presented the problem of finding new workers to fill in for tasks left undone. But whether a serious illness or not, Parkman appears to have asked workers to make up for their lost time, usually by staying for extra days or by decreasing wages accordingly. It must be said that the record on sickness is spotty—so many other factors figured in a final reckoning, including days lost to things like poor weather or military service, that it is difficult to determine with precision the place of illness in a final payment.[27]

The minister seems to have made little distinction between illness and injury. The words he used to describe afflicted workers are ambiguous about the origin of ailments, perhaps an indication that Parkman was more concerned with the consequences of infirmity than with its causes. The terms he applied to ailing laborers like "lame," "indisposed," "weak," or "infirm" were potent because they described not only ill health—a body out of balance—but a worker incapable of sturdy endeavor. It appears that Parkman's male hired hands were more likely to be injured than to fall ill. The heavy work required of hired hands rendered them vulnerable to injury—they suffered strains, ruptures, sprains, cuts, and broken bones, as the following examples illustrate.

A mere two days after he began his term with Parkman, Ebenezer Maynard Jr. suffered a serious injury while he worked alongside John Parkman, the minister's teenage son. As Parkman related the incident, Maynard was "cutt in his Ankle by Johns Ax flying out of his Hands, as he was driving a Post, and glanc'd with great force to *Ebbe* on t'other side the Fence" (April 5, 1769). Despite several visits by a doctor who dressed the wound and the ministrations of Parkman's wife, who applied a dressing, Maynard's ankle did not recover in the following weeks. By the end of the month, a decision had to be made. On the evening of April 28, Parkman met with Ebenezer's father and the two talked of "his Sons sorrowful Case; and therewith the great Disappointment as to my Business."

The link between young Maynard's "sorrowful case" and Parkman's "disappointment" was surely clear to all involved—and awkward. If Maynard had willfully broken his contract, Parkman might have been righteously indignant about the loss.[28] But Maynard had done no such thing, and if anyone were to blame for the injury, it would have been Parkman's loose-handed son. Moreover, the Maynards were friends and neighbors, and Ebenezer's father and other relatives had periodically worked at the parsonage since the injury, no doubt to make up for the minister's loss. In an additional complication, the contract held that Maynard "make allowance if he be not well and able to work." The clause protected Parkman from absorbing the cost of a laborer who was unable to work but also granted a worker some autonomy. Maynard had a say in deciding if and when he would return to the fields—as long as he "made allowance," perhaps through working extra days or accepting a deduction in his wages, he would be honoring the agreement. Even while facing "great disappointment" in his business, Parkman had to show restraint and wait on young Maynard's decision. The minister undoubtedly felt relieved when, a few days after his meeting with the young man's father, Maynard finally determined that he had "no prospect of doing my work," and with the young man's "free consent," Parkman hired another worker for the following four months (April 28, 1769).[29] It was best that the new contract had come with Maynard's blessing.

In other instances, workers suffered injuries that might have slowed them down but did not require that they leave Parkman's service. Asa Ware was one week shy of completing a six-month stint with Parkman when he put "several Bones" out of his ankle climbing over a fence (October 7, 1774). Less than a week after the incident, Parkman noted that "Asa is lame, but husks in the Barn" (October 12, 1774). Ware's time expired two days later. Parkman seemed generally pleased with Ware's performance and talked with him about "helping me further if he gets well of his Lameness; which he consents to" (October 14, 1774). The minister was happy to have Ware return, but only if he was up to speed. Ware was resourceful enough to find tasks like husking corn that could be done with a lame ankle, but a hired hand would have to be able to do more than this if he was to earn his keep. Parkman even appears to have been chagrined by Ware's notion that husking should count toward a full day's work. When the minister agreed that Ware continue on for another six months at the parsonage, he noted dryly that Ware "thinks he made up the time of the first Agreement, the 17th of October" (November 5, 1774). Ware thought he owed Parkman only three days extra of work, though he had been lame at least a week—presumably Ware counted four days of work doing odd jobs that did not require walking, which may have nettled Parkman, though clearly not enough to argue about it. Ware was rehired to work through the winter months.

The cases of Ebenezer Maynard and Asa Ware alert us to the kinds of problems provoked by the intersection of work and affliction. An employer like Parkman needed to assess how long his farm could sustain the absence of work, or work that was not at full speed, and when to go through the arduous process of finding another long-term laborer. The worker had to determine when and whether he would return to work. The longer he held out, the longer other friends and relatives might be called on to lend a hand, or the more days he would have to work at the end of his term. But, as we have seen in the previous chapter, going home ill or injured imposed strains of its own on family life. And for both employer and hired hand, there was the issue of honor. The free labor contract called for a worker to perform certain tasks in exchange for certain pay. As long as work was performed in a competent manner, the contract held. But the delays engendered by affliction and the accommodations necessary to meet its demands gave rise to compromise and contest. When was work done by the injured or ill acceptable in quality and efficiency? When was it no longer sufficient? In affliction, the social met the corporeal, as the concerns of farm, family, wage, and honor pulled at the unstable laborer's body.

These questions were revisited when female help became ill at Parkman's house. Although Parkman was not reliable in recording the daily activities of female workers, he often took special note of their afflictions and the ensuing fallout. Like his male help, female household workers were bedeviled by accidents and succumbed to illness. But Parkman seems to have viewed the maladies of his female workers in a different light. Both the speed with which an ailing female worker was dismissed and the connection the minister made between her suffering and that of his family warrant our attention.

As Ross Beales has illustrated, female workers at the Parkman household came from a variety of circumstances. Some were young women of the "middling sort" who entered service as a regular part of the life cycle. They would work for others, perhaps as an apprenticeship in housewifery, before moving on to become mistresses themselves. Others less fortunate, spinsters or widows and their daughters, worked for wages as a matter of necessity.[30] Regardless of their varied circumstances, however, ailing female help rarely remained long at the parsonage before they either left voluntarily or were sent away. A few instances of such dismissals allow us to speculate on why this was the case.

Like many young couples starting a family, the Parkmans regularly sought female help. In 1726 the young minister and his pregnant wife engaged the services of Silence Bartlett from one Captain Ward, a prosperous farmer in nearby Shrewsbury with whom Parkman was familiar.[31] On March 31, 1726, the two men agreed that Bartlett would live with the Parkmans for the year for £8. The provisions of the exchange are not clear, though it is likely that Silence was under a long-term agreement with Ward and that the captain was hiring out her services to Parkman.[32] After the note of her arrival on April 5, Silence disappears from Parkman's diary for seven weeks, emerging only in affliction on May 31, a day in which Parkman observed that she was "not well" and had gone to the doctor. Still ill two days later, Silence set off to neighboring Marlborough to "take advice of the Phician" (June 2, 1726). Four days passed before the minister sent one of his lads to fetch the young woman. Although Silence apparently had not fully recovered, Parkman needed her back at the parsonage. He had fallen ill and was getting worse, and his wife and young son had also become unwell. It appears, however, that Silence was not up to the task of tending the ailing family while ill herself. Parkman ordered a hired hand to remove Silence from the parsonage two days later, and the family began a search for new help.

Oliver Ward, a kinsman of Captain Ward's (and a fellow townsman with whom Parkman had many business dealings), offered a stopgap measure—his daughter Dinah served the Parkmans for a few days after Bartlett's departure. Another long-term prospect arrived within a week, though affliction cut short her stay as well. As Parkman noted matter-of-factly six days after she came to the parsonage, "Yesterday Rebecca Paddison, apprehending Some Dangerous Tumor in her Breast, returned to her Mother" (June 22, 1726). Only after Paddison's family made provisions for a replacement did the crisis in help came to a close; Hannah Paddison arrived a week later, and one assumes from the absence of further references to her that she was able to stay and caused the minister no vexation.

Silence Bartlett, Rebecca Paddison, and Hannah Paddison had all come from the local economy; they were either daughters from families that Parkman knew in Westborough or neighboring towns, or young women who lived with such families and who could be hired out for a time. Although the pool of such women workers was limited, prior connection to or knowledge of hired help meant that Parkman could make ready substitutions for a worker who through illness or other misfortune was unable to remain at the parsonage; a patchwork of helpers could fill in until one suitable could stay.

But there were times when the minister and family had to turn further afield for assistance, and the sickness of these workers could present problems beyond the need to find new help. After searching in vain for local hired help in 1749, Parkman was finally able to secure the services of the widow Elizabeth Grice of Boston, someone with whom he had no prior connection. Though the family felt fortunate to have found help after weeks of trying, Parkman was soon despondent. Three days after her arrival, he wrote wearily, "Betty Grice, who seems to be but an infirm Body, is indispos'd and lyes by" (August 26, 1749). Grice continued ill and confined for the next several days, tended by Parkman's wife, whose own burdens were made that much heavier now that the "help" had become yet another source of worry. Worse still, Grice had been arrogant and saucy in her affliction. Parkman had offered her "affectionate Words exhorting her to Repentance" and to "Consider her Danger" in illness, only to be met with "unbecoming Answers" by the widow (August 30, 1749). After receiving an assurance from a doctor who maintained that Grice was not "fitt to keep here" and should be returned "to the place from whence she came," Parkman only too happily arranged for her return to Boston, a resolve deepened by Grice's "indecent language" hurled in protest (August 31, 1749). It would be another three weeks before Parkman was able to prevail upon Lydia Champney, his single sister-in-law, to come to the parsonage to help. But the widow Grice was "fitt" neither in temperament nor body to serve, and her immediate return "from whence she came" would absolve the minister of responsibility, legal and otherwise, for her maintenance. Backed by medical opinion, Parkman could claim the matter was out of his hands and send the widow back to Boston (where, incidentally, she would have been an ideal candidate for the poorhouse, a prospect that may explain her recalcitrance).

The lives of Silence Bartlett, Rebecca Paddison, and Elizabeth Grice (and Dinah Ward, Hannah Paddison, and Lydia Champney who filled in for them) fit within the broader context of the improvisational culture of early New England. While some families might have been served by the same female help for long periods of time, women moved rapidly into and out of households across New England throughout the eighteenth century. As Laurel Thatcher Ulrich has put it in her study of Hallowell, Maine, "women exchanged daughters the way they exchanged kettles and sleighs," parting with helpers during slow times, gathering in others as demand dictated.[33] For spinsters like Lydia Champney or widows like Elizabeth Grice, movement could become a way of life, as they shuffled between households to meet family needs or the dictates of the free labor market. Women came and went, binding society together through their ability to meet life's daily urgencies, from household maintenance to care for the afflicted, or—as was often true with the Parkmans—both at once. In this climate, Parkman could readily agree to let ailing female help go or, as with the widow Grice, dismiss others without fear of accusation or reprisal. The work lives of female helpers were understood to be impermanent.

But there were further reasons for Parkman's ready dismissal of ailing female help. Even more than with his sick or injured male workers, Parkman seems to have found a palpable connection between the ailments of his female workers and his own family's sufferings. While it was certainly worrisome for a male worker to fall ill during harvest, as rotting crops in the field meant loss, an unwell female worker meant that the routines of the household would begin to unravel. This was a problem at any time, but most especially when the household was unsettled, as it often was by comings and goings and continual cycles of birth, illness, and death. When Lydia Cutting fell seriously ill for the second time during her nine-month stay with the Parkmans, the minister lamented that, with Lydia sick, "my wife [is] burthened with the Business of the Family" (September 24; 1737). Here was the parallel to the "disappointment" in his own "business" that Parkman registered when a male hand became sick or incapacitated. But in the case of female help, such burdens could not be endured for long. Lydia Cutting was sent away a week later, and Susanna Cutting—perhaps her sister—arrived shortly thereafter.

Finally, concerns about money likely accompanied ailing female workers away from the parsonage. Such an assertion is speculative; in most cases, the diary gives no hint of either the manner or the medium of exchange that brought female help into the household. Because Parkman rarely noted the terms of agreement with hired female help, they cannot be compared to the contracts of his hired seasonal farm laborers. Parkman did, however, watch his purse carefully and could bridle at the work and trouble that came with hiring help. Early in his career as a manager of hired hands, Parkman had occasion to remark, "Perhaps there may be many more Tedious and Chafing things in Hirelings than ever Mention has been made of" (June 2, 1726). Toward the end of his life, Parkman could be less philosophical when confronted with hired help unable to work. Left on his own in 1771 when his wife was visiting family, Parkman made clear he had little endurance for the "tedious" and "chafing." After noting all of the help he had in odd jobs around the house and farm—a neighbor who had fixed some sashes, another who had killed and dressed a pig—he wrote, "But My Young woman, *Anna Batherick* too much indisposed to help us—especially p.m. and Evening" (August 19, 1771). Another woman arrived to help scour the house that afternoon. Anna was paid and let go the following day.

Male farmhands might be asked to make up for their absence by working beyond their time or by taking a cut in wages. But the urgency of the family burdens caused by a sick maid might preclude these options. As with Anna Batherick, it might have seemed best to issue payment and let ailing female workers go. More so than in the case of Parkman's male workers, women's household chores could not brook the interruption. The daily immediacies of female work required a consistently able body.

III. CONCLUSION

Ebenezer Parkman's diary illuminates the politics of family and household competency in eighteenth-century New England. As we have seen in the previous chapter, when they labored in health, outside workers were crucial to a family's competency. But a worker's affliction could all too easily be transferred to his or her master or employer. Those who owned slaves could do very little in such predicaments—they might resort to the rhetoric of reversal, pleading before government officials that they were enslaved through their slave's misfortunes, but would find little sympathy. Those who engaged servants or hired hands had other options when they felt the full impact of a laborer's afflictions. Charged as the governor and protector of all within his house, Parkman nevertheless found times when paternalistic bonds needed to be cut, and those unrelated individuals within the household who threatened his family's survival—those who could not help the family help itself—would have to be let go. He could not risk becoming impotent and lame through the afflictions of those under his charge. Household workers were peeled away from family in the name of competency.[34]

DEPENDENCY

CHAPTER FIVE

Smallpox, Public Health, and Town Governance

Perhaps no other affliction in eighteenth-century New England received the attention given to smallpox. Even the most laconic of diarists noted its presence and charted its approach; others devoted entire journals to its rages. Letters written from infected areas to relatives, friends, and business partners survive despite authors' pleas to burn such material lest the virulent distemper spread further. Newspapers reported on outbreaks throughout the Atlantic world. Chronologies of significant events compiled at the end of almanacs memorialized serious epidemics. Legislative records reveal extensive efforts to stop the communication of the disease, including last-ditch attempts to protect the members of the Massachusetts General Court, who on more than one occasion fled Boston for Charlestown, Cambridge, and Concord, and demanded that guards be posted at the doors of its sessions to keep out the infected.

Smallpox attracted such intense notice because of the threat of contagion. It was considered supreme among a host of "malignant infectious distempers" coursing through New England, diseases that were spread from infected persons (and objects with which they had been in contact) to other persons. "Throat distemper" in the 1730s and 1740s, yellow fever in the 1790s, measles outbreaks throughout the period, and sundry "camp fevers" associated with soldiers returning from colonial wars—debate raged during epidemics about whether they were infectious diseases. There was no such debate on smallpox. Shortly after exposure to infected persons or goods—New Englanders thought anywhere from a few days to a few weeks; present-day epidemiologists would say from ten to eleven days—those who had not already weathered the disease could expect a progression of symptoms: fever, backache, headache, nausea, and listlessness (days 12–14); small pimples that turned to pustules (days 15–

24), which might remain distinct or run together (in a "confluent" and much more deadly form); scabbing (days 25–30); and finally scarring revealed as the scabs dropped off, leaving "pock" marks as evidence of surviving the disease.[1]

Historians have eagerly followed the leads left by smallpox, mapping its trajectory, counting the bodies it infected and claimed (and exploring the ways in which Americans themselves tried to quantify the problem), and charting the public health measures that finally led to its elimination. The arguments surrounding the pox, particularly the practice of inoculation (the act of intentionally infecting people with the disease in an effort to protect them from a full-blown case of smallpox), have been used to reveal dimensions of social and cultural life: the troubled relation between religious, medical, and civil authority; the connection between poverty and disease; and the politics of corporeal identity.[2]

Less attention has been paid to the place of smallpox in everyday life and the social and political relations of contagion. This is not surprising—a decade or more might pass between smallpox outbreaks in New England. But their social significance transcended any particular occurrence, for two reasons. First, the outbreaks that caused disruptions and even terror were fueled by the quotidian world of commerce and sociability. Through much of the eighteenth century, Atlantic trade was a major source of infected persons and goods in New England, and once communities were infected, the social exchange that supported daily life ensured the easy spread of the disease.[3] We need to understand, then, how the specter of contagion integrated the ordinary and the extreme: how consumer goods could be at once alluring and dangerous; how the Atlantic exchange that was critical for markets could also be a source of lethal infection; how the practices of social healing could lead to the spread of disease.

Second, by blending the ordinary and extraordinary, smallpox pushed the affairs of family and household into public life. The fear of contagion— that everyday practices could lead to disaster—led to public regulation and raised broader concerns about civic life: When did the public have a right to intrude upon private affairs? Who belonged to the public? And in the aftermath of outbreaks and epidemics, who was responsible for the social and financial costs of the disease?

These questions had a particular set of answers in New England, which, as we saw in chapter 1, had been at the vanguard of public health measures in the Atlantic world. In Tudor and Stuart England, policies were elaborated over the course of the sixteenth and seventeenth centuries to address plague: marking the houses of the sick; isolating the sick in pesthouses;

and burning clothing, bedding, and other items deemed capable of spreading the disease. Although these ad hoc policies were often honored in the breach for much of the sixteenth century, by the latter sixteenth and early seventeenth century a coherent set of regulations emerged that was more effectively enforced. While Puritan clergymen could balk at regulations as contravening the will of God, key Puritan magistrates understood the public health measures as part of a larger agenda of social reform, which included the eradication of poverty, sin, and disease in godly societies.[4]

Puritans brought their knowledge of the terrors of plague with them to New England. While plague never scourged the region, smallpox came over on the first ships to arrive in Massachusetts Bay in 1630. Drawing on their experience in England, Puritans quickly devised public health measures to resist the pox, achieving success where others failed. In England, the density of settlements and the difficulties of enforcement meant that infectious disease such as smallpox was often endemic, striking frequently and afflicting children and others who had no exposure at regular intervals. In New England, the scattering of settlements and a low immigration rate compared to other regions (particularly in the eighteenth century) meant that diseases such as smallpox broke out less frequently than in other regions.[5]

More importantly, New Englanders enforced public health measures, which were propounded both by provincial legislatures and in local town meetings, with a vigor that proved elusive elsewhere. William Penn's vision for Philadelphia included a carefully arranged layout of streets, houses, and gardens that would ensure the health of the city. But early settlers could not be made to bend to his vision, and within a generation, his beloved city resembled commercial London in its sources of contagion. Steady immigration over the course of the eighteenth century brought fresh cases of smallpox to the city, and a comparatively weak quarantine regime meant that the disease coursed through Philadelphia at intervals of four to six years from 1730 until the Revolution. In Massachusetts, the public health measures designed to isolate the sick and cleanse infected materials were far more robust and successful, although ironically by limiting exposure to diseases like smallpox, increasing numbers of inhabitants were vulnerable to the ravages of epidemic. When Boston was beset by the pox in 1721, for example, it had been a generation since a major outbreak, and more than half of the city's residents became infected by the disease.[6]

This chapter draws on a range of material—diaries, town and legislative records, and the public prints—to sketch social patterns that persisted throughout the eighteenth century. The chapter begins with an outbreak of smallpox in Marblehead, Massachusetts, home of Ashley Bowen, a mariner, ship rigger, painter, poet, husband, and father.[7] Bowen's remarkable diary brings us to the ground level of an epidemic. The following sections of the chapter will elaborate on the threats that smallpox posed to social cohesion and on issues of responsibility and cost, drawing on materials from Massachusetts and the unusually detailed records of smallpox kept by the town councilors in Rhode Island.

The social and political relations of smallpox illuminate just how consuming the burdens of sickness might be for households and towns. Smallpox offers the most vivid view of the province of affliction threatening to overwhelm the metropole of health.

I. OUTBREAK! MARBLEHEAD, MASSACHUSETTS, 1773

Shortly after it became clear that his wife had been infected with smallpox, Ashley Bowen (1728–1813) sat down and wrote a "memorandum," a short narrative that would assemble and inscribe in memory the events that had brought the scourge to his house. Bowen had long kept a meticulous diary of his work life. But smallpox required special attention, a separate journal to chronicle its ravages (and to keep track of other major afflictions, including disasters at sea). Several weeks earlier, on the first of June, a schooner had returned from Newfoundland's fishery to Bowen's hometown of Marblehead, Massachusetts. One of the major fishing communities in eighteenth-century New England with about five thousand residents in 1765, it was the sixth largest town in British North America.[8] While on the schooner's voyage, a crew member, William Mathews, had boarded a French ship, something that Bowen noted was "common for our fishermen to do," and purchased a piece of Castile soap. When Mathews returned home, he gave the soap to his wife, Sarah, who used it to clean his soiled sea clothes. Two weeks later, Sarah Mathews "broke out and swelled to a great degree." At this point a doctor was sent for, and everyone assumed Mathews had been poisoned.[9]

As Sarah Mathews became violently ill during the following week, neighbors and relatives came to visit and help. Her sister Mary ("Mol") Ingalls assumed a large portion of the care, washing her sister with "salt water and the liquor of elder" and perhaps also aiding the doctor who attended. Despite their efforts, Sarah Mathews continued to deteriorate and, worse still, others who had been with Mathews began to feel unwell. Mathews's daughter, who had nursed her mother, fell ill, and she, too, was bathed by Ingalls while more "neighbors all round took their turns to watchings as in any other sickness." Of perhaps greater concern for Mol Ingalls, however, was that her mother, the widow Sarah Shaw, had become dangerously sick. Some openly speculated that it was not poisoning but smallpox that afflicted the women. Ingalls steadfastly maintained that her seventy-nine-year-old mother was laboring under the infirmities of old age and "spaired no pains for to get assistance" to her. As Ashley Bowen later noted dryly, "tis supposed that nearly an hundred or more of Mother Shaw's relations and friends frequented the house all the time from her first complaint."

Bowen had been made privy to the alarming details of the outbreak by his second wife, Mary (Shaw) Bowen, who through her previous marriage to the late James Shaw was a sister-in-law to Sarah Mathews and Mol Ingalls and daughter-in-law to the elderly Sarah Shaw.[10] Although Mary Bowen was not as deeply involved as Mol Ingalls in the care for Mathews and Shaw, she visited both women during their sickness and was especially worried about her mother-in-law. Ashley Bowen, as one of the principal riggers in Marblehead, was particularly harried in the summer months, and as he confessed in his memorandum, when his wife had initially informed him that "her mother was a-dying with old age," he gave it "no great attention." However, Bowen did become deeply concerned when he returned from his loft later that night and found his wife in bed with a fever. Mary Bowen's sisters were summoned.[11] They soon arrived, bound Mary's head, and prepared a balm tea for her, leaving Ashley Bowen to sit up the fore part of the night with his wife to monitor her condition. The following day only one sister, whom Bowen noted "had had the smallpox," came to attend; presumably others not immune to the disease feared that they might be infected if Mary's "poisoning" was in fact the pox. By that night, Bowen could find no one to help. "I sent for a watcher, but the next news it was said to be the smallpox and that five or six was complaining of it at Mother Shaw's, so could get nobody to watch." Under the pressure and special conditions of the smallpox outbreak, the social network of healers who had formed so readily even a week earlier was now coming apart. And here, with smallpox poised to consume the affairs of the household, neighborhood, and town, Ashley Bowen ended his memorandum.

⁂

What struck Ashley Bowen most forcefully was the routine nature of the events that spawned an epidemic. The outbreak had its origins in the everyday commercial relations that sustained maritime life. The pox was brought ashore by a crewman's "common" action in climbing aboard a foreign ship and purchasing goods, in this case some Castile soap. The soap itself reveals something about the domestic life of Marblehead's fishing families. In one sense it was a luxury. Over the course of the eighteenth century, fishermen acquired a variety of amenities, such as featherbeds; linen and cotton sheets and quilt covers; maple and walnut dining tables and chairs; mirrors; pewter and ceramic plates; iron and brass candlesticks; and glassware. Castile soap was part of an "empire of goods" that knit together England and her mainland North American colonies, who eagerly consumed English imports in the decades leading up to the Revolution. The imported soap would have saved the fisherman's wife from the arduous and often complicated task of making her own, which involved boiling the right combination of tallow, lye, and quicklime to produce a bar of the hard soap preferred for laundry. But the Castile soap may have been something more than an indulgence: many fishermen and their families would have owned neither the woodlots nor livestock necessary to create lye from wood ashes or tallow from butchering. In this sense, scarcity itself fueled consumption, driving provincial fishing villages like Marblehead to reach out to Atlantic commerce. In the process, they would enjoy the benefits of acquiring luxuries or time-saving necessities but also suffer afflictions fueled by Atlantic trade. The seeds of epidemic could reside, in the minds of townsfolk, in something as small as a piece of soap.[12]

The piece of Castile soap made its way from a French ship to a Marblehead schooner, and finally into the house of Sarah Mathews. Upon her "poisoning," a remarkable network of concerned relatives, neighbors, and friends sprang into action. To a certain extent, Marblehead differed from other places in the breadth and depth of its healing networks. High mortality rates from the accidents and diseases that attended maritime life meant that many neighbors and friends were also related through marriage; death and remarriage made Marblehead a town peopled by numerous in-laws, half-brothers and -sisters, and other distant relations living in close proximity to one another.[13] On the whole, however, Marblehead folk did not substantially differ from others throughout New England in their strategies for tending the afflicted. Women provided the backbone of care, occasionally aided by men who might help tend family members, fill in for friends and neighbors who had fallen ill, watch with the seriously afflicted, and fetch doctors, nurses, and other healers. Bowen took pains in his memorandum to show that the efforts of his neighbors were customary; they had done as they would have "in any other sickness." The illness of Mary Bowen's mother-in-law, the widowed matriarch Sarah Shaw, had brought forth one hundred or more visitors in just a few days. In ordinary times, such a vast network of helpers would have distributed the time-consuming problem of debilitating sickness into portions small enough that no one person in the community would suffer its full impact. But in the case of contagious disease, the very dynamism of the social healing process could lead to disaster: the more people involved in care, the greater the range and intensity of an ensuing epidemic. In this sense, Ashley Bowen portrays the spread of the pox as the tragic result of well-intentioned townspeople.

Yet the memorandum also lays blame for the outbreak on Mary Bowen's sister-in-law Mol Ingalls, who insisted that her mother had been "struck with old age," not smallpox. How could the pox be confused with the infirmities of age, however serious? One answer is straightforward. In its initial stages—which involved a high fever, headache, and pains in the muscles and back—smallpox was regularly mistaken for any number of other afflictions. Even the swellings and small pimples that appeared several days after onset might reasonably be confused with something like poisoning. Before the body became consumed with the pustules that decisively signified smallpox, the symptoms were subject to varying interpretations.

But as Bowen and others knew well, a diagnosis of smallpox involved more than a reading of its physical signs. To suggest that someone had smallpox had serious social, political, and economic implications that extended well beyond the sick and those closest to them. As one of the few diseases in early America considered to be contagious, smallpox required elaborate rules to contain its assaults, including prolonged confinement of the afflicted and the impressment of caretakers. But even with such procedures, towns might feel an outbreak's effects for years to come through the lives it claimed, the commerce it stifled, and the costs of care it demanded. Mol Ingalls had been prepared for her mother to die, but perhaps she could not bear to usher Sarah Shaw toward such a lonely, costly, and inglorious demise. Would her mother's name be tarnished? Would Ingalls herself be blamed for bringing so many people into her mother's orbit to console and care for her? Might she be made to pay for the spread of the disease? Even if smallpox had physically marked the elderly Shaw's body, the social and political context in which those signs were embedded might have made the pox illegible for her daughter.

For his part, Ashley Bowen soon realized that not only his wife's

mother-in-law but both his wife and son had contracted smallpox. He
would spend the next six weeks dealing with the fallout.

⁣∞⁣

On July 24, 1773, after a night tending his wife without aid, Ashley Bowen
acknowledged the severity of her condition with resigned certitude: "This
day I have the misfortune to find my wife to have the smallpox."[14] Bowen
now had a clear path to follow. Law and custom directed his steps. In Massachusetts, ad hoc regulations imposing quarantine on infected ships in
the seventeenth century gave way to comprehensive acts at the beginning
of the eighteenth. As we saw in chapter 1, suspect ships were made to anchor on outlying islands in Boston Harbor (Spectacle Island in 1717, Rainsford Island in 1737, each of which had a hospital built on it to house the
infected), where they would be kept until the distemper had subsided and
the ship, its men, and all goods could be properly cleansed. Legislation
regulating infection within towns had developed in a similar fashion, allowing local officials to quarantine those suspected of contagious diseases
and, beginning in 1732 with a series of acts "to prevent persons concealing
the small-pox," requiring that the "head" of the family in which the sick
resided to notify local officials and hang a red flag "not under one yard
long and a half a yard wide, from the most publick part of the infected
house" until the house was deemed aired and cleansed by the selectmen.
Failure to comply was to be met with stiff fines or, if one could not pay, a
whipping not exceeding thirty stripes.[15]

Accordingly, at "9 o'clock in morning," Bowen "went and acquainted
the Selectmen" with his situation. Together the selectmen and Bowen
would decide what to do with Mary. She would have to be isolated, but
where was perhaps negotiable. Although Marblehead was a large port
town, it still had no official place to confine the infected sick. At the earliest signs of an outbreak, centers of infectious disease were hastily designated; they would evolve over the course of an epidemic.

Later that afternoon, Bowen removed Mary to Mother Shaw's house.
Whether or not the selectmen had urged or even ordered Bowen to do so,
he clearly thought it was sensible, maintaining in his diary that Mary had
"caught the pox" at the house, and as the dwelling had become the gathering place for other women stricken with the pox and concerned friends
and relatives, his wife would have "some of them to attend" her. Moreover, with Mary at Mother Shaw's, Bowen could still move freely about
the town and attend to his business, something he would not have been

able to do if his house were quarantined, which would have been manda-
tory had Mary remained at home. To stay with an afflicted family member
had its comforts, but in the case of smallpox it was also accompanied by
massive burdens. Perhaps Mol Ingalls, who presided over Mother Shaw's
house, was anticipating these burdens as she evaluated the condition of
the sick women in her midst. As Bowen noted, Ingalls "was very hard
to be persuaded that it was the smallpox although so many was ill with
it." Her reservations aside, the dwelling, which occasionally served as an
almshouse, was a logical place to send the afflicted and became one of the
principal pesthouses in Marblehead during the epidemic.[16]

In the next few days, the Marblehead selectmen implemented measures to contain the outbreak. When Bowen walked to the house of Sarah
Mathews, where she and her daughter were confined with pox, he found "a
fence directed both ways [across] the road," put in place to block all paths
to the afflicted. A Committee of Inspection was appointed and charged
with "daily examining every House in Town" for signs of the spread of the
distemper. Those "suspected" of having smallpox would be identified and
quarantined. A pole flying a red flag would have been attached to all of the
buildings holding the infected, warning passersby of the danger. Guards
were placed at the fences separating the sick from the healthy. Except for
those pressed into service to attend the sick, any contact with the infected
was forbidden; even dogs "running at large" were ordered shot. The response to smallpox constructed a new social landscape, where the sick
were isolated from the healthy and space itself was separated into clean
and infected.[17]

It is tempting to portray in stark terms the inspections, regulations,
and elaborate marking of the sick precipitated by infectious disease. Sometimes individuals and households resisted official orders in ways both flagrant and subtle. Moreover, in the effort to identify the origin and spread
of epidemics, officials and residents alike might be inclined to assign
blame to the most vulnerable, outsiders, and those at the bottom of social
hierarchies. For the moment, however, Ashley Bowen's Marblehead affords
a different picture.

The image of Marblehead during the outbreak is one of order and propriety. Bowen voluntarily identified his wife as a pox victim and removed
her to the pesthouse himself. After his son Nathan fell ill a week later,
Bowen did not object when selectmen took the child from the house, even
as doctors disagreed on whether the boy's symptoms indicated chicken pox
or smallpox.[18] Known for his biting sarcasm and willingness to comment
on the blunders of haughty authority, Bowen never lashed out at officials

during the outbreak, not even within the confines of his diary. The silence is striking. Why had Bowen and others like him so readily complied with the will of town officials? The force of law alone is not sufficient to answer the question.

One answer lies in the moral authority that selectmen gained in safeguarding the "public," an entity that came into sharp relief during a crisis. With the prospect that infection would spread, policies of isolation were justified to protect the many from the few. Public health regulations were part of a larger constellation of provisions that towns made for their residents, including public education, a regulated labor market that favored locals, and allowances for the poor. While the health regulations could be remarkably coercive, literally determining matters of life and death in the placement and sequestering of the afflicted, the goal of the town's measures was, as with other provisions, the protection and well-being of the town. Individuals would need to bend their will to the good of the whole.[19]

Moreover, the economic health of the town was at stake. With robust quarantine and cleansing measures, the selectmen not only sought to prevent further sickness and death within the town but also to preserve the trust of those outside the town's borders. A town like Marblehead, whose economy was based on trade and exchange, could ill afford to let a smallpox outbreak sully its reputation as a safe place to do business. Thus, as rumors spread that as many as five or six thousand persons in Marblehead might become infected with the pox, the selectmen immediately issued their assurances to the "Publick" in the local *Essex Gazette*: "the Small-Pox is in but two Houses, which are near each other, close to the Water-Side, the Passages to which are fenced up, and they are more than a quarter of a Mile below the Market-House, so that the People coming to Market will be in no Danger of taking any Infection." In the following issue of the *Gazette*, the selectmen urged "Market-Men" and "Travellers" to come to the town "as usual," as necessary measures had been taken to prevent the spread of the pox. Isolation regimes and Committees of Inspection not only stemmed infection but also served as theatrical gestures, enabling selectmen to make a case for business "as usual." Extraordinary acts performed in the name of the public were necessary to preserve everyday life, and townspeople like Ashley Bowen undoubtedly knew it.[20]

Bowen and others may also have been more willing to support strict isolation measures because they knew that even when family members were sequestered in pesthouses, it was still possible to keep abreast of their daily progress. Bowen knew when his wife was "quite ill," "poorly," or "in a good way," and he kept informed about the conditions of a variety of others. Some of his knowledge must have been gleaned as he stood guard at the fence outside the pesthouse confining his wife. On other occasions Bowen claimed to be attending the sick, though it seems more likely that he was providing them with provisions than waiting on them personally.[21] Others did decide to stay with loved ones, and some paid dearly for it. Bowen noted that Thomas Dodd, who had not already contracted the pox, was perfectly "indifferent" to the dangers of the scourge and attended within the pesthouse to be with his wife and others. Within a week Dodd was "drooping"; he died a week later. Dodd's indifference may have seemed imprudent to Bowen, but his story indicates that not everyone was gripped by the fear of contagion.[22]

Bowen and others accepted the social segregation of the sick, but the smallpox outbreak did place significant though sometimes subtle strains upon their lives. By 1773 the forty-five-year-old Bowen was accustomed to the demands of sickness. In short and unsentimental entries, Bowen's daybook records afflictions large and small taking hold of his family. In many cases, illnesses lasted for just a few days. But even here, the problem could be exacerbated as ailments spread from one family member to another. With five children in the house, the eldest of whom was only twelve in 1773, childhood diseases posed a particular problem. The year 1773 began with a measles outbreak in the household months before the pox arrived. Bowen himself had been feeling quite ill at the beginning of January, and before he recovered, son Ashley came down with the measles in the middle of the month. As his son convalesced, Bowen's wife became sick. Sensing an impending crisis, Mol Ingalls arrived to help nurse. At the end of the month with his wife still ailing, five-year-old Nathan and nine-year-old Hannah fell ill. And then, three weeks after it started, the measles disappears from Bowen's entries. Apparently everyone's health had been restored enough to be unworthy of comment. Bowen was undoubtedly relieved, but the truth was that his household had seen far worse. In April 1771 Bowen's first wife, Dorothy, became seriously ill after she miscarried at five months. By the time of her death four months later, Bowen had drawn on the help of neighbors, church members, three of his wife's sisters, several hired nurses, a doctress, and two doctors. He knew well the great sacrifices and costs that affliction could command.[23]

Even in a world like Bowen's, accustomed to affliction, smallpox could severely strain households and communities. Helpers like Mol Ingalls who in other circumstances might have come were confined at home with the infected; others who feared contracting the disease may have stayed away. Bowen was compelled to do more for his family and others in the epidemic than he might have in other circumstances, and he marked the disturbances in his journal: "This day so busy about wife could do nothing at rigging" (July 26, 1773); "This day I was confined at home with my son Nathan" (July 31, 1773); "This day do nothing at loft. Employed taking care for the sick of my family" (August 4, 1773); "This day I do not attend Church but the sick" (August 8, 1773). In addition to tending his family, Bowen threw himself into the other tasks deemed necessary to meet the threat of contagion. He watched at the fences blocking paths to infected houses, and he helped to bury the dead, whose corpses were placed in a small boat and carried to "the neck" that jutted out into Marblehead Harbor. On the day smallpox took its first life, that of Mother Shaw, Bowen put it plainly: "This day smallpox day" (July 28, 1773).[24]

Despite these strains, Bowen continued to work as much as possible through the entire epidemic. By 1773, after a decade's labor at his business and craft, Bowen had become one of the principal riggers in Marblehead, having rented his own loft a year earlier and secured contracts with many of the town's most prominent shipbuilders. But success had its costs. Bowen regularly took on more work than he could possibly complete by himself and often had to rely on hired day workers to help him meet deadlines. In ordinary times, the system worked well. Bowen hired workers as needed; chronic underemployment of men in their thirties and older usually yielded a ready supply of men who could be secured at reasonable wages.[25]

Smallpox epidemics complicated matters considerably. When hired hands fell ill or were absent for other reasons, Bowen still had to ensure that he finished work on schedule. Commerce relied upon precise timing, and an artisan who did not deliver on his promises could lose future contracts. Over the years, Bowen had learned to improvise and accommodate some of the inevitable afflictions that befell his workers; he would hire others or find a way to finish their work himself.[26] But smallpox could thwart both of these strategies. Hired hands might be unavailable for weeks, not days. And for those like Bowen whose families had been stricken, it became all the more difficult to make up for delays through personal initiative.

Consumed by the infection of his wife and son, Bowen completed almost no work during the first week of the epidemic. He tried to resume work the following week, delivering rigging, fixing shrouds, and receiving more orders. But his progress was halting, as he spent a large portion of the day "employed" in aiding his wife and tending his family at home. By the following week, when Bowen was ready to hire help to make up for his absence, he encountered additional difficulties: "This day much employed with sick wife. Do little at loft. Would have employed Rimshire but he refused" (August 6, 1773). Bowen had a long history with John Rimshire, having hired him periodically for five years and as recently as the day Mary Bowen was removed to the pesthouse. Whether Rimshire was wary of someone in such close contact with the infected is unknown, but Rimshire had never refused Bowen's many offers before. Bowen apparently had equally little success hiring other familiar hands, and a week later he secured the services of someone entirely new, a Mr. Humphreys. Within days Bowen was obliged to depart from routine once again. Rather than hiring Humphreys by the hour and day, Bowen offered him a contract for the month. To do so meant a certain loss; even at his busiest, Bowen simply did not have enough work to warrant hiring hands on a monthly basis. But with his family ill and so few others about who were willing or able to work, it may have seemed the most prudent course. In times of epidemic, one had to absorb such losses and hope that their accumulation would not become unbearable.[27]

❦

Four weeks after she was removed to the pesthouse, Mary Bowen was allowed to return home; son Nathan followed two weeks later. For Ashley Bowen, their return brought an end to his family's immediate involvement in the smallpox outbreak. The coming weeks saw a reckoning, an assessment of the credits and debts accrued during the outbreak.

Some clearly benefited from the outbreak. Smallpox constructed its own economy, and many would be compensated for their efforts during the crisis. Bowen was one of thirty persons listed on an account presented by two of the town's selectmen for services that they had hired during the epidemic. While the account merely states that Bowen was to be paid for "labor" (and the amount due is not listed), Bowen could expect to collect for his work on behalf of the town: standing guard, burying the dead, even gathering the corn of a townsman who had been quarantined. It was not at all uncommon for towns to consider these sorts of services chargeable, and accounts submitted in the wake of epidemics bore the names of persons like Bowen who had aided their towns in similar ways during the crisis. Others, including at least five women in town, were hired as nurses; along with caring for the poor, smallpox epidemics were one of the ways women entered the money economy. Still others, such as Mr. Humphreys, would benefit indirectly from the pox, using the labor shortages caused by the affliction to secure favorable contracts. In a town facing chronic underemployment, an outbreak of smallpox created jobs and opportunities.[28]

Yet there were also many debts to be paid in the wake of the smallpox epidemic. Towns would dip into the treasury to pay laborers like Bowen, but would then ask the afflicted or those responsible for them to contribute a share of the costs. If Bowen could expect payment from the town for his service during the emergency, he also owed the town for his family's involvement in the epidemic. Bowen most certainly would have been asked to pay for at least a portion of the nursing, attendance, medicine, and food that were provided for his wife and son Nathan. Individual items would be negotiated. Bowen was able to send his son to the pesthouse with many of the basic items deemed necessary for a patient: a bed, sheet, blanket, and clothing. He would not be charged for these provisions, but he might be expected to pay for the airing and cleansing necessary to remove all threat of distemper that might lay hidden in the material. In the meantime, Bowen and his family would have to do without these items; it was a full month after son Nathan returned home before Bowen was able to collect the load from the pesthouse. To these costs would be added those harder to assess. How would Bowen make up for six weeks of delays? With his oldest son still several years away from entering the workforce as a fisherman, Bowen would have to depend on his own efforts to secure the money necessary for rent and the procurement of commercial goods. As an established artisan, he had the wherewithal to weather the crisis; business was booming, and he would have the opportunity to recover his losses. Had Bowen and family been stricken two years later, when his business had come to a complete standstill under the restrictions that attended the imperial crisis, he would have been in serious trouble. As things stood in 1773, he would survive with his competency intact.

⚬

Ashley Bowen's diary and the few town records that pertain to the early days of the epidemic in Marblehead provide us with at least a partial picture of an artisan and his family making their way through the crises that grew out of the contagious distemper. Was Ashley Bowen's experience typical of New Englanders' confrontations with smallpox? The answer must be equivocal.

As a port town, Marblehead was more familiar with contagious disease than many rural areas but less equipped than a metropolitan center like Boston with the infrastructure to contain an outbreak. Yet the town had managed to contain the ravages of the initial outbreak. The stringency of public health provisions in New England, provided in law and carried out dutifully by towns like Marblehead, had ensured that large swaths of the population in the region might be vulnerable to the pox. The fact that the seventy-nine-year-old Mother Shaw had been vulnerable to the disease was a measure of the incredible success of public health measures followed in the years prior to the outbreak. Bowen noted in his journal twenty-three cases of smallpox and thirteen deaths by August; by the following February, forty-seven residents had been stricken and twenty-seven had succumbed. Despite the appalling death rate, the episode paled in comparison to large epidemics in Boston in 1721, 1730, 1752, and 1764, when thousands were stricken.[29] When larger numbers of persons were involved, daily life could be severely affected for months on end. In its initial approach to the outbreak, Marblehead had escaped this fate, in large part because of following the sometimes severe requirements of quarantine. As for Bowen, not a leading man in town, his family would weather the storm with its competency in place.[30]

At the same time, the robust response to contagion could threaten the interlocking economic and social relations sustaining and perpetuating everyday life. How could society continue to function when contact between individuals might be deadly? And equally troubling, who was to assume the responsibility for the spread of contagious disease and the costly responses devised to contain its destruction?

II. THE DYNAMICS OF CONTAGION: INTEGRATING THE EVERYDAY AND THE EXTREME

If we step back from the particular circumstances that made each outbreak of smallpox unique, a more general social and political script for smallpox throughout the eighteenth century comes into view, from the manner of its entrance into society to the steps to identify and eliminate it and the final measures deemed necessary to incorporate the infected back into everyday life. Smallpox animated a familiar set of rituals in New England that had been in play for over a century. Moreover, as a form of affliction, the pox was a call to change one's ways, a chance for self-examination, repentance, cleansing, and finally renewal. Through such rituals, that which was tarnished could be redeemed.[31]

1. COMMUNICATION

It was often said that smallpox was "communicated" to individuals and communities. The term highlights the connections that made the expansion of the distemper possible. Spread directly through face-to-face meetings or indirectly through exposure to objects that had been in contact with the infected, smallpox provides a map of the full range of communications in eighteenth-century society.[32]

Outbreaks of smallpox lay at the intersection of two realms of communication, the provincial and that of the world outside its borders. As noted above, smallpox epidemics raged when a large number of persons who had not previously been exposed to the distemper were suddenly placed in contact with it, as was often the case in British North America. Thus the origin of epidemics invariably could be traced to elements outside a stricken community.

Chief among the forces that pulled the pox into households and town were war and commerce. Throughout the century, smallpox was known to devastate troops and frustrate carefully conceived plans of attack. In the early stages of the Revolution, John Adams commented that the "small Pox has done Us more harm than British Armies, Canadians, Indians, Negroes, Hannoverians, Hessians, and all the rest."[33] Conceived of as a "formidable Enemy" during war, the pox continued to rage on the domestic front as soldiers returned home. Infected soldiers were regularly released by armies that had neither the supplies nor the personnel to tend the afflicted. Veterans who were fortunate enough to make it home before they succumbed to the disease might well find that they were regarded with suspicion if not outright hostility.[34]

If war ensured periodic outbursts of epidemic, the diffusion of Atlantic commerce throughout the colonies posed a more serious problem. War was episodic; commerce was inscribed in daily routines. Every element of a healthy commercial economy—from the continual arrival of ships in ports to the dispersal of goods throughout the countryside—could be transformed from the mundane and harmless to the extraordinary and deadly through an infectious disease like smallpox. Any goods that provided a soft surface to hide the pox were especially suspect. Hats, coats, shirts, and other garments; sheets, blankets, beds, pillows; finished cloth and bales of cotton—these were the items of comfort and necessity that might now be considered dangerous. Even paper money was thought to carry the pox, a vivid metaphor for the special dangers of commerce.[35]

To the forces of war and commerce might be added other modes of communication that brought smallpox into provincial life: expansion and conquest (which involved both war and commerce); long-distance travel and visiting; and even letters from infected areas. Whatever the means, once the pox arrived, every dimension of everyday life that brought individuals into contact with one another fueled epidemic. Worse still, the very process of meeting the demands of ordinary sickness could spread the contagious distemper through towns before anyone could arrest its progress.

How did New Englanders cope with a world in which everyday life could suddenly turn lethal? We must imagine modes of perception and structures of social organization flexible enough to shift in an instant to meet the demands of contagion and then, just as quickly, to return to everyday life once the threat of infection subsided. Special routines would have to be put in place to identify, contain, and finally eliminate infection. Extraordinary measures were required to ensure a return to everyday life as quickly as possible.

2. SUSPICION

On the day that Ashley Bowen had the misfortune to discover his wife in bed with smallpox, he wrote in his diary that "many more are much suspected to have it" (July 24, 1773). Suspicion was often given this passive voice construction; we don't know who is doing the suspecting. People like Bowen might gather information on the wharves, along the streets, or at the houses of neighbors, and share or elaborate on suspicions. But suspicion, particularly in a time of smallpox, had more force than rumor or gossip, as powerful as those could be in New England life.[36] The imperatives of suspicion were codified in legislative acts to meet contagious distempers. Anyone coming from places outside the town's borders known to have been recently infected by the pox, or suspected of the same, would have to identify themselves to selectmen or face fines. Towns had the right and duty to act on suspicion; even if the suspicion proved unwarranted, the suspected were asked to pay the costs of their own isolation. If a party could prove in court that they had been wrongly suspected, their accusers could be excused from paying court fees through an appeal to the General Court. Finally, individual citizens might be given incentives to be informants. With towns given broad authority to enact their own preventative legislation, it was not unheard of for informants to be paid half the fees assessed on the suspected, the other half to go to the town poor. In times of contagion, suspicion was encouraged.[37]

Two cases from the small town of Richmond, Rhode Island, show suspicion at work. Sometime in the spring of 1754, James Harvey arrived in Richmond with his family and took up residence at the house of the widow Grant. A laborer from Scotland, Harvey undoubtedly hoped to find work in the inland town but soon found himself embroiled in controversy. Late in June, the Richmond town council observed that there was "a family of Scotch People, lately Settled who is Suspected to be Infected with the Small pox," and promptly dispatched two men to "Cleanse and air the whole family with all their Cloathing and Goods According to Law. . . ." The family would be confined to their quarters at "Widow Grants" and supported with the "Necessaries of Life" by others in the town. Within three weeks, the care for the Scotsman and his family had amounted to a little over £37 old tenor: Jeremiah Rogers and David Nickels asked for the costs of airing and cleansing clothes; Joseph Tefft and the widow Alice Potter asked for the provisions they supplied the family; and Simeon Perry put in a request for a jug of liquor he donated to the cause. In September the council called James Harvey before it and asked to be paid for the town's efforts on his behalf. When he had not paid in full by December, the town threatened to sue Harvey at the next meeting of the court of common pleas. Finally, in June 1755, fully a year after he and his family had been placed under suspicion, Harvey struck a bargain with the town council. He would pay them £30, all that he owned, and they would drop the remaining £7 1s. 6d. in charges.[38]

Harvey and his family had, in one sense, been lucky. The town might have thrown him in debtor's prison or placed him in the service of someone else in town until his debt had been paid. Harvey's family might have been split up, his children bound out. But the town appears to have had some sympathy for the stranger. When Harvey implored the council that he "being a poor Man & was Entirely unacquainted with the Circumstance of this Country Consering the Small Pox," they must have found some truth to it. In the end, Harvey would be allowed to remain in town. But the cost of his unfamiliarity with local custom would likely be his life's savings.[39]

Suspicion was not only directed at outsiders. In January 1760, the town of Richmond had reason to suspect that John Holloway was infected with the pox. It appears that John Holloway had become quite ill at his own house while enjoying a visit by his siblings and other relatives. Nicholas Holloway, John's father, was ordered to keep all members of his own brood who had been in contact with son John from leaving the infected house until the council allowed them to return home. In the meantime, both Nicholas Holloway and another of his sons, George, were ordered to appear before the council to give an account of John Holloway's circumstances. Clearly irritated by the request, young George told the town sergeant, "If the Council has any thing to Do with him the Council may Come to him"; he would have to be taken into custody to answer questions. Father Nicholas, more obliging, answered questions voluntarily. After both men had sat before the council and town inspectors had corroborated their story, it was determined that John Holloway was not, in fact, suffering from the pox. Father Nicholas was immediately allowed to move his goods and family back to the Holloway house. But the costs of suspicion would have to be paid. As the patriarch of the family, Nicholas Holloway promised to reimburse the town £42 12s. old tenor for the "charge Relating to his Son John Holloways Being Suspected of having the Small Pox."[40]

The stories of the Harvey and Holloway families reveal how suspicion affected the lives of quite different people. James Harvey was a poor stranger in town, a laborer who had to rent out a room for his family; the Holloways were fixtures in community life, owning at least two houses in Richmond. James Harvey came to the town council as a supplicant; George Holloway, at least, felt entitled to rebuke authority. Harvey strained for over a year to pay his fine to the town; Nicholas Holloway immediately promised to reimburse the town for its trouble on behalf of his son. What the Harveys and the Holloways shared was their subjection to the prerogatives of suspicion. In a world of uncertainties, rumor, and partial information, and fearing contagion would be unleashed, town officials had to act decisively to determine the particulars of individual cases. That they fumbled and made false determinations is not surprising. What is remarkable about the entire process is that persons like James Harvey and Nicholas Holloway complied with its demands. Both men submitted to inspection, and both paid their fines. Holloway did so even though his son was, in effect, innocent of carrying the pox. The legal and cultural power of suspicion commanded acquiescence.

3. RENEWAL

Suspicion was the first step in identifying and isolating potential carriers of smallpox. In the wake of charges of suspicion, New Englanders would construct barriers between the healthy and infected; not only law but custom and rhetoric would be used to create a new social geography. Yet far from creating a lasting wedge between the healthy and contaminated, such barriers in fact enabled tainted persons, places, and objects to be absorbed back into daily life. Only after the trials of isolation and cleansing could the infected be incorporated back into society. Communication of the pox and suspicion gave way to renewal.

New England's vigorous policies of quarantine illustrate this phenomenon at work. Every ship suspected of carrying the pox was supposed to be detained, inspected, isolated, cleansed, and finally certified as being free of the distemper.[41] Quarantine policies mediated between the fear, on the one hand, that each arriving ship posed a potential threat to public health, and the desire, on the other, to sustain Atlantic commerce. New Englanders lived in a culture well attuned to the connections between the foreign and the perilous. If the content of newspapers and almanacs may be taken to represent popular interest, provincial residents were fascinated by the marvelous, strange, and tragic circumstances of life in other lands, including narratives of the epidemics that raged there. Oral culture also told of ships hailing from places rife with infectious distempers like the pox; selectmen and legislatures often quarantined ships based on anonymous sources. However, in many cases, quick inspections of ships rumored to be carrying the pox sufficed to allow entry into ports. And for those ships found to be smitten with the pox, persons and goods were allowed to enter ports after quarantine and steps to cleanse infectious material were completed.[42]

Isolation and cleansing could remove the threat posed by incoming ships, but what could be done about local places tarnished by the pox, particularly ports where trade was crucial and where, not coincidentally, outbreaks often became most severe? The very intensity of human contact in the ports that allowed commerce to thrive could also fire the distemper; when the pox was afoot, centers of trade were to be avoided. In times of epidemic, the ports became "cities," fearsome and sinful sites that had drawn the frowns of Providence. While the great metropolitan centers of Europe differed greatly from the tiny port towns dotting New England's coast, New Englanders were ever ready to repent for the evils of city life when smallpox reared its head. When Ashley Bowen memorialized in verse the outbreak that swept through Marblehead in 1773, he chose to describe the fishing town that was one-third the size of Boston as a "city," a word he undoubtedly thought commensurate with the affliction visited upon it:

> In the Scripture we may plainly see
> And read such words as these
> Can evil in the city be
> Except the Lord be Pleased.

Marblehead itself had suffered the ravages of New England's largest city when epidemics spread from Boston up the coast in 1721, 1730, 1752, and 1764. It was not enough that "the city" suffer in afflictions of its own making; it expelled the distemper, infecting the country at large.[43]

During and after epidemics of the pox, places like Marblehead and Boston would have to move quickly to restore their reputations as safe areas to enter and trade and as good neighbors to the vulnerable countryside. As we have seen in Marblehead in 1773, the relatively small number of persons infected with the pox enabled selectmen to argue in local papers (and no doubt by word of mouth as well) that there was no danger in town. Larger epidemics, such as Boston's major outbreak in 1721/22, posed greater challenges. Lacking plausible claims that the city was safe for incomers, the city would need to draw outsiders with special enticements. Boston's selectmen offered reluctant sloopmen the option of leaving their loads on outlying islands, a measure necessary to keep city folk supplied with even basic materials such as firewood. The city would also do its best to court its "country neighbors," as the selectmen put it, especially in the waning days of an epidemic. In addition to a rigorous and well-publicized regimen of isolation, inspection, and policing the sick, the selectmen took other measures to restore civility to the city. The ringing of funeral bells that announced the death of another victim was curtailed. The burial of the dead was scheduled late at night and along deserted streets. Hawkers and peddlers who traveled about the city were forbidden to ply their goods at large, lest the pox spread generally through the country. Thus, places like Boston purged themselves of the distemper's stains, hoping to return to normalcy as quickly as possible.[44]

Infected individuals who survived could also be restored to society through ritual, emerging from the trials of the pox to face the world anew. The terrors and disruptions of the distemper would flow into a new beginning, a new self. Some would be reborn through the experience. Brought to the brink of eternity through the awful visitation, the stricken might leave the bed of sickness with a purified soul and the determination to do the Lord's work.[45] Others became ensnared in the endless worries and obligations created by smallpox. As we have seen, the extraordinary measures deemed necessary to meet the demands of contagion were accompanied by severe financial and social costs. Who would pay for the massive response deemed necessary to meet contagion? What were the rights and responsibilities of the infected and those who cared for them? We turn to these questions now, and to the politics of contagion.

III. THE POLITICS OF CONTAGION

If the communication of the pox was merely a matter of will, it would have been far easier to address and comprehend. To be sure, there were cases in which the pox was communicated in a decidedly sinister fashion, the willful act of contagion. Jeffrey Amherst's suggestion in 1763 that rebel Indians be subdued through the generous gift of blankets infected with the pox is the best known instance, but there were other persons in eighteenth-century America perceived to have similar intent.[46] In most instances, however, the matter was more complex. On the one hand, smallpox most often spread through something less odious than base designs, and thus could not be relegated to the realm of unmitigated evil. On the other hand, outbreaks and epidemics were often born of something more than naïveté, and thus invited questions about responsibility for the pox's dissemination. In this ambiguous territory between intentionality and innocence, the meaning and consequences of communication were debated.

As smallpox worked its way into everyday life, it rendered dangerous and unacceptable the ordinary and expected. Order would eventually emerge, but in the process the very building blocks of society would be shaped and defined.

1. THE STRUCTURE OF AUTHORITY: HOUSEHOLD AND TOWN

The pox was most often identified as being "at the house" of a given individual, and thus the public gaze during epidemics frequently fell upon household heads. To be sure, it was common for nurses and watchers to bear some relation to the afflicted. And as we have seen in the case of suspicion, a parent could be made to pay for an infected child even after he had left home. Family ties could also be drawn on when towns were faced with debts to be paid. But the operative term used in cases of smallpox was less often the family than the household. The boundaries between household and town—and, in particular, the responsibility of the household head for all who resided within the house or on the property as a whole— were cast into sharp relief during times of epidemic.

The unfortunate circumstances of John Rogers Jr. of New London, Connecticut, will serve as a case in point. His father, the seventy-two-year-old John Rogers Sr., had achieved notoriety in New London as a leader of the Rogerenes, a dissenting sect that had broken from the Seventh Day Baptists in the late seventeenth century. The elder Rogers had been in Boston during the devastating smallpox epidemic of 1721 and carried the pox with him on his return home to New London. He fell ill at the house that he shared with his son John Jr. and died two weeks later. From this point onward, public attention was directed toward John Jr.; as the new head of the household and of the larger compound including other Rogerenes, he would bear the ultimate responsibility for those within his purview. This was no small task. It was reported to the governor and council that there were "upwards of twenty persons" residing at the household when infection arrived. Some were family members, others were boarders, and at least one person appears to have been a transient passing through.[47]

John Rogers Jr. was to ensure that none of these persons would leave the household and infect the neighborhood in the ensuing months. Laws that forbade communication with the infected and guards charged with enforcing these laws certainly aided Rogers, whether he wanted the quarantine or not, but he was understood to be the ultimate authority within the bounds of his house and property. On November 27, 1721, a full month after the pox had been brought to his house, the governor and council issued the following injunction against Rogers:

> John Rogers will become bound . . . in the sum of one hundred pounds, with the condition that neither the said John Rogers nor any of his family, or any other person that has been sick there with the small pox, shall come to any house in this town, or go out of the limits of the farm on which the said John Rogers lives, or suffer any persons to come into their company, until such time as they are recovered to a good state of health and have taken effectual care to purge and cleanse themselves, and their cloathing, and bedding, and the house or place where the sick have been tended, from all dregs of the said distemper. . . .[48]

The crisis illuminated both the power and the vulnerability of the patriarch's position. The same laws, customs, and cultural expectations that enabled the patriarch to stand in for his family in public life demanded that he reign supreme at home—or pay the price for his ineffectuality.

If smallpox raised questions about patriarchal authority over the household, it also led to an examination of the unwieldy relationships within the household. The household in eighteenth-century New England could be populated by a complex of individuals and groups, combinations of family members, distant relations, single renters, apprentices, and sundry hired laborers and servants. Despite living in a common space, however, they did not necessarily share common interests; two families living under the same roof could very well follow separate agendas to suit their own priorities. In this loosely connected world, the contagious distemper united in affliction all who shared the same space. When the pox swept through households, it branded the persons within it with a common identity—they became the infected or those in danger of infection. When the pox was identified in its earliest stages within a given household, towns made serious efforts to protect the vulnerable within, either by removing the sick or those not yet infected. But in many instances, town officials were informed of outbreaks after the infection was already under way, in which case everyone within the stricken household was sequestered. Boundaries would be drawn around the household, constituting the household as its own society.

The impact of this enforced social identity on household members is difficult to assess. Reports of life inside stricken households comes to us in fragmentary rumors and rarely from the mouths of sufferers themselves. In most cases, we have only hints of the special trials of the afflicted within the household. When Hannah Greenman of South Kingston, Rhode Island, became infected with the pox in 1760, town officials appear to have asked Elizabeth Bull to watch, as Bull and her family lived with Greenman. But within two weeks, the costs of household affiliation became apparent; the town council reported that the pox had spread to Bull's family as well.[49] James Potter tried to avoid a similar fate. When one Miss Abigail Stoddard of Middletown, Rhode Island, fell ill of the pox in 1785, Potter immediately made plans to protect his family residing at Stoddard's house. Potter applied to the town council for permission to inoculate members of his family. The council considered and debated the proposition, but ultimately refused. While inoculation potentially would have saved Potter's family, the process was still suspect in the late eighteenth century, as inoculated persons often walked about communities while they were still infectious to others, thus fueling epidemics. Given a choice between endangering the lives of the few or protecting the lives of the many, the interests of persons like Potter and family would be sacrificed.[50]

The pox created and exposed links between household members, many of which were surely unwelcome. Individuals and families who shared shelter and resources also had to confront the possibility that they would be implicated in each other's infirmities. Under normal circumstances, these connections were often a blessing; household members might well help each other through times of sickness. But in the case of contagious diseases such as smallpox, it was feared that the bonds of affliction might lead to severe illness and painful death. Town officials were not unsympathetic to such situations. But if removal from the household was thought dangerous to the public at large, officials would create and reinforce household boundaries, defining what was permissible for its members and determining the fates of those within it.

Smallpox created a world in which towns became deeply enmeshed in the affairs of households, becoming the occasion for town authorities to reach into the lives of all residents. Even as the distemper afflicted individuals with its disruptions and threats of death, towns asked that the stricken and those who cared for them think of themselves not as smitten individuals but as members of a greater whole. As we have seen in Marblehead, townspeople would be called on to meet the needs of the public to which they belonged. Selectmen and councilors were granted extraordinary powers to effect this transformation. In the absence of willing and able caretakers, nurses and watchers would be forced into service or face prison and fines. In the absence of appropriate shelter to isolate the sick, houses would be turned into pesthouses and makeshift hospitals. In the absence of strict adherence to rules, surveillance measures would be put in place. And finally, in the absence of a clear narrative that identified the cause and course of the epidemic, authorities would investigate rumors, require oaths, and conduct examinations to reach an ultimate determination of culpability. In these ways, they managed the fear and confusion that surrounded the contagious distemper.

The actions performed in the name of preserving the public health inevitably created invidious distinctions among townspeople; some would be impressed or required to relinquish property, while others would suffer no such losses. Even though town records are not swollen with accounts objecting to the perceived injustices of official policy, there are enough to warrant our attention.

Consider the case of William Wever of East Greenwich, Rhode Island. Wever served as a soldier during the Seven Years' War, and when he returned to his hometown in the winter of 1757, he was suspected of carrying the pox. Wever and his wife and children were immediately isolated. When it became apparent that the house holding them was unsatisfactory—it was said to be so leaky that no one could remain dry in it as the December rain poured in—the town council endeavored to move Wever to another building (though his family was ordered to remain in the ramshackle shelter until further notice). James Fowler's house was selected as a likely site to place the infected Wever. But Fowler would have none of it. The council reported that Fowler "refuses or Neglects to Remove himself and family," and so two men were sent off to remove Fowler from his house. Several weeks later, a different problem arose. On January 23,

1758, the council reported that Wever "has near Got Well" of smallpox and "is Now Contrary to the order of this Council astroling about from place to place." The town sergeant was summoned to bring Wever before the council, where he was promptly ordered to pay for the care given his family while sick, and presumably made to stop his unlawful wanderings about town.[51]

Of the two incidents, Fowler's was the more flagrant violation of town rule, a flat denial of official orders. Fowler acted as the protector of his family, refusing to relinquish his property and dislodge his family. The town fathers appealed to Fowler for his own safety and that of his family; their removal was necessary to place them in a house "more Remote from the Danger of Taking Said Infection Whilst in Helth." But lest Fowler think of his family alone, the town councilors reminded him of his larger obligations. By preventing sickness in his own family, the councilors argued, Fowler would stifle "the Farther Spreading" of the distemper and protect others in town. Even if persons like Fowler might prevail in some instances, the odds were stacked in favor of towns, which had the authority to fine their recalcitrant members and to commission others to forcibly remove them from their property.

Although less confrontational, Wever's disregard of quarantine measures after he had "near got well" was perhaps a more difficult transgression to address. Officials had to convince townspeople of the fundamental similarity between the slightest violation of policy and the most serious; the potential for contagion had to be contained in every instance for isolation to work. When persons like Fowler refused to house and isolate the contagious, everyone might agree on the gravity of the offense. But when officials tried to exercise their prerogatives in cases that might have seemed harmless or trivial, they encouraged infraction. Authorities could meet these sorts of infractions with fines but could not stop them from happening in the first place. It was at the margins of their power that town officials must have felt most vulnerable.

What emerges from town records is a curious blend of anxiety and mastery. Viewed up close, selectmen and councilors seem to have tried to anticipate possible infractions. Every possible behavior that connected the sick and the healthy—from visits and the provision of food and supplies to the building of caskets and funeral processions—had to be carefully choreographed and policed. Viewed at a distance, order seems to have prevailed. Town officials might be tested in bold outbursts aimed squarely at their policies or in the more subtle resistance of their authority at its margins. But given the major demands placed on residents, overt and sustained violations of town authority were rare.

2. Hierarchy

As the pox worked its way through society, it painted everyone with the same brush, subjecting all to communication, suspicion, and the requirements for successful restoration into everyday life. Though the burdens placed on afflicted individuals and those in their care could be extreme, the pox did not instigate major protest. Rather, household, town, and General Court became implicated in a shared task.

At the same time, the pox created and maintained fundamental differences upon which society was based. Although eighteenth-century New England was one of the most egalitarian places in the Western world, it was a society bound together by inequalities. The deference and allegiance that wives owed husbands, children owed parents, and servants and slaves owed masters were enshrined in custom and law. However, the pox distinguished only between those who were vulnerable and those who were immune. And so the question arises: How were the leveling tendencies of the contagious distemper grafted onto a hierarchical social order?

Much of the work of officials during smallpox outbreaks and epidemics consisted in spreading the burdens of affliction as evenly as possible, or at least in creating this impression. Particularly for the vulnerable population that resided in the vicinity of the infected, care was taken to adopt measures that would appear equitable. Present throughout an epidemic, the problem became particularly acute at the point of death; those who succumbed to the pox would have to be removed from the household, and as bodies were taken to their final resting place, infection threatened all who lay along the path to the grave. When Captain Benjamin Smith of Providence, Rhode Island, died of the pox in 1759, due care was taken to contain his infected essence. Smith was wrapped in a tarred sheet, placed in a coffin "Tard within and without" that was covered with yet another tarred sheet, and then the entire coffin was put into a larger coffin which was itself tarred from within. Lest townspeople complain of unfair exposure to the pox on the way to the grave, the council plotted a route that would equally distribute the contagious threat posed by Smith's body. In its final approach to the graveyard, the town council instructed the funeral party to make sure to keep "an Equel Distance betwen the houses of Luther and Dexter" even though a slight deviation was unlikely to bring illness to one of the houses. But the principle of the equal diffusion of potential risk was important to uphold in a time of crisis; it anticipated and removed the threat of controversy as the pox extended its reach through towns.[52]

For all the town's efforts to be fair to its residents, the case of Benjamin Smith also reveals the ways in which many of the decisions made by town officials presumed and reinforced hierarchical social relations. Although selectmen and councilors never formally stated in their records that some individuals were entitled to special treatment, they arranged it through special provision and exemption. When Benjamin Smith became sick with the pox, the town council had him removed to a pesthouse. But in a departure from procedure, Benjamin's father, Daniel, was allowed to choose a person to carry necessaries to his son, and fourteen persons were given certificates to visit and watch with Benjamin, including Obadiah Brown, one of the most prominent residents in Providence, who was on his way to becoming a leading merchant in the colony. The number of guests allowed was highly unusual, and the increased volume of visitors would be a nuisance for officials. Everyone leaving the pesthouse would have to wash themselves with vinegar, and an attendant would have to be appointed to make sure that they followed directions. Nevertheless, when persons such as Obadiah Brown were involved in smallpox cases, their needs would have to be accommodated. The privileges of genteel sociability (and, perhaps with it, the commercial relations of the elite) could trump public health concerns.[53]

Yet even elites could face clear limits in times of epidemic, perhaps nowhere more so than in considerations over whether to inoculate residents. Inoculation raised questions about the rights and responsibilities of individuals in relation to their towns and larger communities. What special provision should be made for the poor? And what prerogatives might elites exert?

The practice of inoculation consisted of gathering matter from the pustules and scabs of active cases and introducing them to the inoculee via an incision, usually in the arm or leg. Those patients who were successfully inoculated could hope to undergo a less virulent form of the disease and, if they survived, to be protected from future smallpox infection. Beginning with its first large-scale introduction during Boston's smallpox epidemic in 1721, inoculation ignited controversy. Alongside arguments about whether the practice contravened the will of God and whether it was in fact efficacious and supported by expert medical knowledge, the decision to inoculate raised difficult concerns about the texture of community life. Patients undergoing the treatment often had milder symptoms than those who were infected the "natural way," and because inoculees might feel better even while they were still infectious, there was widespread fear that the inoculated might walk about, socialize, and thereby infect others in town, generating further outbreaks and inflaming epidemics.[54]

A steady stream of legislative restrictions tried to minimize this possibility. The Massachusetts General Court forbade inoculations unless towns were overwhelmed with smallpox cases. In contrast to Philadelphia, which allowed the practice between outbreaks for those who could afford it, Massachusetts preferred to rely on its strict regimes of quarantine, isolation, and cleansing. Through the 1730s and 1740s, as the General Court steadily elaborated laws that identified, contained, and cleansed sick persons and goods from infected areas, it forbade inoculation, provided that the distemper was present in fewer than twenty houses in a town. When infections exceeded that number, towns could instruct their selectmen to devise inoculation hospitals, and by general consent these were placed in areas deemed "convenient and safe," most often in more remote areas or outside the town proper. Finally, when infections threatened to overwhelm towns, a general inoculation was allowed. Red flags identifying infected households came down, guards were dismissed, and the town itself became, in effect, a hospital.[55]

During Boston's epidemic in 1764, for example, when the selectmen approved a general inoculation, thousands underwent the procedure, including hundreds of outsiders allowed to enter the city. An official count taken toward the end of the epidemic registered 699 "natural" cases (with 124 deaths) and 4,977 inoculations (with 46 deaths). While the overall numbers of deaths was lower than prior epidemics, the prospect of future inoculations in the town threatened further outbreaks, not only in Boston but in neighboring towns. The General Court therefore passed a new law restricting inoculation in the wake of the epidemic and, more importantly, it lay the onus of further infections on the sick themselves, whether they contracted the pox naturally or through inoculation. Before patients were allowed to leave their places of confinement, they were required to obtain a certification from a physician stating that they were no longer infectious. Anyone who violated the law—and thereby exposed neighbors, townsfolk, and others in adjacent towns to the risk of infection—was charged with the "willful" communication of the pox and subjected to a £50 fine.[56]

In addition to this restrictive legislation, towns across Massachusetts grappled with the possibility that inoculation might be available only to those with means. As a practical matter, inoculation could reduce the number of people vulnerable to the infection and hence the likelihood that outbreaks became epidemics. And so towns wrestled with the problem that the costs could put inoculation out of range for the middling and, especially, the poorer sorts. It required isolation for a month, which meant a potentially devastating disruption in wages and work. Beyond that, the costs to prepare for the procedure, to pay the inoculator, and finally to secure nursing, lodging, and food for a month of isolation could be prohibitive. A critical part of deliberations by towns over whether to offer a general inoculation turned on provision for the poor. In the wake of Boston's epidemic in 1721, the town spent a whopping £1,000 on the sick poor and asked the legislature to help. Not until the overseers of the poor agreed to treat the poor gratis was inoculation permitted in Boston's 1764 epidemic. By the time the epidemic waned, some 1,025 poor inhabitants had been treated.[57]

Over the course of the eighteenth century, Boston increasingly stood out in the Atlantic world in the concern its governing bodies had for inoculating the poor. In Philadelphia, for example, quarantine and isolation measures were lax and residents were left to their own means to seek inoculation until 1774, when a charity was created to inoculate the poor for free and local physicians promised the same. The city was known to be hospitable for inoculations, and those with means traveled there to undertake the procedure. But in Massachusetts, the backing of governing bodies meant that larger numbers of persons, and especially the poor, could be treated. In Boston, general inoculations ensured that increasingly large percentages of the population had been inoculated over the course of the eighteenth century. In 1764, with provision made to support the poor, fully 87% of the smallpox cases in the town were by inoculation (4,977 inoculated), up from 2% in 1721 (247 inoculated), 10% in 1730 (400 inoculated), and 28% in 1752 (2,109 inoculated).[58]

Provisions to support the inoculation of the poor were intended, like other measures, to protect the town as a whole from the risk that any given individual might pose. Were any special privileges to be afforded the gentry? We have seen above how elites might be given special dispensation for visits during outbreaks, a bending of the rules that would accommodate their special station. Accommodation for the privileged became a fraught topic in debates over quarantine for inoculees.

Ashley Bowen's Marblehead offers a vivid example of the ways in which inoculation raised concerns about elite privilege. In the wake of the outbreak of 1773 (discussed above), the town debated whether to build an inoculation hospital with public or private funds, settling finally on the latter. The private inoculation hospital would be funded by four proprietors, prominent merchants and Whigs in the town. Fearing that inoculation at the hospital might unintentionally spread the pox, the town adopted strict rules requiring the selectmen's permission to approach and leave the hospital.[59]

Before long, many townspeople began to have regrets. First, when it was revealed that the hospital would be located on an island close to town, Marblehead residents feared that this proximity would increase the chances of spreading infection. Second, when the costs of the inoculation procedure and provision at the private institution were established, they exceeded what most of the town residents could afford. Finally, after the hospital was built and accepted its first patients, it became clear that inoculees felt at ease to travel more freely outside the hospital than isolation measures allowed.[60]

For his part, Ashley Bowen began a narrative in his diary to detail with sarcasm the follies of the hospital patients, whom he called the "Enockulation Gentry." People were irked by rumors of wine flowing and carefree socializing, and they deemed unacceptable the patients' seeming disregard of regulations limiting their access to the mainland. In the end, the transgressions of inoculees and the hospital were met by the mob. As in other crowd actions during the imperial crisis, the crowd acted in the name of defending liberties and directed its ire at specific persons and the institution directly implicated in offenses. Four men accused of stealing clothes of inoculees and bringing the goods back to Marblehead were tarred and feathered. When a new outbreak of the pox was discovered in town, the loose ways of the hospital were suspected. Some twenty men rowed to the island and burned the three-story hospital to the ground.[61]

The riot in Marblehead was not about inoculation per se but rather the possibility that the private inoculation hospital, and the privileged persons within it, might act against the greater interests of the town. When Marblehead considered inoculation again, this time backed by the town meeting and with a price that could be met by most inhabitants, the measure passed and further inoculations were undertaken without incident.[62] Yet the hospital riot also signaled a rift in town life in Massachusetts that would continue to grow over the course of the century. Inoculation hospitals developed steadily during the late eighteenth century, despite concerns about whether they inflamed epidemics. In the wake of an outbreak in 1788, Watertown, Newton, Medford, and Brookline established inoculation hospitals. The most famous of these, presided over by Dr. Aspinwall in Brookline, promised genteel sociability, including visits with family and friends and musical entertainment in the first days after inoculation. The physician Benjamin Waterhouse, in reporting on the hospital, noted that no paupers were present in the hospital's early days. Over time, as the gentry secured more options for inoculation in hospitals, a rift developed between the elite who could afford more comfortable means of taking inoculation and the poor who favored general inoculation with the support of towns.[63]

In outbreaks and epidemics, the lower orders of society could be weighted with extra restrictions, burdens, and other markers of inferiority that reinforced social hierarchy. One of the central fault lines that developed was between whites and persons of color. Several examples from Boston will illustrate the point. Even in the absence of a public health crisis, numerous restrictions were applied to the lives of free blacks in eighteenth-century New England, including limitations on their access to credit and the right to buy land. Epidemics highlighted the disadvantages of free blacks. At the inception of Boston's smallpox epidemic of 1721, the selectmen warned "all free Male Negros. Mollatos & c." to take up carts and cleanse the streets and lanes of the city of the filth that was thought to aid and harbor the distemper.[64] No other group was singled out in this fashion. Free black men in the city had long been forced to clean the streets, a task required in lieu of service in the militia (which was forbidden to them). But in a time of smallpox, cleaning the streets of the refuse that poured out from houses placed these men in close contact with the dregs of the distemper, something no one wanted to endure.[65]

As if to recognize the differential treatment accorded whites and blacks, morbidity and mortality statistics during epidemics became part of a racialized numeracy. When overseers of the poor and the selectmen of Boston walked through the wards of the city in an effort to take "an exact count of the number of persons who have had the small pox," they neatly divided their totals into "whites" and "blacks." The surveyors might have sorted the population in any other number of ways, such as by sex or age. But nothing was deemed as important to tally as race; black and white were the most salient categories in the public analysis of the distemper.[66]

As the numbers of dead climbed during the epidemic of 1721, the Boston selectmen tried to restore some semblance of order to their noisy streets by limiting the tolling of bells that announced funerals, especially for Indians, blacks, and mulattos:

Ordered. [T]hat at Each funeral there Shal be but one Bell tolled, and that but a first and a Second time, and that it Shal be at the Election of the Person or persons ordering the funeral which Bell they will haue tolled . . . and non of the Said Bells are to Toll longer then Six minuets, and that for the funeral of Indians, Negros & mcllattos the Bel shall toll but once for each. . . .[67]

For those listening on the streets of Boston, the sounds signaling death were racialized, separating whites from all others and obliterating the distinctions among those of color, placing freedman and slave in the same category. Not ignored entirely, their deaths would be marked through a diminishment, a final signal of their rank in society. No other divide emerges from official records of smallpox in eighteenth-century New England with the same force and clarity as race.

3. Dependency

The issue of how individual residents and their families would cope in the wake of epidemics could be of grave importance to towns. In the best of times, towns across New England were populated by significant numbers of persons fighting to preserve a modest competency and others simply trying to keep poverty at bay. The pox threatened a broad section of the population with costs that were difficult, if not impossible, to pay altogether. To the extent that afflicted individuals were unable to reimburse towns for the costs of their care, the town would have to absorb the loss. And to further compound the problem, the death and destruction that inevitably attended the pox would mean that some in town would be reduced to poverty, swelling the ranks of the town poor, and further increasing the town's financial burdens. Smallpox fueled a vicious cycle: the very conditions that created massive costs were the same conditions that made those costs difficult to pay.[68]

The stories of those overburdened by smallpox are muted in town records. Left with only a name and a simple request for relief in many instances, we must imagine the events that led up to the crisis. Fortunately for us, in certain circumstances individuals felt compelled and entitled to present their cases before the General Court and, in so doing, recorded a narrative of their afflictions. Wartime losses often prompted such petitions; the following chapter will explore the connection between war and sickness. But a few examples from cases in which war, though the justification for a petition, was only tangentially related to the petition's content will illuminate the strains that smallpox could place on individual lives.

Obadiah Sampson of Middleborough, Massachusetts, petitioned the

General Court that his son Samuel, returning from an assault on Crown Point during the Seven Years' War, had brought the pox back with him. Sampson argued that the costs of the sickness had mired the family in debt. The charges went beyond the need to pay for the care of son Samuel (who ultimately died) and another son who contracted the distemper and survived. Because others in the family were vulnerable to the disease, Sampson had been forced to move out of his house while his sons lay ill there. The General Court recognized that the costs of the illness and the dislocations it had occasioned were "very Expensive" and had caused "much loss and damage in his [Sampson's] business, which he is unable to Support." Sampson was allowed £20 5s. 1d. to pay off his debts.[69]

Twenty years later, Alexander Thompson sounded a variation on this theme. James White, a soldier belonging to the Continental army, had been wounded at the Battle of Bunker Hill and had returned to his hometown in the western part of Massachusetts. When White came down with the pox shortly thereafter, he was placed in the care of Thompson, which had proven extremely burdensome. Thompson had been forced to send his own children, who had not already contracted the disease, out of the house and to hire a woman to care for them while White lay ill. And worse still, Thompson argued that he and his wife "were taken from their daily calling for the space of thirty one days before his House was cleansed; and this happen'd at a time of the Year, when his Husbandry Business should have been done, and few would come near his House for fear of the Distemper whereby he has lost most of the produce of his Farm for this Season." Thompson concluded that these unfortunate occurrences, coupled with his "advanced age" and already "low Circumstances," warranted due consideration. Thompson asked for £10 10s., an amount certified by his selectmen as "very reasonable." He was granted two-thirds of the request.[70]

As both Sampson and Thompson pointed out, there were extraordinary charges associated with the pox: removing oneself or one's children from a household; cleansing the same; being called on to nurse the afflicted or pay for nursing. But what added to the severity of these costs was that all of the actions required to meet the threat of contagion could seriously hamper, if not destroy, the normal means used to pay off debts. Both men maintained that the pox threatened their "business." Moreover, Thompson, in suggesting that both he and his wife were taken from their "calling," recognized the costs of losing the full range of labors necessary to sustain the integrated household.

In a sense, Sampson and Thompson were fortunate that the cause of the pox entering their lives could be traced to the war. Others who suffered similar losses, would not, in most instances, have the same option of petitioning the highest levels of government for relief. Nor could the afflicted necessarily turn to their towns for help. From the perspective of the town, it was bad enough that smallpox could tear through the households of the poor, adding to the public outlays needed for their support. No one in the town was prepared to assume the far more costly burden of aiding large numbers of newly impoverished residents who had formerly supported themselves. Towns could ill afford to stand by as residents slipped from competency to dependency.

In the wake of smallpox epidemics, towns pleaded with the General Court for relief that would prop up their residents who could no longer withstand the financial burdens of affliction. Towns highlighted the circumstances that would give them special consideration. Selectmen might plead that the pox had been brought in by an outsider, such as a soldier. Or they might detail all of the circumstances that had damaged commerce. But the bottom line, for both the town and the General Court, was the alarming increase in the impoverishment of town residents. The petition set before the General Court by the selectmen of Boston in 1752 is illustrative. The selectmen represented the "distressed State" of the town in great detail. The court was informed of "the great Increase of the Poor. Decay of their Trade & the removal of many of their Inhabitants to other Towns. . . ." In the end, however, the court was most moved by the threat of growing dependency. In explaining its resolve to grant the town £600 out of the public treasury, the General Court stated that it allowed the money because with the pox "so generally prevailing" in Boston, "many Persons are reduced to very great Streights & necesitous Circumstances who otherwise would have been in a Capacity to have Subsisted, their Familys in Comfortable Circumstances." The overseers of the poor would be allowed to distribute the sum as they saw fit. The enduring poor of the town would be granted some form of relief; those who stood on the brink of dependency would be shored up, their competency preserved by the benevolent hand of government.[71]

IV. CONCLUSION

In one of the first studies of epidemics in early America, John Duffy cautioned his readers that smallpox stood out in the historical record beyond its "real significance," by which he meant its role in colonial mortality rates. Duffy noted that malaria, dysentery, and a variety of respiratory diseases unquestionably claimed more lives than the pox. But as a disease that was understood to be contagious and fatal, smallpox "aroused the most consternation among the colonists."[72] Duffy's basic claim for the special anxieties caused by smallpox still stands. In many ways, the pox must be viewed as a special sort of affliction. It could rip through households and communities with a ferocious speed and intensity. And the measures designed to contain its destruction—a regime of suspicion, isolation, inspection, impressment, and cleansing—could be equally unsettling.

Yet despite its unique horrors and costs, smallpox also represents an extreme example of the workings of affliction in daily life. The pox was emblematic of the power of affliction, its capacity to structure authority, dictate routines, devastate lives, and exact costs that could not be easily retrieved. The force of affliction lay not only in what it did but in its potential. No one knew when, where, and whom it would strike. Nor was it clear how long it would last. The only certainty was that afflictions like smallpox would arise in daily life, and that somehow they would have to be accommodated and endured.

As outbreaks and epidemics quieted, New Englanders like Ashley Bowen would sift through the events of the past weeks and find expression in the language of affliction. His poem, entitled "On Small Pox," suggests the ways in which the social tensions animated by smallpox could at once be articulated and absorbed by a providential understanding of disease and death:

> A sore distemper is crept in
> It seized on all both old and young
> But by what means I cannot tell
> And very fatal proves to some.
>
> In Scripture we may plainly see
> And read such words as these
> Can evil in the city be
> Except the Lord be Pleased.
>
> Short-sighted creatures as we are
> Could not our danger see
> Tho often-times distressed with fear
> What this disease should be.
>
> Surely the hand of Providence
> Over us did bear a sway

> Tho we so much distressed with fear
> Must fall an easy prey.
>
> The 24 day of July
> We were all fenced around
> Before the 17 of August came
> Eight bodies are lain in the ground.

The disturbing blending of the everyday and the extreme—that smallpox had "crept in," hiding itself in daily routines—all made sense within the providential frame; God's hand lay behind it all. Immersed in the frenzied activities and nervous anticipation that accompanied smallpox, one could lose sight of the comforts of true helplessness. Fear and bereavement obscured providential design. It was all too easy to become distracted by fences, the wracked bodies of old and young, the corpses borne out of houses of affliction. The ravages of the pox were entirely too visible in the foreground, obscuring God's hand that lay behind the dreary scene. With God in the fore, the everyday and the extreme were all of a piece.

Possible tensions between private and public, between friends and strangers, were subsumed as well in Bowen's concluding thoughts.

> How do you think dear friends
> What we must feel within
> To see so many carried out
> That had our neighbors been.
>
> Not only neighbors unto some
> But their dear friends likewise
> Which makes our very hearts relent
> And draws tears from our eyes.
>
> Let's not impute it all to chance
> Nor merely second cause
> But let us view the hand of God
> And what we do deserve.[73]

There are hints here of the ways in which a circumscribed public could be called into being in an epidemic. Bowen calls out to "friends," who, in turn, can sympathize with the loss of their own friends and neighbors; the possibility of feeling, of the softened heart and the sentimental tear, are reserved for the intimate, not the host of others that Bowen also knew were taken from their homes, the anonymous "gal," "child," and "stranger," who rumor had it were removed to the pesthouse. Bowen's public consists of persons well-ensconced in society. But if the poem suggests degrees of attachment, Bowen concludes by joining all in the brotherhood of righteous suffering. Sinful man—which is to say, all persons—had received what he justly deserved. Even in the severity of divine rebuke, there was a source of consolation. All was not random carnage and disorder, but part of a larger purpose and scheme, however difficult to apprehend.

CHAPTER SIX

The Domestic Costs of War: Wartime Afflictions

It would be hard to overestimate the importance of warfare in late seventeenth- and eighteenth-century New England. In the century that followed the Glorious Revolution, war insinuated itself into the social, economic, and political life of the region to an extraordinary degree. Between 1689 and 1763, New Englanders played a crucial role in Britain's enduring battle with the French and Indians for control over North America. Each generation of New Englanders struggled with the burdens of wartime mobilization and strained to raise and provision troops. They watched political and economic fortunes rise and fall with cycles of war and peace. They were immersed in the contradictions of war—its honors and humiliations, its opportunities and devastating losses. By the time of the Revolution, New Englanders were well accustomed to a martial way of life.[1]

Over the last several decades, the "new military history" has moved from a study of the strategy and tactics of battle into a broader consideration of the tangled relationship between warfare and society. Taken as a whole, these works tell us much about the implications of converting a civilian into a military population.[2] But we know far less about the conversion in the opposite direction, that is, the movement from a military to a civilian population. What effects did war have on households and towns that absorbed soldiers back into civilian society?[3] Wartime sickness offers one approach to this problem.

For the purposes of this chapter, we might conceive of war as a force that manufactured affliction in eighteenth-century New England, not that all wars during the period, nor even individual campaigns, were equally disruptive. Nor was affliction the sole or even primary result of war. Soldiers who survived the hardships of battle used the bounties and wages of war to move toward the goal of achieving a competency. Enterprising farmers and merchants were able to capitalize on the army's need for a wide range of goods and services. Though war could entail costly taxes and inflation, Britain's reimbursement policies could soften the blow, as was the case during the latter years of the Seven Years' War under the administration of William Pitt.[4] Despite these possible benefits, however, an abundance of records left in the wake of war depict a world of affliction. With relentless persistence throughout the century, war removed healthy persons from households and towns and returned them injured, desperately ill, or chronically infirm. As a massive engine of affliction, war had the power to pull soldiers and their families into dependency, leading them to call on government for protection and relief.

This chapter and the following address war and its aftermath. In this chapter, we will follow soldiers into the military through their service, and finally back home again, focusing on how illness figured into their life stories and tracing broad patterns over the course of the eighteenth century. The following chapter examines ongoing negotiations between soldiers, the Massachusetts General Court, and finally the federal Congress over long-term provision for disabled veterans, revealing change in what constituted "disability" over the century.

Writing nearly a half century after the close of the American Revolution, Joseph Plumb Martin reminded his readers that if the late rebellion was spiritually and ideologically charged, the war was also an event grounded in the trials of the body: "The period of the Revolution has repeatedly been styled 'the times that tried men's souls.' I have found that those times not only tried men's souls, but their bodies too; I know they did mine, and that effectually."[5]

Whether they captured their immediate experience in diaries and letters, published petitions before general assemblies at the end of their service, or composed memoirs as Martin did many years later, soldiers of the eighteenth century created a remarkable catalogue of their sufferings and misfortunes. The scope and intensity of afflictions facing them resist ready comprehension, even defy imagination. Soldiers lived with a poor diet and the chronic fear of starvation, insufficient and decaying clothing, exposure to the elements during days of marching and river crossings, and broken nights of sleep pressed to the wet or frozen ground. These conditions alone were enough to fuel indisposition. But it was the wretched environment of camp life that seems to have pushed many into the realm of dire illness. Soldiers who had rarely traveled far from home—along with the men, women, and children who followed the army—were gathered together from across New England and funneled into military camps. This assembled mass of humanity created what one scholar has aptly characterized as cities in the wilderness, and camps soon became ridden with the problems that plagued the metropolitan centers of early America. The smell of camps alone—the thick smoke, the stench of rotting refuse and human excrement—was thought to cause exhalations that poisoned the local environment. When outbreaks of typhus, dysentery, smallpox, camp fevers, and other maladies erupted, few were surprised by the turn of events. With war came the expectation of disease.[6]

Scholars have explored the causes of wartime sickness and its most extreme consequence, death. Given that severe casualties were uncommon in the wars that wracked eighteenth-century New England, most scholars argue that disease was the primary cause of high wartime mortality rates, especially in garrisons and camps, which were among the most lethal places in all of early America.[7] Even the more mundane moments of war produced mortality rates far in excess of what could be expected on the domestic front. Fred Anderson has found that in some regiments, in a period of only three to five months, soldiers in Massachusetts in the Seven Years' War died at two to four times the yearly mortality rate in Boston. Harold Selesky reports similar results in his study of Connecticut soldiers during the same period. And Howard Peckham, in an admittedly speculative assessment of total deaths during the Revolution, argues that as many as 12.5% of soldiers in the Continental army died, a figure comparable to the losses suffered by Union troops during the Civil War. The combined trials of warfare—battle, imprisonment, and the woeful conditions of camp life—killed soldiers with a ferocity rarely seen in civilian life.[8]

One is hard-pressed, however, to find scholarly exploration of the consequences of illness aside from death.[9] Despite the intimate link between sickness and mortality, one needs to be careful not to equate the two. While severe illness could lead to death, in many cases soldiers languished for weeks or even months. These ailing men posed as great a challenge, if not a greater one, as the dead did to the prosecution of war. To put it starkly, while death ended the hope that a soldier might be reincorporated into the war effort, it also put an end to the need to care for him. The sick consumed costly resources—food, shelter, clothing, and medicine, as well as the attention of surgeons, nurses, attendants, and friends—that might go for naught if the afflicted did not recover. Moreover, a soldier's sickness continued to pose difficult questions that only death or full restoration to health could put to rest. To what extent could the sick be counted on to perform the full range of duties asked of soldiers? What was reasonable to expect of them? What was beyond their means? At a time when both officers and enlisted men might be tempted to use sickness as an excuse for furlough or dismissal, how could the truly sick be separated from malingerers? And these questions, originating in a military setting, could be brought home by the afflicted and revisited in civilian life. The answers depended on who asked them, setting the stage for confusion and contest over the social and cultural meanings of the sick soldier in war.

I. THE SCOPE OF THE PROBLEM: NUMBERS AND THE DIFFICULTY OF COUNTING

War created an abundance of sick bodies—but how many? The problem of terminology complicates the answer. Most inhabitants of eighteenth-century America used a vocabulary to describe ailments that may have made sense within the framework of humoral medicine, but confounds any attempt to distinguish among what we might think of as illness, injury, and disability. Consider the case of John Dent, who addressed the New Hampshire Assembly in 1759:

> [H]aving been for more than seven years in the service of his King & Country . . . where by hard & Incessant Labour (in January the very dead of winter) in wet & cold; being obliged to work, in water, snow, & Ice, & extream cold; and when Nights come on; then to Lodge between the Heavens & the Earth; and besides this; and not a Sufficiency of the Common & Necessary supports of life & c—which exceeding Difficultys bro't upon your poor Petitioner such sore disorders & diseases of Body as caused a long & tedious sickness which at length fell into his feet; for which both of his feet have been cut off & yet are not healed; and in this distressed state your petitioner was obliged to spend all his wages . . . & is ever entirely Incapacitated for Labor. . . .[10]

In Dent's world, the assaults of the environment, the hardships of labor, the inadequacies of provisions and shelter, the diseases of the body, the wounds of amputation, and the incapacities that ensue from all of these maladies are blended together in a narrative of affliction that spans several years. In phrases repeatedly employed by soldiers, the combined trials of warfare "assaulted" or "injured" or "exposed" their "health." The healthy body was conceived of as a system in perfect balance, and once this equilibrium had been violently disturbed, it resisted easy restoration. Whatever the cause of the "unhealthful condition," soldiers were more interested in addressing their overall state of poor health than in identifying a precise source of their afflictions.

Even if one created criteria for differentiating injury, sickness, and incapacity, official tallies of the sick during war would frustrate the classification effort. Throughout the eighteenth century, soldiers who were sick were lumped together with a variety of others wounded or incapacitated by battle in the category of those "unfit" to serve. Troop returns from the Revolution subsumed both the ill and the injured into the categories of those who were "sick," distinguishing only between those able to remain in camp (the "sick present") and those sent off to hospitals or on furlough to recover (the "sick absent"). Synonymous with incapacity, "sickness" in these records is a category far broader than what we might associate with the term. Even the use of official records to obtain a morbidity rate during a given campaign is problematic: because soldiers moved into and out of sickness, the exact count of the sick varied over time. The end-of-the-year returns that tallied the cumulative number of dead cannot be replicated for the sick; at best, the records offer a snapshot of sickness at one place and time.

Despite these qualifications, a few observations may be offered. First, morbidity rates, though variable, were often several times higher than mortality rates from the same period. For example, Fred Anderson has found that at the end of 1756 four times as many soldiers from Massachusetts were sick as had died. In Connecticut, at the end of the same year, some troops registered that three-quarters of their men were unfit to serve. Although the mortality rate that year was 8%, a figure slightly above average for Connecticut's troops during the entire Seven Years' War, it was dwarfed by the rate of sickness. In other words, for many soldiers, to get sick or wounded did not necessarily mean that they would die—or, at least, that they would die before leaving the service and disappearing from official records.[11]

The second, related observation is that while rates of sickness could vary considerably according to the season or placement of troops, it was likely that a significant portion of soldiers, perhaps as many as 20–30%, would be sick during a campaign. To use Anderson's figures again, 21.3% (650 men) of Massachusetts troops were either sick or wounded at the end of the campaign of 1756. Charles Lesser has compiled a more complete set of data from Continental troop returns during the Revolution, yielding average rates of sickness that suggest Anderson's figures are not an aberration. The percentage of "sick present" and "sick absent" ranged from 5.4% to 35.5% of the total numbers of rank and file during the war years, peaking during the smallpox epidemic of 1776 and Valley Forge in the winter of 1777–78. Over one-quarter of the war years saw rates of sickness between 20% and 35%, which must be considered low estimates because they do not include data from the Canadian expedition that regularly registered higher rates of sickness. Moreover, because Lesser bases his figures on the average rate of sickness throughout the entire Continental army, it masks the higher rates of sickness in individual regiments and companies, which could run as high as nearly 50% of the total rank and file.[12]

These rates of illness, scholarship has shown, presented special difficulties both to those executing war and to those living in the middle of it. They point to the structural challenges inherent in addressing affliction on a large scale, indicating the struggles to contain sickness and provide medical care and supplies to the ailing. Other sources yield portraits of soldiers suffering in camps and hospitals, particularly during times of epidemic. Rather than follow either of these lines of inquiry in any detail, the following discussion explores the troubled connection forged between the military and the domestic front during sickness and its aftermath. More than an obstacle to the prosecution of war, more than misery and terror in hospitals and camps, wartime sickness reached beyond the soldier's life into the life of his family and town. Ever demanding, sickness visited upon the individual body of the soldier in fact implicated many others.

II. SOURCES OF THE PROBLEM: SCARCITY AND CONFLICTING TEMPOS IN EXPEDITIONARY WARFARE

In order to appreciate the link that sickness created between civilian and military life, one must understand the scarcity of military resources available to care for the ailing or incapacitated. At many times and places, there were simply too many soldiers who needed attention and too few facilities, supplies, or personnel to attend to them. In theory, the sick and wounded could be tended to in field, regimental, and general hospitals. But despite some advances in the organization of medical care over the course of the century, the numbers of sick and wounded often overwhelmed the military's best efforts. Field and even regimental hospitals were often hastily arranged shelters, perhaps barns or houses appropriated for medical use. General hospitals, ostensibly equipped to see more serious cases, were few and far between. By the time of the Revolution, a concerted effort to rationalize medical care was hampered by chronic fights between regimental and general hospitals, as allies of one or the other battled over lines of authority and access to limited supplies. Sickness could leave a soldier on his own to recover.[13]

As Joseph Martin recalled, medical attention could be notable for its absence. After spending the night in a trench, Martin and several others in his detachment "took violent colds by being exposed upon the wet ground after a profuse perspiration" and were sent back to the company's baggage (where the portable equipment was kept) to recover. Martin quipped that he had only "the canopy of heaven for my hospital and the ground for my hammock." He was left to his own devices, receiving the attention only of a messmate who brought him some "boiled hog's flesh" and turnips, neither of which Martin had the stomach to eat. In the absence of medical care, those like Martin would have to count on the goodwill of comrades.

Even in more serious situations, soldiers might find that their last hope lay with persons who had only informal healing experience. On a tour of duty through the South in 1781 with the Fifth Connecticut Regiment, Josiah Atkins discovered that his skills in letting blood and drawing teeth made him a much sought-after man. As Atkins explained with due humility in his diary, his popularity was no doubt a result of "there being not a nother tooth-drawer in the whole army" and "because few doctors have tools to let blood." No doctor himself, Atkins nevertheless tended to those whom beleaguered medical men passed by. In one instance, Atkins came across a soldier "continaully groaning, rolling over, & screaming out horribly" after receiving a spider bite. Atkins thought the man should be bled but deferred to the company physician. When the latter claimed that nothing could be done for the soldier, Atkins took matters into his own hands and bled him immediately. Approaching Atkins the next day, the man told him that he had no money "to reward me for what I had done, but he was sure he owed his life to me."[14]

If scarcity of facilities, supplies, and qualified medical personnel created hardships for ailing soldiers, these men also were put at risk by the very different tempos dictated by expeditionary warfare, on the one hand, and sickness, on the other. Movement characterized much of eighteenth-century military life from the inception of service through the close of each campaign: there was the journey to meet the army, guard duty that sent men to outposts or to scout or forage, fatigue duty spent constructing or repairing roads and bridges, hasty attacks and retreats during the heat of battle, and finally travel home again. These often rapid rhythms of the soldier's life conflicted with the slow tempo of sickness. How was the army to deal with the sick, who might move sluggishly or not at all?

Expeditionary warfare meant constant motion, and the body in sickness was not easily moved.[15]

For the sick, one of the most troubling effects of their infirmities was abandonment. The ailing soldier might be unable to keep pace with a hurried attack or a swift retreat. Or the constraints of expeditionary warfare might require that the sick be left behind deliberately. Jeremiah Greenman, a seventeen-year-old private from Rhode Island, recorded in his diary the strained efforts to care for the sick during the grueling Quebec campaign in the fall of 1775. By September, Greenman's company was exhausted. The men had struggled to move north along the Kennebec River but had found the water too rough for travel or even crossing in many places and the dense and unforgiving wilderness difficult to negotiate with their battered boats and unwieldy supplies. On September 24, Greenman noted that "our provision growing scant sum of our men being sick held a Counsel / agreed to send the Sick and we[a]kly men back" and to dispatch a detachment of men ahead to try to secure and bring back provisions. Two days later the men began to talk of killing and eating some of the dogs that traveled with the company. A week later the plan to send the sick downriver had failed miserably; the water was "so [rapid] and swift that thay could no batto [bateau] go down the river," and the company had lost one boat carrying ammunition, guns, and money in the process. The next day the sick men were jettisoned. Greenman wrote, "Set out this morn very early/ left 5 sick men in the woods that was not abel to march." Two "well men" were left with the sick, and the departing men each gave the ailing soldiers a small portion of their remaining provisions. But Greenman was not optimistic about their prospects. In the name of survival, the company had been "obliged to leave them to the mercy of wild beast."[16]

The scarcity of resources and support placed sick soldiers in a vulnerable position. In civilian life, many would have had a social safety net to hold them. Family, household, neighborhood, and town wrapped an individual in an intricate web of social credits and debts that proved remarkably resilient in times of need, as we have seen in chapter 2. But in war, the soldier was separated from his steady means of support, and in its absence, he would have to compensate, which often required money. The soldier whose spider bite made him beg Josiah Atkins for help was lucky to have found a sympathetic healer. Atkins was apparently satisfied with the man's gesture of offering a hearty thanks for saving his life—as the man said, "He had no money." Yet the sick man's expectation was that the issue of money had to be broached. Sickness called for immediate attention, and there simply wasn't the opportunity to build social credit in war. In many cases, those who tended the sick did, in fact, ask for money or some other means of payment. Men like Atkins's patient or the suffering soldiers left behind on Greenman's ill-fated expedition to Quebec might find their sickness chargeable.

The theme of indebtedness runs through petitions and pension applications filed by soldiers who had fallen sick: they accumulated a long list of debts as they lay ill—some of gratitude, others that they had been able to satisfy through barter, and still others that lingered and threatened to force them into dependency. The narratives of these soldiers provide us with a map of their travels in sickness and the debts they accrued. The winding journeys of these men as they moved into and out of camps, along the frontier, through towns that lay in the path of war, and finally home again were often costly, as their suffering bodies relentlessly generated expenses that could be stopped only by death or restoration to health.

III. NEW ENGLAND'S SONS ALONG TRAILS OF SICKNESS

When sickness required more sustained attention and provisions than the military could provide or when the sick were unable to keep up with the pace of expeditionary warfare, it was common for these soldiers to be sent on furlough or to be discharged early. Samuel Larrabee of North Yarmouth, Maine, served with a Massachusetts regiment of the Continental army during the siege of Boston. In August, several months after the British had evacuated the city, Larrabee's regiment was one of three selected to be inoculated with smallpox. His inoculation did not take, and on the day his regiment marched to Ticonderoga, he broke out with the pox. Larrabee recalled, "Not having anyone to take care of me, there being no hospitals, I was ordered back to Widow Dimond's, with whom I was quartered when inoculated, who nursed me and got me well of the smallpox though I was long after very feeble and afflicted with boils." Upon recovery, the weakened Larrabee paid the widow with his watch, returned his gun and equipment, and traveled home to Maine by boat, "not being able to walk that distance."[17]

Larrabee's trail in sickness was a short one. He had found refuge at the fringes of camp, where one could find healers, particularly women like the widow Dimond, used to dealing with sick soldiers.[18] The combination of an experienced healer and a disease that, while serious, was relatively predictable made for a straightforward exchange between Larrabee and Dimond. Informal rules defined what was required of both nurse and patient. The widow Dimond would have provided a place to sleep and perhaps a special diet and medicines. She would have kept close watch to make sure that no one who had not already had smallpox was exposed to Larrabee. And when Larrabee recovered, she would have cleaned or aired her house and bedding to make it safe for others to occupy. There was no question that Larrabee would have to pay for these services, and given the frequency of smallpox during this period, Larrabee and Dimond would have had an idea of what the prevailing costs were. They settled on Larrabee's watch as payment, perhaps a sure medium of exchange at a time when soldiers like Larrabee might have received little or no money for their service, and when what money they had was declining in value. One has no way of knowing if either Larrabee or the widow Dimond felt that they had been bested in the exchange; if either did, Larrabee was silent on the issue.

As trails of sickness stretched further from camp, the encounters between ailing soldiers and civilians could become strained. At the end of annual campaigns, companies and regiments regularly dismissed invalids whose growing numbers proved too burdensome for ill-equipped and understaffed operations.[19] As these soldiers tried to make it home before becoming completely incapacitated, they encountered a wary civilian population. Even in ordinary circumstances, a soldier on furlough might be suspect. One who welcomed a soldier into his or her house could wake to find food, livestock, or tools missing.[20] Sickness complicated this problem considerably, both recommending itself through the innocence of vulnerability and, at the same time, threatening its own brand of plunder. On the one hand, it was not easy to turn away a desperate and sick soldier who arrived at the front door. On the other hand, sickness was mysterious and dangerous. The stranger's sick body could not be read in the same way that one might discern the meaning of a wounded body, whose bandages, torn flesh, and missing appendages marked the nature and severity of its injuries. A soldier might arrive appearing to be mildly unwell only to fall violently ill. And although most illness in eighteenth-century America was not thought to be contagious, it was well known that the soldier might well have been exposed to smallpox and camp distempers.[21]

Henry Hallowell's journey back to Lynn, Massachusetts, at the end of his term with the Continental army illustrates the mixture of generosity and suspicion reserved for the sick soldier. Hallowell fell ill at Philadelphia late in the winter of 1776 and was dismissed at the end of December. Begging as he made his journey north, Hallowell later remembered that "people generaly was very kind But some was afraid of me. The people was willing to let me lay by the fire or on wheat straw; on my way I would have gone into a house but they refused my going in But brought me to the Barn some broth thicknd with cabbage."[22] Although the people along his journey had not rejected Hallowell, many had kept him at a safe distance. Perhaps they noticed his lice, bad enough that the flesh underneath his soiled shirt was "much gone," or feared the diseases that Hallowell might have been carrying from Philadelphia, where several of his mates from Lynn had recently succumbed to illness and died. Or perhaps they were afraid to let Hallowell into their houses because he looked like a man who might well cost them money. The stranger was always feared for the financial havoc he could bring upon a house. Although Hallowell's town of birth or permanent residence would have been legally obliged to pay for him should he fall into poverty through illness, New Englanders knew that recovering such costs often involved protracted legal battles. Better to let Hallowell stay in the barn, or to allow him to eat and get warm and then move on as quickly as possible.

Hallowell eventually made it home, as did many other sick soldiers. They paid for their food and care when they could, begged and counted on the generosity of those they encountered when they could not. For others, however, the severity of their sickness thwarted their efforts to return. Some lay abandoned along the frontier to the north or west; others made it partway home, only to be forced to stop for weeks or months while they recovered. Released from a military with neither the time nor the resources to cope with their ailments, the plight of these men soon put a strain on the households to which they hoped to return.

When John Waldron Smith fell ill in the wake of the Crown Point expedition in 1756, his sickness frustrated the efforts of both the military and his family. Smith's petition to the New Hampshire General Court details his troubled odyssey:

> I went to fort Edward and there was Taken Sick & Returned Down To ye half moon In a Waggon & there Laid Sick Three weaks & Senceless in which Time my Gun was Stolen from me: & from thence was Carried To ye flats in a Battoo [bateau] & there Laid Sick three months att ye Point of Death in which tim my Brother obediah Came up to see if he Could Gett me home If I was alive But I was so Bad I could not Come for which I paid him fifty five pounds old Tenor. . . .

After "a long & Tedious sickness & Grate Expenc[e]," Smith managed to get home the following January. But for a period of several months, the extreme condition of Smith's sick body had resisted efforts to remove him from the theater of war and return him home, causing more than mild inconvenience. In an effort to retrieve Smith, his brother had traveled from southern New Hampshire into New York, only to return empty-handed. In his incapacity, Smith was also vulnerable: like many others in his position, he was robbed as he lay "senceless." The sick body's power to demand attention and resist help and its vulnerability to theft and invasion was a potent combination that generated a series of costs for the afflicted and those who cared for them.[23]

In his petition to the legislature, Smith carefully illuminated the connection between the expenses he had incurred and the sickness he had endured, hoping to secure maximum compensation for his sufferings. He assumed that he should not be held responsible for the consequences of his sickness: he had become ill through helping the country in war, and the government should pay for his affliction and its attendant costs. A year and a half after he returned home, Smith was granted £9 and allowed for his missing gun.[24]

Many petitions recount the difficulties of retrieving sick soldiers and bringing them home. Some soldiers, like Smith, waited until after the war to document their costs and present their case to the general assembly. Others, in the desperation of the moment, filed for immediate redress, hoping to convert their stories of sickness into cash. As the widow Bridget Clifford pleaded to the New Hampshire governor and assembly in March 1762, her twenty-year-old son, Nathan Smith, had enlisted in the summer of 1760 and was taken sick and left behind when his company was released at the end of the campaign against Crown Point in 1761. Although her grandson, apparently also on the expedition, had been able to stay with Nathan for some time, he was forced eventually to come home without him, leaving Nathan in Albany. Nathan finally arrived home in July 1762, four months after his mother's initial petition, which the legislature had "ordered to lay." Nathan subsequently applied to the assembly for his pay during his sickness, which was eventually granted in February 1763.[25]

John Smith and Nathan Smith had both been successful in petitioning for at least some of the costs of their sickness. But a number of petitions were filed not by the sick soldier himself, but by those responsible for caring for him, most commonly parents. In 1753 Joshua Prescott asked for an allowance for nursing and doctoring his son who had fought at Louisbourg, was taken ill, and subsequently died. Sixty-five years old, Joshua could not pay the bills generated in his son's sickness. Joshua Bean spelled out the costs of his son's illness in greater detail. Bean's seventeen-year-old son had enlisted in the army in 1758 and served with New Hampshire's forces for the following thirteen months. "In his return home, said Son was taken and Continued Sick for a long time, by means whereof the said Joshua was at great Cost in defraying the Expences of his Said Sons Sickness; in cloathing him (who returned almost naked) and in hiring other Persons to perform the service and labor which his said son might have done, during his Absence." It was not uncommon for a son to go off to war and return sick or disabled—or die—leaving his parents to find ways to pay for his care and replace his labor as a member of the household.[26]

There was an irony here. War had served as a safety valve for New England's surplus sons, young men who were old enough to be within reach of a competency but who had not yet received an inheritance to let them grasp it. These young men, the "life-cycle poor," were joined in the military by others, poorer, who also counted on the wages and bounties of war to better their status. War had been a means of improvement for these men, and perhaps a relief to households that did not have the wherewithal to lift them into positions of independence. But wounds or disease transformed these men into sources of debt that could far outweigh the wages of war. From the limited data available, we know that young men in their twenties were far less likely to die in war than the older, more marginal men in New England's forces. Although contemporaries did not cast the problem in these terms, the most costly element of war for civilian society may have been the disabling of healthy men. Returning soldiers might well have to fight disease and infection incurred at the front—if they survived, or lingered before dying, they might amass costs that neither they nor their families could pay.[27]

IV. DISTRESSED FAMILIES AND DERIVATIVE DEPENDENCIES

In times of peace, the family attended to the calamities of everyday life, the illnesses, injuries, and other misfortunes that struck its members. War asked more of the family, requiring that it extend its reach well beyond the local circumstances of daily life. When a soldier fell ill, the army would do what it could, but the family was finally responsible for caring for its own. As we have seen, members of the family might make the trek to retrieve the ill soldier. In other cases, the family could count on the help of friends, neighbors, or connections they may have had to persons closer to the lines of battle. Still other situations required the aid of strangers who minded the sick and saw to it that they arrived home. Whether involved directly or not in these efforts, most often the family was forced to pay for bringing back those who could not return on their own. In due time, sick soldiers or those who petitioned on their behalf would try to recoup these costs. But there was a long hiatus between petitioning and receiving funds, with no guarantee that such funds would be forthcoming. In the meantime, the afflictions of war had imposed additional demands on the family.

Having arranged for retrieval, the family had to cope with the disabled and impoverished body that bore the marks of the violence of battle and the wretched conditions of military life. Alongside the finished goods that the household had worked to purchase from the wider world of Atlantic commerce lay the ailing soldier, a battered product of distant war. In turn, the soldier's sick body would create its own economy of consumption. If the soldier's illness was severe enough, as petitions by household heads pleaded, it could drain family resources, pushing those hovering on the edge of dependency into poverty.

Rowland Thomas's petition to the Massachusetts General Court provides a good example of how this argument was made. On December 18, 1760, one month after his son Samuel died following a yearlong bout with camp fever, Thomas submitted an account of his distressed circumstances:

> [H]aving no means to support himself his wife and children but his hands Labour (and them allmost wore out) by which means Through Divine goodness he has hetherto Supported himself and Family without being chargable to the Town or County but by reason of a sickness befalling his son Sam[ue]l Thomas who was a Soldier in Capt Israel Hutchinsons company which at the isle of orleans in the year Past, Thence he came home sick in vesel commanded by Capt Hunford of Ipswitch on the 11th of November of 1759, and on the 12th or 13th of said month Twas Brought to my Place of abode in Danvers aforesaid very ill of a camp fever of which fever and weakness Subsequent to it he lay Confined untill the 13th Day of November next at which Time he Died of the aforesaid illness after enduring Twelve months Extreem Poverty, Sickness, & weakness, & c and as your Petitioner is a poor man as abovesaid and utterly unable to Pay the charges which has arose by the sickness & Death of his abovesaid son with out the Charitable assistance of others he flatters himself that he may obtain a Reasonable Consideration of the Excellency and Honrable by the above Representation of his Distressed Surcumstances (which is but Part) and to that End has Exhibitted an acct of the Charges with this his Petition.[28]

Thomas's "Representation of his Distressed Surcumstances" neatly ties his son's plight to his own. The narrative begins with Thomas's life as an honorable man living on the edge of poverty; his well-worn hands are all that keep his family from plunging into the pool of the town poor. But when his son Samuel gets sick, the burden is too much. The narrative makes it clear that it is not sickness alone but the entire cluster of corporeal and financial consequences surrounding severe illness that weakens Thomas's grip on independence. The combination of "Twelve months Extreem Poverty, Sickness, & weakness" brought on by his son's illness is simply too much weight to be transferred from son to father. In order to fend off charitable assistance and the disgrace that accompanies it, Thomas turns to the General Court. There he can ask for "Reasonable Consideration" without shame, "flatter[ing] himself" that the wise men of the court will understand the intimate connection between the government's war, his son Samuel's sickness, and Thomas's present distressed circumstances.

The financial account attached to Thomas's narrative arranges the items in such a fashion that they speak for themselves. The account maps the costs of Samuel Thomas's sickness as he is carried home from war, lies ill in the petitioner's house, and is finally laid in the ground. The bill reads: "to a journey of a man & horse to Bring the said Saml from [the town of] Ipswitch" (6s.); "to Nursing and Tendance 52 weeks" at 4d. per week (£10 8s.); "to firewood candles sugar & c & c" at 8d. per week (£20 16s.); and "to Funeral Charges," "Diging a grave" (5s. 4d.), "7 p[ai]r gloves" (16s.), and "Toleing the Bell."

In the end, Thomas's appeal to the court was only partially successful. The committee reviewing the case agreed to approximately half of what Thomas asked, or £15 18s. that was to be paid to a town official "for the use of the petitioner." Would this money have been enough to keep Thomas and his family from entering the ranks of the town poor? Or did the disbursement, paid not to Thomas directly but to another man now in charge of overseeing Thomas's distressed circumstances, indicate that Thomas was already in those ranks, raising the question of whether he and his family would have the strength and support to climb out?

We might think of Rowland Thomas's responsibility to care for his son's sickness as a particular form of dependency, what Martha Fineman has called "derivative dependency." Derivative dependency is the dependent status derived from caring for dependents. Fineman writes, "The very process of assuming caretaking creates dependency in the caretaker," for she needs "someone to provide for her so she can fulfill her tasks."[29] While Fineman uses derivative dependency as a tool to critique the construction of motherhood and family in modern society, the term is helpful in thinking about eighteenth-century society as well.

Rowland Thomas's case shows a different kind of derivative dependency at work. Thomas was most likely not the primary caretaker for his son; women in the household performed this considerable task. But when we consider Thomas's responsibility as a financial caretaker for his son, his derivative dependence becomes clear. As the head of the household and an independent man, Thomas is charged with caring for his dependents. But through paying for his son's care, Thomas fears that he may be forced to rely on charity, and in so doing, he will be pulled across the boundary separating the independent and dependent members of society. Thomas's dilemma exposes the fragility of his identity as an independent man and patriarch; it is based on a fiction that unravels in his son's illness. Addressing the public through the medium of the petition, Thomas maintains that it is his work alone—the labor of his worn hands—that is the only means of support for himself and family. This is the script that he must follow as an independent man in eighteenth-century public life: he demonstrates his independent status in large part through his claim of supporting a household of dependents. Yet when we move from public discourse to the mechanics of household maintenance and production, this image needs to be almost entirely turned on its head. In eighteenth-century New England, it was the composite labor of husbands, wives, children, and servants that enabled the household to function. These two realms—the public realm in which Thomas stood as the sole support for his family household and the realm of household maintenance and production in which he labored along with them—usually existed alongside each other without incident. Law and custom funneled the productive labors of all in the household into the figure of the independent man and patriarch, making it possible for him to represent not only himself but all of the dependents assigned to him in public life.[30]

But when Thomas's son Samuel fell desperately ill, Thomas's dependence on the labors of others within—and outside—the household was revealed. If Samuel's case had been less severe, his care might have been able to be contained largely within the household economy. Women in the household—perhaps Thomas's wife, an older daughter, a relative, a servant (less likely in this case), or even a neighbor—would have nursed Samuel. But in the case of a serious and long-term illness, such as Samuel Thomas's yearlong bout with camp fever, the ministrations of women within the family and their support network of "social healers" might not suffice.[31] Caring for the sick young man would simply take too much time, forcing a choice to be made between nursing Samuel and the performance of other tasks that were vital to the family's maintenance and survival. This is why Rowland Thomas had been forced to hire a nurse and attendant for fifty-two weeks. Unlike the unremunerated labor of family caregivers upon which he could rely in ordinary circumstances, hired help would cost money. And with money came debt and the specter of dependency. Rowland Thomas was forced into debt because the system of household maintenance on which he relied for his support as an independent man had crumbled under the weight of catastrophic illness.

V. EPIDEMICAL DEPENDENCY

The most destructive cases of wartime illness combined the contagion of dependency with the contagion of infectious disease, spreading dependence to large numbers of persons and institutions in the wake of an epidemic. We might think of this phenomenon as epidemical dependency. As soldiers and camp followers returned home, they brought with them an array of ailments that had wreaked havoc on camp life. Called "camp distempers," "camp fevers," and "camp disorders," diseases like dysentery, typhus, and typhoid fever could devastate towns, killing civilians in large numbers. During the month of November 1775, for example, the minister of Danbury, Connecticut's First Church reported that of his flock of four hundred families, one hundred parishioners had been carried off by a virulent camp distemper. Other towns in the area evidently suffered similar fates.[32] We have to imagine the same process repeating itself during the century, as soldiers came back from war.

But the death wrought by these diseases is only part of the story. In the aftermath of outbreaks, households and towns were left to cope with the costs that infectious illness exacted from the living. As we saw in chapter 5, smallpox left not only death in its wake but also enormous accounts that might mean poverty for its living victims or those responsible for them.[33] Consider the plight of Brentwood, a parish in the southeast corner of New Hampshire. In 1762 its selectmen petitioned the governor and assembly, seeking reimbursement for the damage caused by a single "Soldier In the Comon defence" of the colony. Brentwood's Joseph Moody enlisted in the army in 1760. Sometime during the following year, he was exposed to smallpox and returned to the parish to recover. The petitioners claimed that "he secreatly brought" the infection to the parish. Had Moody informed the selectmen of his infection, as he was bound to do, the distemper might have been contained. But Moody had remained silent, perhaps fearing the costs that he would have to pay for his quarantine. Whatever his motivation, Moody's secrecy meant that the pox began to spread. First, it moved through his family, left "naked" and with "nothing for their Support" after Moody died. Next it extended throughout the parish, hitting the poorest members of the community the hardest, and causing several others "Great Cost" as well.[34]

In the end, at least seventeen Brentwood residents died and many more were infected, leaving the parish to bear costs that the selectmen detailed in an account submitted with their petition. A special pesthouse had to be constructed for the infected, which meant paying for wood, nails, and labor. Guards had to be hired to make sure that the infected did not come into contact with anyone who had not been exposed to the disease. Nurses had to be secured to care for the sick. Food and drink had to be provided for all parties involved. Finally, coffins had to be built and the dead buried. The cost of caring for Moody's family alone had amounted to £228 6d. old tenor; the parish claimed that it had expended some £1900.[35]

Brentwood's selectmen knew that they were legally bound to support the parish's poor, but warfare called for a reexamination of the rules of poverty. As they argued in the petition, "Inasmuch as these things Came upon them by the means of a Soldier In the Comon defence," they humbly prayed that they would be "allowed an oppertunety of making their Case more fully known and a proper Remedy applied" to the town. Wartime created its own afflictions and called for its own "proper remedies." A smallpox epidemic did not have to start with the sickness of a soldier, of course. But Joseph Moody had been asked by a community far larger than Brentwood to participate in war. He had been part of a "common defence," representing Brentwood's efforts on behalf of the colony of New Hampshire. And it was only proper for that larger community to pay for the costs that his sickness had exacted from the parish. A remedy was needed to stave off a crisis of widespread or epidemical dependency, social suffering on an immense scale.

As smallpox spread, it generated costs beyond the means of many Brentwood residents. These costs, in turn, were shifted to the parish. And the parish, arguing that it could not pay, turned to the New Hampshire General Assembly. Sickness incurred in warfare set in motion a chain of dependency that moved up through the basic units of social and political organization, from individual to household to parish or town to the legislature. Burdened with more affliction than they could handle on their own, New Englanders were offered the hope that the costs could be broken into small enough pieces that no one person, household, or town would lose everything in the process. If war created affliction, it also opened channels of compensation through the aid of government. In this case, the selectmen of Brentwood were able to recoup at least some of their extraordinary expenses stemming from the epidemic. A little over a year after the epidemic had ended, the selectmen were granted "the amount of the several accounts presented," or £23 19s. 8d. sterling, to be drawn from the fund used to pay off New Hampshire's troops.[36]

Thus far we have explored a range of costs that war imposed on sick soldiers and those who cared for them: the costs of fetching and returning the soldier to the household; the costs of doctor's visits, nursing, watching, and medicine; the costs of food and other necessaries. These expenses were compelled by the power of the soldier's ailing body, which resided not in its physical strength, but in its weakness and extremity. The incapacity of the sick soldier acted as a kind of magnet drawing persons and objects closer to him; his individual suffering became a social suffering. At its most extreme, a soldier's incapacity could be transferred to those responsible for caring for him; his dependency might mire his caregivers in derivative dependencies. And in cases of infectious disease, the sickness of a soldier might spread to others, initiating derivative dependencies that worked their way through households, neighborhoods, and towns, and finally erupted in epidemics of dependence that could swell the ranks of the poor.

When sick soldiers or those who cared for them petitioned for the immediate costs of wartime affliction, they appear to have been able to recover at least some of their expenses. Soldiers and their families were regularly allowed back wages, money that the soldier had been unable to collect in his affliction. Many medical accounts were allowed as well, most especially those in which payments to doctors and nurses were carefully documented. At the same time, it also appears clear that legislatures regularly paid less than the overall amount petitioners requested, and that petitioners received proportionately less of their total request as the amount of those requests grew in size. But even the prospect of limited compensation for the costs of wartime affliction justified the effort for many. The reimbursements that government could provide might be enough to allow soldiers and their families to preserve a modest competency.

Over the course of the century, warfare thus became the occasion for the distressed to turn to government for aid. In Massachusetts alone, the numbers asking for compensation were significant. Major campaigns throughout the century produced large numbers of claimants, particularly in the wake of widespread illness, sending many dozens of petitions to the General Court from soldiers, their families, and others charged with their care. As one example of many, consider the fallout from the Crown Point expedition in early September 1755. After 3,500 provincial soldiers and 400 Indians battled the French at Lake George, there were heavy casualties on both sides (the French lost 230 and the provincials 262). But it was the sickness that descended on the troops shortly thereafter that turned what had been considered a provincial victory into a dizzying malaise. Within ten days of the battle, wagonloads of the sick were sent on furlough in an effort to finally reach home. The General Court recognized that the journey would be fraught, as sick soldiers might suffer without any ready provision for care. In October, it voted that "all needfull and Necessary support be allowed such Sick & wounded Soldiers as shall have liberty to return home . . . (who belong to this Province) who shall desire relief, until they shall get to their respective homes. . . ." The court expected that ordinary persons in the commonwealth would provide care and asked that "every Person that shall supply such Sick or Wounded Soldier shall keep a fair and particular Acco[un]t of each and every Man's name," along with his Company, and return the account with a certification of the relieved soldier to the Commissary-General"; the court would find a way reimburse costs later.[37]

In the meantime, petitions to the General Court flooded in during the court's 1755–56 sessions. Some fifty-four petitions arrived, issued by sick soldiers and their families from all over the province: Essex County generated the most petitions, but there were also petitioners from western and central Massachusetts, from Plymouth County, and from Boston (and a few petitions from New York, Connecticut, and Rhode Island). The vast majority of soldiers petitioned for themselves. But thirteen of the soldiers had died, and others were incapacitated; five widows, five fathers, two masters, and an executor brought forward their stories and asked for compensation. The court offered reimbursements on a case-by-case basis, allowing anywhere from around £1 to £8. In 1756 the average wages and bounties paid to private soldiers ranged between £15 4d. to £18 4d. for an eight-month campaign, and so the bills that accrued during a soldier's sickness might run as high as 50% of what a soldier could hope to earn as pay. It is easy to understand why so many would come to the General Court and, with head down and hand out, ask that their distressed circumstances be relieved for themselves and their families. In the impulse behind these petitions, one sees the ways in which social welfare bound members of the commonwealth to their government. Along with providing for recruitment, pay, billeting, munitions, and a host of other sundry and pressing concerns, sickness must be seen as a major element in which government, in asking for service of its inhabitants, became obliged to soldiers and those who cared for them for their sufferings during war.[38]

We close with one of those wartime claimants, Ashley Bowen, the sailor and soon-to-be ship rigger from Marblehead, Massachusetts, whom we have met earlier. He had served during the siege of Quebec in 1759, and would later claim to have surveyed the St. Lawrence River while acting as a midshipman under the shipmaster James Cook, the famed explorer and circumnavigator. Writing to the Reverend William Bentley in 1809, Bowen maintained that while friend and patron Cook was duly "entitled to all that character that the World has given him," Bowen should have received credit for his part in the survey. Bowen had never been properly reimbursed for his 1759 service in the war, and his failure to receive his wages still rankled. His payment had been delayed until the outbreak of the Revolution, and when Bowen failed to side with the rebels, he lost his best chance of garnering what he was due.[39]

But Bowen *had* been paid in 1760, not for his eminently able surveying or for engaging the enemy, but rather for tending the ill. After the siege, Bowen and 160 others were bound for Boston on a transport ship that was struck by a severe distemper. Thirty-five men died. Some six weeks after he arrived back onshore, Bowen petitioned the General Court for his troubles. He had been "exposed to great Difficulty & Danger in tending the Sick, and taking care of them (who must otherwise have greatly suffered) and in Burying the Dead by reason of the foulness of the Distemper" onboard. Bowen had done this without pay or any special commission. Others, such as surgeons and their mates, were contracted for such work. But their scarcity in war meant that men like Bowen were often forced to step into the breach. Bowen asked the General Court for consideration, whatever in their "great Wisdom shall seem Meet. . . ." The General Court considered the case and passed a resolve in April to pay Bowen £3 4s. out of the public treasury.[40]

Warfare in eighteenth-century New England made stories like this one common. In obligating men to serve and placing them in harm's way, the provincial and later state governments of New England became obligated to compensate the people for the misfortunes of war. If those who had been touched by the afflictions of war—the sick, their families, caregivers who helped along the way—could document their losses, and if those losses were discrete, the General Court recognized its responsibility.

In the aftermath of war, a different sort of petitioner arose, concerned not so much with the immediate costs of wartime sickness as with its enduring effects. These soldiers struggled with newfound and unsettling limitations, unable to work as they had in the past or as they had expected to in the future. And thus they petitioned the General Court for the recovery of something that was necessarily more abstract than the visit from a doctor, back wages, or funeral costs—they asked for the costs of no longer being capable of supporting themselves and their families. War had taken from them something that only government could make whole. We turn now to these invalid soldiers and their efforts to obtain disability pensions.

AGENCY

Colonial Pensioners, the Revolutionary Invalid Corps, and the Advent of "Decisive Disability"

Wars in early New England raised urgent and often vexing questions about ability and disability. The overarching criterion for wartime service was that a man had to be "able-bodied," which required attending to the porous border separating the able-bodied from the disabled, the fit from the unfit. In recruiting soldiers, there were "objective" guidelines to follow—men had to be of a certain age and height, for example. But these criteria might be finessed by soldiers eager to reap the rewards of service or by officers who needed to enhance or maintain the size of their troops. During expeditions and longer campaigns, continual assessments had to be made of men's fitness, whether they were able to fight or to perform some lesser duty, such as manning garrisons. And finally, in the wake of war, there were lingering questions about men who returned injured or infirm. After enlisting soldiers to fight in dangerous and harsh environments, to what extent did government become obligated to attend to veterans' health? Where did government's responsibility for the soldier end and where did the personal responsibility of the soldier begin?

In the previous chapter, we saw these issues play out as soldiers and their families requested allowances for medical bills and nursing for their acute ills. We turn now to a much smaller group of soldiers, veterans asking for disability pensions, as a way to think about the enduring legacy of warfare over the course of the eighteenth century. Drawing on the petitions for pensions of Massachusetts veterans of the colonial wars and veterans of the Revolution, the chapter traces a long arc of change in political culture over the century. By examining the shift in locus of responsibility for the incapacitated soldier, we see a larger change from a form of governance that accepted responsibility for a wide range of bodily woes facing the disabled veteran to a form of governance that increasingly placed responsibility for ailments on the invalid himself.[1]

The chapter begins by examining petitions to the Massachusetts General Court in which veterans of England's imperial wars in America asked for compensation for their "service and suffering." For much of the century, those narratives told an integrated story of injuries and illness on the battlefield, recurrent episodes of incapacity in the years that followed, and difficulties facing soldiers in supporting themselves and their families. The chapter argues that behind the legislature's willingness to hear and act upon these petitions lay a fundamental assumption of early modern governance: that the world was filled with afflictive forces beyond anyone's immediate control, and that it was therefore the business of government, as the protector of the people, to respond where it could to misfortune and the problem of extremity. The interweaving of personal, social, and corporeal detail in colonial soldiers' petitions was embedded in a political culture that invited government to consider an array of sufferings.

The second half of the chapter turns to the very different political culture in which veterans of the Revolutionary War asked for invalid pensions in the 1780s and 1790s. Massachusetts continued to allow state pensions in the wake of the Revolution, but the ambivalence about "pensioners" and the possibility that pensions might mask idle habits was revealed in the requirements that soldiers serve garrison duty in a corps of invalids, if possible. Finally, in the 1790s, Secretary of War Henry Knox went further, taking aim at the undifferentiated stories of affliction that had been commonly heard by provincial and state governments. Knox demanded that soldiers asking for federal disability pensions demonstrate that they had incurred a "decisive disability" on the battlefield: a discrete, documented wound that made it impossible for veterans to support themselves upon their return to domestic life. The development of criteria for decisive disability was an effort to limit sharply the claims that veterans could make on government, and it represents an important shift in governance, a distancing of the emerging "early American state" from the personal and bodily sufferings that local governments had regularly considered.[2]

I. TO BE "DISENABLED": COLONIAL
PENSIONS AND PENSIONERS

By the eighteenth century, there was ample precedent for government's role in compensating disabled soldiers. Pension laws for soldiers originated in the reign of Queen Elizabeth, when soldiers who had served against the

Spanish Armada and had "adventured their lives and lost their limbs or disabled their bodies" were financially rewarded. A century later, Chelsea Hospital was opened in 1692 as a soldier's home to house invalid noncommissioned officers and men; Greenwich Hospital for disabled seamen followed in 1705.[3]

Britain's North American colonies never provided hospitals for veterans on the order of Chelsea or Greenwich, but they did pass laws throughout the seventeenth century compensating soldiers who were hurt or maimed in war with Indians. Under its new charter in the wake of the Glorious Revolution, the Massachusetts General Court promised in 1693 to honor any past pensions awarded by the former government (provided pensioners remained in the Bay Colony), and it offered soldiers and seamen "at any time hereafter" who "shall be maimed or otherwise disabled by any wound received in their majesties' service within this province" to be relieved out of the public treasury. In an effort to find volunteers willing to pursue "the Indian Enemy and rebels" on their own accord, the court offered a grim schedule of rewards and payments, bound together in the same clause of a 1697 statute: all the plunder that could be had of the enemy; £5 for every man or woman "slain in the defense of any house or garrison," proof of which consisted in producing the scalps of the killed Indians; and the promise that any persons "wounded in the aforesaid service" would be "cured at the charge of the publick" or "if maimed or otherwise disabled[,] shall have such stipend or pension allowed unto him or them as the general court or assembly shall think meet." The statute betrayed frank recognition of the physical violence inherent in warfare—that it involved killing, maiming, and dismembering. But adjudicating claims stemming from that violence was another matter. Even the presentation of the enemy's scalp, which would seem to have been straightforward, if gruesome, led to accusations of fraud and to fines and imprisonment for those who tried to deceive the General Court by producing scalps of Indians not slain in battle. For the soldiers who were impaired in war, the law left open the most fundamental of questions: What did it mean to be disabled? Who would make the determination? What constituted a "meet" settlement? And on what grounds?[4]

A single, well-documented case from the early eighteenth century opens a window onto the ambiguous political, medical, and social terrain that early pensioners had to negotiate. John Baker, a weaver from Swansea, Massachusetts (on the border of Rhode Island), petitioned the General Court in 1699 and again in 1700. He had been pressed into service during King Philip's War (1675–76), which left a dozen English towns in ashes and led to the death of some 5,000 Indians and 2,500 colonists. Baker had been "sorely Wounded" in December 1675, when the English stormed the Great Swamp Fort of the Narragansetts in Rhode Island, refuge for as many as 3,000 or 4,000 natives (mostly women and children hidden for protection in the swamp). The English burned hundreds of wigwams and killed those who fled. Baker's arm was "broak by a shott" he received from the enemy, and he was sent to seek a doctor in Rhode Island. After he had recovered sufficiently, his father fetched him home, and he was able to pursue a modest competency: he married in 1682, learned "ye trade of A weauer, wrought hard, earned money, bought a bitt of land, [and] built a small house" in Woburn, Massachusetts.[5]

But finding that "now and then my arme would break out," Baker sold what he had and moved back to Swansea (and presumably back to family who could aid in his care). His condition worsened when he was again pressed into service during King William's War (1689–97). As he explained in the petition, "being late in ye yeare and Cold, I got cold in my old wound, it swelld exceedingly, [and] I vnderwent more paine then at first." Baker was forced to put himself "vnder the hand of severall doctors" who tried to cure his arm, and he found himself in debt and in need of protection from the General Court. He pleaded that his father was dead, "my mother a poor widow," and so "I have nothing to help my selfe withal." And "being disabled to work at my trade," having "a greate famaly to maintain," and facing the prospect of being "thrown into Gaol by ye doctors," his last best hope was payment of his bills by the General Court, and "A small pention Allowed me Annualy," which would not, in any case, amount to much: "many skillful do think this wound will be my death at last." In the end, Baker was successful, garnering a lump sum of £10 to pay his medical bills and an annual pension of £4 that would last until "this court shall see cause to order otherwise."[6]

Within the petition and behind the scenes, Baker's request for a pension illuminates the political, medical, and social dimensions that combined to produce his disabled state. There was a good deal of uncertainty on his part. In the first place, it was not clear to whom he should apply for aid. The principle underlying the petition was that, through protecting the people, their governors earned the people's allegiance. But whether one approached the General Court as a whole, or particular assembly members, or, indeed, the governor himself was not certain. Baker initially approached the governor directly. Sometime in 1699, he presented himself to the Earl of Bellomont, the governor of Massachusetts, who was touring the colony shortly after his arrival. "His Lordship" handed the petition to his traveling companion, the secretary of the province, and ordered the humble supplicant "to com down to boston to him" at a later time. But when Baker arrived in Boston, the governor was suffering from the gout—a disease often associated with the elite—and not accepting visitors.[7]

The result of the journey was "greatly to my Damige in respect of my wound," Baker later claimed in correspondence with another patron, James Converse, from whom Baker sought advice after the episode with Bellomont. Baker hoped the "Noble hardy and Well beloued Majer James Converse," who had served as an officer in King Philip's War, might "shew my condition to the great and generall Court theare assembled" for the March 1699 session, given that Baker's injury prevented his travel. While Converse does not appear to have approached the General Court in person, he did write to both the governor and speaker of the house, urging them to be compassionate with a "poore wounded soldier." In the uncertain world of patronage politics, in which the exact province of the governor and the legislature were ill-defined, Baker was fortunate to have found an insistent and conscientious benefactor.[8]

To explain how his debility had resulted from war, Baker both advanced his own theory and sought the support of other people who could advance his case. Evincing a conception of the body and its perils characteristic of early modernity, he claimed that as he had been exposed to the elements, a cold had seeped into his old wound, reawakening and enlivening its latent powers of growth and decay. To return to Charles Rosenberg's evocative phrase, the "body was always in a state of becoming—and thus always in jeopardy." Like others, Baker understood that the bodily equilibrium that constituted health could be all too easily disturbed, and he believed wounds that had been "cured" could reemerge with new vitality. The dangers facing one's health called for vigilance, a continual assessment of risks and moments when one was imprudently exposed. But the soldier had little choice in his environment and routines, nor could he control the "non-naturals" of sleep, exercise, and diet thought critical to the maintenance of health. In this sense, soldiers claiming chronic impairment by wounds or other means could point to forces beyond their control—not just the savagery of the enemy, but the harshness of the environment—to make the case for their just compensation.[9]

To further bolster his claims, Baker added the testimonies of two healers who had treated him. Major Converse may have suggested doing so—Baker obtained the certificates after his initial correspondence with Converse—but personal experience would have made it a prudent measure in any case. Baker had been offered just one award of money as compensation for his earliest wound and his initial visit to a doctor, but the General Court had refused to issue him more because, he was told, his father "had fetchd me away before I was well."[10] Now, many years later, having undergone a second round of visits to doctors and surgeons, Baker made sure to include their written testimony. And like Baker's own description of his wound, their reports projected an image of a "body in a state of becoming," and now likely in decline. Thomas Estabrooke testified "yt 3 years agoe I cured the arme of John Baker," which "now is badd againe and a very great sore hauing 3 holes wch is constantly running" and Edward Pratt, "Chururgion," added that he "toock Joh[n] Bakers Arm in hand" several months earlier, and that "when I toock it to Cure," it "was Hollow from the shoulder to the Elboe the Boane ffoul the arm had five holes in it aboue and vnder his Armpit Alwayes runing. . . ."[11]

However, the point raised most insistently by Baker, his healers, and Converse was not the physical condition of his wound as such, but rather the wide-ranging implications of being physically impaired, particularly the ways in which his injuries had imperiled his masculinity. Albeit from different angles, each returned to the idea that Baker could no longer be expected to labor for his support, that he would forever be poor without his labor, and that he was not, then, able to be a complete man. As Converse wrote in a note to the governor, the "poore Wounded soldier" had "spent all he hath" and is thought "not to be worth a Groat, by Reason of his Wound yt he Recd in his Majts service." Estabrooke argued that Baker was "very vncapable of labor an[d] questionable whether he can be his own man any more." Pratt, the surgeon, found that there was some hope in that his arm was "Almost fild up with flesh and there are now but three holes in it," but he questioned "whether ever hee will Bee A sound man any more. . . ." And Baker agreed. He was "never like to be my own man." There was nothing definitive here; Baker's future state was a matter of prediction. But the stories pointed to the same conclusion: Baker's wounds threatened to make him something less than a competent man.

Disability fit into narratives like Baker's not as an immutable identity but as a contingent, contextual state. Petitioners wrote that they were "disabled" *from* something: from working the land, from a particular trade, and thus from supporting themselves and their families, a fundamental component of manhood in New England—the ability to be "useful" or "of use."[12] In a related word used by pensioners that captures this meaning (and is consonant with recent rethinking of the meanings of "disability"), other petitioners claimed to have been "disenabled": applicants claimed to be "disenabled from helping myself," for example, or "in Great foar yt I shall be utterly disenabled for ye mentainance of my wife & family."[13] One was disenabled now, but that did not mean that the condition would last if another means of survival could be found; cne person's disenablement would not necessarily have been another's.

What united those pleading that they had been disabled or disenabled was the impossibility of separating a wartime impairment from the economic and social consequences of that impairment. Blending the physical and the economic, petitioners presented themselves as being in "weak & low condition of person & purse," or as "exceeding low in . . . health as well as otherwise."[14] The connection between the want of money and an able body found its most poignant expression in petitioners' claims to have been made unable to pursue their calling. As Thomas Philips wrote of his wounds in 1707, "The Occupation ye Petitioner Exercised, was a Blacksmith, whic he has little hopes ere to be in a capacity to follow again, and has no other, to help himself by." Josiah Jones put it more simply in 1739. He had been "very much wounded, and thereby So Disabled that he has laboured under very Great Difficulties," "not being able to Earn his Dayly Bread, much less to Maintain his family."[15]

To be disabled from labor was a problem whose social ramifications reached well beyond the suffering veteran. The vast majority of pensioners noted that they had wives and children, "great" and "growing" families, that they could not "support" and "maintain" in their impaired state. This was the refrain, repeated with minor variations, running through the petitions throughout the colonial period and into the early republic—that claimants were "unable of doing any labour for the support of my selfe or famely."[16] Not simply a physical impairment, disability was also a social impairment that produced social suffering. Government was asked to protect men who, through their wartime service, could no longer protect their own dependents.

As a political solution, the General Court could apply the healing balm of money to the pensioner's social wounds, which, if it could not restore him to the realm of the fully useful, could at least prevent him from becoming his neighbor's burden or a ward of his town. As we saw in the preceding chapter, threats to the ability of the patriarch to provide for his family could pry money loose from public coffers. Over the course of the eighteenth century until the conclusion of the colonial period, the range of conditions that the General Court might consider in granting assistance expanded and the practice of petitioning became more common than in the tentative days of John Baker. In response to this expansion, the federal government felt obliged to restrict grants of assistance in the wake of the Revolution.

II. EXPANSIONS, 1740s–1760s

John Baker's request for a pension, issued at the beginning of the eighteenth century, would have been familiar to pensioners and members of the General Court alike several decades later in both the basic form of the petition and its narration of disenablement. But there were two important midcentury developments that extended both the number and the range of applicants.

The first development concerned the "rise of the assembly." With an eye toward explaining the political and constitutional origins of the American Revolution, early histories of the assemblies in the colonies traced their pursuit of power over the course of the eighteenth century, their increasing conflicts with royal governors and the Crown and Parliament, and their critical role in the eventual rupture with the mother country. More recently, studies have considered the ways in which the assemblies in the eighteenth century became increasingly enmeshed in the daily lives of the colonists. Through the power of the purse, through the adjudication of disputes, and through the invitation to the people to petition the legislature to bring private sufferings to light, the assemblies became a potent force in mediating social and economic relations.[17]

Throughout the colonies, legislatures fielded more petitions over the century covering a greater range of topics as they tried to meet the needs of their constituents. From 1715 to 1765, the Massachusetts House of Representatives accepted more than twice the number of petitions as other colonies, with an average of 95 a year between 1715 and 1720, and 257 a year between 1760 and 1765. With increasing number of petitioners came greater ease and certainty in presenting personal stories before the assembly. Whereas someone like John Baker had tried several avenues to get his story heard, initially approaching the governor and then corresponding with Major Converse, later petitioners could be more assured that the General Court had both the greatest authority and interest in hearing their claims.[18]

A second, related development at midcentury was that two new sorts of soldiers began to take advantage of easier access to the General Court. Pension rolls continued to be dominated by wounded soldiers who secured pensions within a few years after their service ended. But they were now joined by aged veterans applying for pensions many years after they had been discharged as well as veterans of all ages who maintained that they had been disabled from labor by sickness and the hardships of war.

The aged veterans tried to establish the link between their present distressed circumstances and wars long past. Their stories take us into the politics surrounding poor relief for the elderly infirm and reveal the many parties who had an interest in awarding the aged a disability pension. The case of Benjamin Rockwood of Wrentham, Massachusetts, although extreme in the passage of time between service and a pension request, nevertheless sounds several common themes.

Rockwood was ninety-three years old when his son-in-law petitioned the General Court on his behalf. The year was 1742, and Rockwood maintained that his present state of ill health could be directly linked to his service during King Philip's War, nearly seventy years earlier. Rockwood claimed that during his service he was "Sevaralley or Twice Wounded" and that when he "He Took a Sudan Colde" in addition to his other maladies, he was sent off to recover his health. It was "a Quarter of a year Before" he was able to return home, but "He Not having a Parfict Cure An ill state of Helth to Him Became Habituoall," and he was thus "Redust to A very low Condition Driven to A dependance upon oathers for His subsistance and supleys." Rockwood argued that it was only fitting that he be allowed some compensation for his "loss of time and long suffarings," especially because he had received no wages or any other benefit for his distressed circumstances. In conclusion, Rockwood asked that his anticipated benefits go to his son-in-law, William Man, who had cared for him for a "Long Time," hoping that the court would offer Man "A Grant of so Much of the unapropriated Land of the Province" as it thought reasonable.[19]

To support his father-in-law's petition, William Man added a note of his own. He claimed that his "Father Rockwood Hass Alleways and for a long time Been Estemd as a Man of Grat verety and Truth," and that Rockwood's "Most Aged" friends could swear to the authenticity of his story. Accordingly, it appears that Man arranged for several of these friends to sign a statement of their own. They urged that "from what we have heard Seen & Known Do verily Beleve that the ill Estate of Health Which [Rockwood] has Laboured under for a long time" was occasioned by his war service. The General Court did not grant Man any lands but, finding that Rockwood had been "much disabled" by his "wounds and sickness," it voted to allow him £4 a year for life for his service and sufferings. Man assumed control of the funds with the implicit intention of using them toward Rockwood's support.[20]

Had William Man adequately discharged his duty, Rockwood's public history might have ended with his pension in 1742. But four years later a selectman from Wrentham, Eleazar Metcalf Jr., complained that Rockwood had become a public nuisance despite his pension. Metcalf maintained that William Man had pocketed his father-in-law's pension and "converted it to his own use," leaving the town to support the ailing Rockwood. Metcalf had personally taken on this burden, perhaps as a stopgap measure to keep Rockwood afloat without draining the town's funds for the poor. William Man apparently offered no explanation to counter the selectman's charges. Did he feel the pension was his due after supporting Rockwood for many years? Whatever the case, the General Court ordered Rockwood's pension to be transferred from Man to the town's overseers of the poor, who would arrange for Rockwood's "Support & Comfort" until he died. Governance of the poor was concerned primarily with providing for dependents, not for those who cared for them.[21]

Cases like Rockwood's show the collective effort necessary to bring about a disability pension. The form of the petition itself demanded a collective effort. First, there was the need to convert an oral story into writing, and to perform the necessary expressions of deference that began and ended such petitions. Especially for poorer New Englanders like Rockwood, this effort would require assistance. And so Rockwood relied on his son-in-law, and some interaction between the two yielded the petition that Rockwood signed with his mark. Then others added their stories. William Man attested to the probity of his father-in-law. Friends and neighbors of Rockwood were called in to state what they had "heard Seen & Known," to represent the knowledge arising from the daily inspections of community life. And finally, the selectman spoke up when Rockwood's poverty threatened to become a public problem.

Each of these players had a stake in Rockwood's disability claims. When the General Court responded favorably to the assembled stories concerning a veteran like Rockwood, his afflictions could be transformed into money. And in a cash-poor society, even limited amounts of money mattered. William Man wanted to recoup his losses in supporting his father-in-law. For the selectmen, Rockwood's pension lessened the town's burden in paying for its own poor, allowing limited funds for poor relief to be directed elsewhere. And any decrease in those supported at the town's expense meant lower taxes, a fact that surely pleased taxpayers, including, perhaps, Rockwood's friends, whose bonds with him certainly did not preclude an interest in their own affairs.

While Rockwood's seventy-year gap between his service and pension request was unusual, several factors insured a steady growth of aged pensioners over the course of the century. In the first place, annual pensions were hard to get and might be received only after years of trying. The General Court was frugal with public expenditures, and it was not uncommon for a veteran to receive a lump sum for medical bills on his first try, an annual pension for a limited number of years (usually between three and five) on subsequent efforts, and finally, if a convincing case could be made, an annual pension for life.

Second, once an annual pension was awarded, it might be inadequate to the task of preserving the aged veteran in anything like a comfortable subsistence. The gratuity remained the same, a problem that became quite significant as money depreciated over time, and dramatically so when Massachusetts tried to discharge its public debts by issuing paper money unsecured by specie (a solution, in part, to paying for a war without overtaxing the people). As Peter Rich noted in 1748, the "good intention" of the generous pension he had been issued thirty years earlier "is manifestly frustrated in a great Measure, by the Depreciation of the Province Bills, wherein He has been paid it of late years. . . ." Rich assured the General Court that his wartime wound still "render'd [him] uncapable of performing the ordinary Labour of a Man," that "through the hardships he Sustained . . . he is So broken, and become the Constant Subject of So much pain and Illness ever Since his Return . . . that he is Scarcely able to do any thing forwards the Support of himself and his Family." On top of it all, the limited payments made him "a great Sufferer in his Advanced Age."[22]

Aging petitioners also relied on the general plausibility of the claim that past wounds could lead to a life of pain and suffering, making the point that "wasting wars" had taken their vitality. John Green wrote in 1741 that "In his youth he was able bodied and Effective and according to his ability was servicable and faithfull In his Majesties Service against the Common Enemy." But his service had led to "many and Greivous hardships," and though pleased to have a yearly pension, he was "now aged and Cripled and Under low Circumstances In the world." He argued that his pension was "In no measure Equal to what he received from year to year" after his initial grant, and (more tentatively) that he had not shared with recent soldiers the "Common Bounties" offered by the General Court, including free land grants. Dutifully following the form of the petition, he concluded with a humble prayer, begging the "Pity and Compassion" of the court, for which he was awarded an increase in his allotment.[23]

For the General Court, war came with its narrow immediacies: the need to recruit and provision officers and soldiers; the need to address all of the discrete charges that accompanied battle—of billeting, of lost guns, of sundry special services performed for His Majesty. But the aged veterans were a reminder of the long history of warfare in the region, whose effects lingered and even increased over time. Each legislative session dedicated to the fallout from the most recent battle could also expect to encounter the residue of the region's past history of violence. When the storming of Louisbourg was in the public eye in 1745, veterans from King Philip's War still asked for compensation; when the injured from Bunker Hill were making fresh applications for pensions from a new state in a new nation in 1780, one-third of the claimants before the General Court were trying to secure their pensions and payments due from the colonial wars.[24]

In addition to aged veterans, a second class of pensioners emerged at midcentury. While the legal criteria for pensions privileged wounds as a cause of disability (offering payments for those "wounded or otherwise disabled"), and while the majority of pensioners claimed to have been disabled by wounds, diseases brought home from the battlefront and the more mysterious ailments generated by the "hardships" of war joined the musket and cannonball as grounds for disability pensions.

We have seen in chapter 6 the ways in which wartime illness, particularly epidemics in the wake of large-scale campaigns, could send many soldiers, along with their families and other caregivers, to the General Court in hopes of recouping their losses. The most spectacular of those diseases was smallpox, and we see in that dreaded distemper one of the ways in which persons initially stricken with the disease could later claim to be disabled by it. After the campaigns in 1759 and 1760 in the Seven Years' War, the General Court heard from pox-afflicted soldiers and their families in some eighteen towns in central and eastern Massachusetts who asked for the costs of nursing, medical attendance, the "loss of time" to quarantine, and the loss of property to smoking and cleansing. While the impact of smallpox for the smitten and their families was most often concentrated in a few months of costly care, the pox, it was well known, could also lead to chronic ailments such as blindness and ulcers.[25]

When Daniel Druce petitioned the General Court in 1765, he recounted how he had been taken sick of smallpox as a servant five years earlier. Initially enlisting in 1759 to serve "at the Westward," Druce reenlisted the following year and marched to St. Johns, contracting smallpox on his return. That illness, coupled with "wading through Cold Rivers so Called he took a Great Cold which Settled in one of his Leggs," had disabled him from labor. Druce's master at the time had been able to secure costs from the General Court that paid for the seventeen-year-old to get home. But two years after having been set free, Druce complained that the "Sore grows worse dayly"; he was continually in pain, and he was in debt for doctoring and nursing that had been "all to no Purpose." And he was destitute. His father had been captured in the war and taken to Canada and subsequently died on his way home, leaving the young man "fatherless, and without any Estate to help him Self." Druce's leg continued to be so swollen that Druce repeatedly claimed it "unfits him from a Business." Awarded an initial annual pension in 1766 for four years, Druce petitioned again in 1770 and 1772, each time making the case that he was lame, incurable, and without means. He had been obliged to count on his neighbors and townsfolk, with "nothing left but depending upon the Charity of all good People his Neighbours to assist him," something confirmed by his minister and selectmen who signed his petitions.[26]

In Druce's later petitions, he added to his litany of misfortunes that he suffered "many Fatigues and hardships" in war that "very much Impaired his health. . . ." It was, no doubt, a way of explaining the weakened state that left him vulnerable to the ravages of smallpox and the debilitating ulcers that he had suffered thereafter. But it also invoked wartime experience, distinct from wounds, as grounds to claim a pension. Part of the hardship was attributed to poor provisions, limited equipment, and exposure to the elements. As William Clemens wrote in 1761, he had served the province three times, at Fort William Henry, at Ticonderoga, and at Fort Cumberland. He had, until his final tour, been "well & free from fits," but in Nova Scotia he had been forced to lie "on the ground cold and wet," and there being "Grate foggs & Raines," he took "Severall Grate Cold which Brought on me terrible fits that remaine to this time." It was not a wound, but Clemens argued that it had so "Impaired my Health that I am unable to labor, & have no other way to suport my Self." With no estate from his father, who had died twenty years earlier, and dwindling savings, Clemens surmised that soon "I shall have Nothing to live on, and no Relations able to help me," all compounded by medical bills and the fact that "the Doctors Give me litle Incouragement of a Cure after so long and to me Expensive triall."[27]

And so it went for others: hardships led to sickness and finally to lasting debility and debt. Nathaniel Conant wrote that in 1762 he had served in Halifax and Newfoundland, and "thro the Difficulties & Hardships he underwent, he lost his Health, and returned home poorly," lying sick for several months until "his bodily Disorders Semd to enter in One of his Knees, and render'd him very lame." After "loosing much Time" in trying to obtain a cure, he grew "Something better" and was able to farm, but his knee soon failed him, and he asked the court to consider a pension, or possibly the offer of garrison duty, for "a Miserable Cripple not able to Labour and nothing to live on."[28] William Snell had also been in Halifax and Newfoundland in 1762, and on his return home was "cast away at Cape Sables" (Nova Scotia) and "there taken Sick and came Home so, and confin'd to his Bed with Sore Sickness for Seven Months and after that confin'd to his House Fourteen Months longer with weakness and distressing Pain in his Limbs . . . and finaly has almost lost the use of both his Legs." Snell found hope in a "kind Providence" that "restord his Health" in part, allowing him to walk with a crutch and staff, but despite "frugal living" he had spent most of the allotment that the General Court had "in great Goodness, done for him," and now asked for consideration.[29]

As accounts of the visitation of disease, these narratives represented nothing new. In a fluid economy of correspondences within the body, an assault upon one part could easily manifest itself in another. It was not at all far-fetched to claim, as these men did, that sickness circulated about the body and then descended into the knees and legs. Nor was it unusual to claim that a harsh new environment could cause sickness; the cold and fog of Nova Scotia could enfeeble the constitution of even the heartiest of New Englanders, unaccustomed to the severity of the northern climate. Nor was it out of the ordinary for these accounts to be general in their depiction of disease. Petitioners were comfortable in claiming to suffer from generic "sickness." Like others in the eighteenth century (and earlier), they registered an understanding less of "diseases" (although smallpox was an exception here) than of "dis-ease": the sense of unsettling changes in their interior, the intensity and extent of their pain, and the ongoing effort to alleviate their suffering.[30]

What *was* new here was the political accommodation of these stories. As the Seven Years' War developed, the volume of petitions increased that asked for onetime payments to discharge debts for medicine, nursing, and "loss of time" occasioned by "sick soldiers" returning from the field. While many of these were claims for the costs of attending those with smallpox, some resulted from camp fevers and unnamed "sicknesses" carried home with the soldiers, afflicting both them and their families, often for many months. Veterans and their caregivers had enjoyed the right to petition for reimbursement for medical costs since at least 1703, when the General Court allowed soldiers sickened in warfare to be relieved at public charge. But not until the 1740s was it common for soldiers and their families to submit such claims, and the numbers of these petitions grew during the Seven Years' War.[31]

The massive mobilization of Massachusetts men required by the war, the increase in bounties to attract soldiers, and the overall number of men who served—perhaps a third of those eligible—had brought the force of government into the homes of Bay colonists in an unprecedented fashion. In obliging subjects to fight and sacrifice, government had itself became obligated for their care. When veterans like Nathaniel Conant and William Snell claimed that their wartime sicknesses had caused lasting debility, they were taking advantage of the provincial government's expanding sense of its responsibility to compensate its subjects for their wartime sacrifices. Both men were awarded annual pensions.[32]

In these ways—in the claims of aged pensioners who pleaded that their wartime afflictions had intensified over time; in the claims of veterans who pointed out that they had been vital youths before the war but were now decrepit old men and unable to act the part of patriarchs who would protect their dependents; in the claims of soldiers who, though not wounded, were, through sickness and the hardships of war, "otherwise disabled"—the grounds for petitioning the General Court for an annual pension were expanding at the end of the colonial period. Pensions were neither automatic nor easy to obtain, nor were the numbers of pensioners great; they represented a small fraction of the overall numbers of persons asking for wartime compensation. But the expanded grounds for compensation in the colonial period played a critical role in the ideas and practices of the federal government to come as it considered veterans' welfare. Faced with the potential burden of supporting pensioners from every state in the new nation, federal officials would rethink government's responsibility for individual citizens and their bodily suffering.

III. THE REVOLUTIONARY INVALID CORPS AND THE AMBIGUITIES OF COMPENSATION

Following a precedent set in the colonial wars, disability pensions were used as one means of recruiting soldiers during the Revolution. Officers and soldiers "so disabled in the service of the United States of America" as to render them "incapable, afterwards, of getting a livelihood" were to be allowed half of their monthly pay for life. Those with lesser disabilities, which might render them unable to serve in the army or navy, and which might hinder, though not totally disable, them from future work, would be awarded a proportion of half pay. The states were put in charge of making the disability determination as well as ensuring proper evidence was produced, including certificates from commanding officers and the attending surgeons, in keeping with colonial precedent. But Revolutionary pensions would differ in one significant way: unless a soldier could prove total disability, payment was contingent on continued service during the war in a corps of invalids.

The Invalid Corps was first introduced in Congress on August 26, 1776, as part of pension provisions for disabled officers and soldiers who might still be made "of use" in the war effort. All officers and soldiers "found to be capable of doing guard or garrison duty" would be employed. How men would be recruited, what their precise obligations would entail, and what the size and extent of the corps itself would be were not specified initially, but it was crucial that all would-be pensioners understand that injuries and other disabling conditions did not necessarily mean an end to their service.[33]

There were practical reasons for the development of an Invalid Corps, particularly after the initial *rage militaire* of the war had passed and the Continental army was wanting for troops. George Washington was particularly troubled by the numbers of men who claimed to be unfit for duty. In 1777 he complained that many men accounted for as "sick absent" in monthly strength reports might be malingerers searching for ways of getting dismissed (or even colluding with others who would collect their wages), an observation borne out by scholarship on New England's forces in the war. Malingerers or not, there were surely men listed as "sick present," as Washington noted in a 1778 council of war, who "might be capable of acting on an emergency." The Invalid Corps, in this practical sense, was one way of retaining soldiers at a time when Washington had to fight with an army of men, many of whom were not able-bodied.[34]

But the development of the Invalid Corps was also a response to ideological concerns growing out of the Revolution. Before the imperial crisis, the pensioner seemed untroubling to colonials. One finds, for example, favorable reports in colonial newspapers of the coronation of George III in 1761, celebrated with an elaborate procession displaying the different ranks in the kingdom, including "Gentlemen pensioners" who closely followed the king (behind only the "supporters of the train" and the "master of the robes"), a symbol of the hierarchy and patronage that infused monarchical society and politics. However, the Revolution called into question the very category of "pensioner." Living idly at the expense of taxpayers and entirely dependent on their patrons for support, pensioners were seized on as a vivid example of the moral corruption of the mother country that threatened to ruin the colonies. As John Adams suggested in February 1775 to a friend in London, "the reduction of placemen and pensioners," along with "shorter parliaments," the "annihilation of bribery and corruption, the reformation of luxury," and a host of other measures would be required to "restore your country to a free government, and to a safe, honourable, and happy life. . . ." These reforms, Adams thought, would take nothing short of "miraculous change" to effect. And without such change, there would be no stopping the onslaught of taxes and duties extracted from industrious colonials, driven by the need to feed the idle habits of their dissipated brethren overseas and their minions in the colonies.[35]

There was a sharp contrast, of course, between the pensioners and placemen seen as emblematic of the ancien regime and the invalid veteran pensioners who were recompensed for their disabilities. Figures like Governor Thomas Hutchinson, who was hated to an almost pathological degree by Adams and others as a cunning and unworthy beneficiary of patronage, differed greatly from soldiers whose pensions were compensation for harm incurred in service to country. But the larger discussion over pensioners and placemen spilled over into the consideration of pensions for invalid soldiers. In New England, particularly, the question of whether Revolutionary War officers should be granted lifetime pensions for their service, which was hotly debated in the region, had implications for the assessment of the worthiness of invalid pensioners. Arguments on both sides of that debate weakened the case for invalid pensions and fueled the logic of requiring disabled veterans to continue serving in an Invalid Corps, even after the war, in order to receive compensation.[36]

Washington delivered one of the most forceful statements supporting pensions for officers. His celebrated "circular," written from Newburgh, New York, on June 11, 1783, and sent to the governors of each state, in what he imagined as a final communication before retiring from public service, was reprinted many times in New England newspapers. Washington took up both the case of compensation for officers and the need to support invalid veterans, framing each as a matter of "public justice," the overarching theme of his circular. But he differed in his manner of presenting how and why each group warranted consideration.[37]

Regarding officers, Washington explicitly denied that their compensation—initially planned by Congress as a lifetime payment, and later, after protest, commuted to a promise of half pay for five years—should be construed as a pension. Half pay, Washington argued, should not be seen in "the odious light of a pension," because it was a means of completing their just payment, "a part of their hire. . . ." But more importantly, it was "the price of their blood, and of your Independency." Washington scolded; "more than a common debt, it is a debt of honor, it can never be considered as a pension or gratuity, nor be cancelled untill it is fairly discharged." There was no discretion where a debt of honor was concerned, as there might be in the case of a pension, which could be awarded as a special means of offering appreciation. Officers deserved half pay for service as a matter of honor and right.[38]

When Washington turned to those disabled in war and receiving pensions, to the "obligations this Country is under, to that meritorious Class of veteran Non-Commissioned Officers and Privates who have been discharged for inability," he pursued a different line of reasoning, observing that "their peculiar sufferings, their singular Merits and claims to that provision, need only be known, to interest all the feelings of humanity in their behalf." To do otherwise would be to mire these worthies in "the most complicated misery" that would be only too visible if payment was not forthcoming. The "melancholly and distressing sight" of these men who had "shed their blood or lost their limbs in the service of their County, without a shelter, without a Friend, and without the means of obtaining any of the necessaries or comforts of life, compelled to beg their daily bread" should have been enough to excite the "warmest patronage" of the states.[39]

Washington's distinction between officers asking for half pay and invalid soldiers in need of disability pensions is striking. On the one hand stood the officer, who had earned compensation by virtue of his service, bravery, and blood that had secured independence. On the other stood the invalid pensioner, who might be awarded a pension to ameliorate his present and future misery. To support the officers, Washington drew on the language of honor, which had a deep history; in fact, the rhetoric and rituals of honor were providing one source of political stability in the early republic. To support the invalid enlisted men, however, Washington drew on a newer language of sensibility. Although he invoked an idea central to monarchical political culture—the duty of the governors to protect the people—he wrapped the principle of protection in this new language by evoking the spectacle of the invalid soldier's suffering and the sentiments it should inspire in men of feeling. Washington could hope that the image of the miserable, lonely, homeless veteran would excite the "feelings of humanity" and persuade state legislatures to acquit themselves admirably.[40]

For Washington to write as a man of feeling about invalid soldiers extended a mode of discourse that had been drawn on heavily in the war. The delicacy of military men, their keen sense of the feelings of others, and their ease in shedding tears at the sight of misfortune were prized qualities attributed to gentlemen officers during the war. In addition to martial prowess, a rational ability to feel was considered essential to the exercise of sound military judgment.[41]

But there was a danger in continuing to use the language of feeling to address the invalid soldiers' plight. In the world of colonial pensions, when supplicants approached their governors with their head down and hand out, asking for compassionate consideration and the protection of their betters, they expected a price to be placed on their suffering. Governors and the people alike understood the act of "commiseration" to be inseparable from allowance; soldiers asked that their claims be "commiserated," that is, recognized by the act of bestowing money. Washington's appeal to feeling ran the risk that the invalid soldier might become the object of sympathy but not necessarily the recipient of money. In the new economy of feeling, it would be possible to respond to misery with a display of humane sympathy—the horror excited by the spectacle of present and future suffering—without the money to accompany it.[42] Washington could "recommend" to the governor and legislature of each state that they exercise their "warmest patronage" in regard to the suffering soldiers, but he could not compel it through the language of feeling. The debt of honor owed officers was a sturdier basis on which to ask for compensation than the invalids' evident suffering.

Those who opposed the pensions for Revolutionary War officers offered other arguments that would have unfortunate implications for invalid soldiers. A piece written by "Freedom" to the *Boston Gazette* in June 1783 neatly encapsulated the broader debate, first summarizing the arguments of the officers and then rebutting them. "I suppose, the gentlemen [officers] will begin to say, we have spent a great deal of time, impaired our health, and exhausted our estates in the service of our country, and we think it no more than right to have a reward for it." Under careful study, each argument withered. Having taken out a commission, Freedom observed, officers should have found full satisfaction in "the noble reward" of their elevation in the service of the country. To suggest now, in the wake of war, that they deserved more than others was an outrage. Had not the private also "spent as much time as you?" Had not others similarly been afflicted with the enormous sufferings of war? How could "the inhabitants of Falmouth, Charlestown, New-London, and New-Haven with others, almost numberless to count, suffered by fire and sword, cold and nakedness, and almost every other cruelty which the malice of hell could invent," be asked to "pay a pension out of their scanty remains, which you proudly touch not the burden of with one of your fingers?"[43]

At the heart of Freedom's arguments against pensions for officers lay an understanding about ability and disability predicated on the notion of agency—that in a free society, one had a personal responsibility to labor for one's maintenance as well as a personal responsibility for the failings of one's own body. For officers to receive pensions when still capable of employment posed the threat of idleness that was the bane of free societies. "[D]id not you leave some domestic employment by which you used to obtain a support?—And are not most of you as capable of following it now, as ever? And if so, why ought we to raise you to this elevation, and thereby make you not only useless cumberers of the ground, but dangerous birds of prey, whose interest it is now become to be picking out the very vitals of that liberty and freedom, which we have obtained. . . ." But even for those who were presumably not "capable of employment," Freedom believed that pensions were not warranted. "And as to your health," Freedom wrote, "did you suppose the community became accountable for your health? Which of you, having agreed with a person to perform a hard piece of service, and paid him a large price for it, shall think yourself obliged to be accountable for his health if the service should prove too hard for his constitution. I believe not anyone."[44]

Here was an argument with significant implications for the invalid soldier. Earlier pensions from the colonial wars—and exemption and compensation by provincial government for accidents, sickness, and a host of other afflictions—were based on an understanding that misfortune was the lot of those living in a community of peril; when one had been devastated by life's assaults, it was possible to turn to government for protection. In arguing against half-pay pensions as compensation for the impaired constitutions of gentlemen officers, Freedom was, in effect, suggesting that the burden of risk, of being placed in harm's way in warfare, lay with the sufferer. Military service was conceived of as a contract, and in an anticipation of arguments later used by employers regarding industrial accidents in the early nineteenth century, Freedom maintained that the market absolved the employer from a paternalist regard for his employee's health; freedom to buy and sell labor meant that the laborer, not the employer, was responsible when his body failed.[45] Government had fulfilled its obligation to officers through salaries, just as employers fulfilled their obligation to workers through payment, even when a "hard piece of service" proved too difficult. There was nothing compelling the workers, or the officers, to undertake special burdens; but once they had, the onus of their physical sufferings was placed squarely upon themselves.

Taken together, the arguments waged for and against pensions for Revolutionary War officers pointed to new vulnerabilities that invalid pensioners would face in the wake of the war. Like officers asking for half pay, the invalid had spilled his blood for the country and deserved compensation for his *past* injuries and other incapacities incurred. But the language of sensibility that was used to make the case for the invalid soldier was not as strong a tool as the language of honor. Further, in thinking about the invalid soldier's *future* welfare, the arguments regarding officers' personal responsibility for their health raised the problem of where the government's obligation for wartime suffering ended and personal obligation began. We take up this question now in looking at the law and practice of awarding pensions to soldiers in post-Revolutionary Massachusetts.

The development of invalid pensions in the final years of the Revolution and the years immediately thereafter both reached back to colonial precedent and responded to new ideas about individuals' responsibility for their own welfare. New policies subjected soldiers' requests for disability pensions to further scrutiny and the additional requirement that, in order to receive compensation, the soldier might be made to labor in an Invalid Corps. But even with the new scrutiny, pension claims continued to be accepted for a wide array of conditions, from wounds to diseases and general states of weakness and "dis-ease." Nothing in the medical thinking of the time argued against such claims, and once they had been accepted, it was difficult to shut them down during and immediately after the war.

We will first consider the ways in which invalid pensions in Massachusetts reflected changes in thinking about the personal responsibility of veterans for their own suffering, seen most clearly in the elaboration of pension law and the requirement that disabled veterans serve in an Invalid Corps; we will then turn to the practices of the colonial period that were carried forward into the 1780s, shown in the range of physical conditions that were considered disabling enough to place men on the invalid rolls. The broad range of physical conditions that might warrant a pension would come into question in the 1790s and help to propel a bureaucratic turn in social welfare provision.

In 1782, a year before the war was concluded, the Massachusetts General Court issued a resolve declaring that while "many persons, by reason of their having met with misfortunes while engaged in public service, have become pensioners," it was now possible to imagine that "the reason on which such pensions were granted, in some instances [may] have ceased." The General Court encouraged freeholders to inform justices of the court of general sessions if they suspected that their fellow townsmen no longer deserved a pension. The allegations were to be followed by an examination by the justices, and if determined to be well-founded, the pensioner would be stricken from the rolls.[46]

Four years later, in the wake of congressional legislation stipulating federal oversight of the Revolutionary pensions, the Massachusetts General Court required all pensioners to submit to an examination and obtain annually a certificate validating their claims. The rules for authentication had some flexibility: pensioners had to produce a certificate from either a commanding officer or surgeon of their regiment, ship, corps, or company, or from a physician or surgeon of a military hospital, or to provide "other good and sufficient testimony" setting forth their disability. Without newly obtained certificates, former Revolutionary pensioners could expect no further compensation. And, most significantly, those deemed capable were assigned to garrison duty at Castle Island, which in 1785 had been turned into a prison for state criminals.[47]

Massachusetts was the only state after the war to insist that its disabled pensioners serve garrison duty in an Invalid Corps. Legislators likely had the promise and potential of the Revolutionary Invalid Corps in mind, rather than its actual record of success during the war, which was mixed at best. After its tentative beginnings in 1776, the Invalid Corps was taken over by Lewis Nicola (1717–1807). The son of a British army officer, Nicola served in the armed forces in Ireland (where he had been born) and Flanders before immigrating to Philadelphia in 1766. Nicola worked diligently to break into that city's cosmopolitan community of letters, founding a circulating library in 1767, joining the American Society for Promoting Useful Knowledge (and serving on the committee that facilitated that group's merger with the American Philosophical Society), and establishing the short-lived *American Magazine, or General Repository* in 1769. The outbreak of hostilities with England allowed Nicola an opportunity to merge his literary and martial talents. He composed *A Treatise of Military Exercise, Calculated for the Use of Americans* (1776), translated two French works on military affairs, and accepted the position of barrack master and town major of Philadelphia, which had him organize men who were not fit for militia marches to serve guard and watch duty. But Nicola was frustrated by his recruits, older men wanting in military experience, and he urged Congress to establish a more robust corps consisting of invalid veterans, who though unfit for expeditionary warfare might still be of great use to the country.[48]

Congress obliged in 1777, electing Nicola as colonel of a corps to consist of eight companies, totaling one thousand officers and enlisted men. For officers, the corps was envisioned as a training ground and a necessary means of self-improvement, "a military school for young gentlemen, previous to their being appointed to marching regiments." For enlisted men, the corps held out the possibility of full pay for injured soldiers (twice what invalids would receive for disability pensions in the absence of service). The men would be "employed in garrisons, and as guards in cities and other places, where magazines or arsenals, or hospitals" were placed, which would free up other soldiers for the field. In theory, at least, the Invalid Corps also offered a means for disabled soldiers to remain "of use" and to justify their compensation by their continuing service.[49]

But despite Nicola's protests to the contrary, the corps never seems to have reached the goals that he envisioned. At its height, it never had more than five hundred men, half the number that Nicola had requested. Its troops were stationed at Philadelphia and Boston for much of the war, and then moved to West Point in 1781.[50]

Both officers and enlisted men from Massachusetts had found cause for complaint in the Revolutionary Invalid Corps. As Lieutenant Osgood Carlton noted in a petition to the Massachusetts General Court, he desired "Cloathing for the Year 1778" so that "he may be put upon an equal Footing with other Continental Officers." In 1778, at age thirty-seven, Carlton had been awarded a full disability pension (half pay) "in consequence of general debility." A seasoned military man, he had served as a private in the Seven Years' War and lived in Nova Scotia for five years with the chief engineer of the British Army in North America, learning mathematics and astronomy (which he taught in Boston after the war). He knew enough of the military to ask for his just deserts. The court responded sympathetically, resolving that all officers and soldiers in the Invalid Corps receive the "same Privileges and Gratuities" as other officers and soldiers in the fifteen battalions representing the state. Despite good intentions, however, the corps was never properly provisioned. When the Boston detachment received orders from Washington to go to West Point in 1781, the court was informed that the troops were "very bare of cloathing," and quickly tried to order 146 pairs of overalls, hunting-frocks, hats, knapsacks, and stockings for the troops. At a time when the Continental army as a whole was suffering severe shortages of this sort, it is hardly surprising that the Invalid Corps was in similar straits. But petitions to the General Court, and the court's response, recognized that the corps was perceived to be at the bottom of the heap.[51]

It is no wonder, then, that the Invalid Corps had trouble attracting men. In a newspaper advertisement for Massachusetts recruits in July 1781, several months after a detachment of the Invalid Corps had been ordered to West Point, Moses McFarland, captain of the Invalid Corps stationed at the Boston garrison, noted that there were in Massachusetts "and neighboring States, a number of idle soldiers who have long since been transferred to the corps of invalids in Boston, but have neglected their duty in not joining the camp." The task of guarding the town required "immediate recruits," this task being impossible for those who remained in the city. He asked the assistance of selectmen throughout Massachusetts to "take up and send to their duty all such delinquents as shall be found within their respective towns." Enthusiasm for sending men to Boston was likely dampened by the benefit the towns stood to gain from a soldier's pension, which, if he were one of the town poor, would be used for his maintenance. Extant returns for the late years of the war list no troops of the Invalid Corps in Boston whatsoever, in part because many had left for West Point, but also because of the limited enthusiasm for the corps among those remaining.[52]

Towns may already have sent along to garrison duty in Boston persons whom the Continental army had deemed unfit. A return of "Recruits unfit for service sent by the State of Massachusetts" affords a view of the range of persons sent by towns across the state as of January 1781. Next to the name of the recruit was listed his age, height, the county and town that had sent him, and the amount of the bounty he had received. At the end of the line were brief notes detailing why each man was unfit: "Dropsical," "Subject to the falling Sickness," "Been in the hospital," "Rheumatic," "Deaf," "Lame," "Blind," "lunatic," "Ruptured," "Bodily deform'd," "Idiot," and "old & infirm." Some men were "small & weak," "too small to bear the weight of a Musket," "unable to bear the fatigue of Camp." And then there were simply "children."[53]

Its existence prolonged by Colonel Nicola's lobbying, the Revolutionary Invalid Corps was formally dismissed by Congress in May 1783, a month after Congress proclaimed the end of the war. Secretary of War Benjamin Lincoln (a Massachusetts man) had argued in 1782 that the Invalid Corps was too expensive, of too little help to the war effort, and in such a "miserable state" as to warrant embarrassment. Colonel Nicola countered that, save for the marching and fighting of the expeditionary forces, the Invalid Corps had done all that other regiments had done and more; the "duties and fatigues" of the corps were strenuous enough that enlisted men feared being transferred to it. In his formulation, we see the ambiguous moral terrain of the corps: the debilitated would have to labor more assiduously than their healthy comrades to demonstrate their worth; their redemption lay in labor that others would view as punitive.[54]

Despite what would seem at best tepid success, the Massachusetts legislature revived the idea of the Invalid Corps in 1786, insisting that its pensioners serve in it if able. Although some in the state claimed that garrison duty was a cruel punishment for men who deserved better, many in the legislature, and certainly the governor, James Bowdoin, were notably impatient with requests for protection from the state government. Farmers in western Massachusetts, laboring under taxes to redeem the state's war debt, had requested that stays be granted, in-kind payments be permitted, and other kinds of common exemptions be revived, all of which claims were denied. Construing rural poverty as the consequence of a want of industry and too keen a desire for luxuries, the legislature could in a similar vein ask that invalid soldiers work toward their improvement by joining an Invalid Corps.[55]

Occasional pieces in the public prints on the invalids and garrison duty argued that it was not only an obligation for the invalids to work, but rather an opportunity, which they could be denied only through callous disregard. "A Soldier" writing in the *Massachusetts Centinel* in November 1787 made the case that it was the critics of the garrison policy who were cruel and unthinking. Those who objected to the garrison duty must have felt that "none of this class of men can be trusted with such an important post; and consequently will be a dishonour to the State." But these men's service and sacrifice had entitled them to industrious and honorable work, which labor in the garrison would provide. "I confess I never had an idea, that a man's bleeding in defense of his injured country, was proof of his disloyalty." "A Soldier" presumably spoke from personal experience. To deny him the opportunity to labor in the garrisons was to call into question his loyalty and honor.[56]

Massachusetts's revival of the Invalid Corps had had been informed by the concern that "equal justice may be done the said Pensioners & the Publick." Pensions were an act of redistributive justice, taking money from the taxpayers to provide security for the incapacitated. At a minimum, the soldiers might be asked to labor for their support, if at all possible (and those who were no longer deemed incapacitated by wounds or other debilities—those "otherwise disabled"—would be denied "any further compensation from the Public").[57]

A careful look at the examination certificates, mandated in 1786 for all invalid pensioners, reveals that a wide range of physical conditions were deemed worthy of a disability pension. Many invalid soldiers would be recommended to serve garrison duty; others would be exempted altogether and allowed to receive a disability pension at home. But whether they were asked to serve garrison duty or not, the broad category of "disability" continued to be as capacious as it was in the colonial period. In other words, even with new efforts to ferret out veterans who had recovered sufficiently enough that they no longer needed a pension, and even with pressures imposed on disabled veterans to labor at garrisons and be "of use," the examination certificates from the period reveal a world in which a wide range of conditions—including "dis-ease"—might be considered at least partially disabling and worth public consideration.[58]

We can see the range of physical conditions considered worthy of a disability pension in a surviving notebook of "certificates" granted by the commissioner of invalid pensions for Massachusetts, John Lucas. Each certificate consists of a short paragraph describing the soldier, recording his age, cause of disability, and evaluation of fitness for garrison duty. There are 233 applicants in the notebook, which covers the years 1786 to 1792, a limited sample to be sure, but large enough to reveal some general patterns.[59]

As in the colonial pensions, the chaotic violence of war emerges in the certificates: limbs shattered and lost; musket balls having struck every conceivable part of soldiers' bodies (fingers and toes, arms and thighs, ankles and wrists, head and neck, lungs, bowels, and groin); and some musket balls still lodged within. Just how much pressure pensioners were under to continue to be "of use" can be glimpsed in the records of pensioners asked to keep working for the state. Lieutenant Bartlett Hinds (age thirty-one), who had a musket ball pass through his lungs; Samuel Angier (age forty-nine), disabled by a "musket ball entering the left side of his neck, passing thro' to his right"; Richard Moore (age fifty-five), disabled by his "left hip being put out": these veterans and many more were deemed fit for guard duty. Exemptions were granted in severe cases—to those who had lost a limb or lost both eyes, or for whom a musket ball had wrought enough damage to make it impossible to move. But accounts of soldiers who preferred to simply receive their pension payouts without serving on guard duty in their present state reminds us of the thresholds of pain and discomfort that early moderns found intolerable. When Josiah Rumrill (age thirty) was told he was able to serve garrison duty despite a "ball through his face and Tongue," he opted for a discharge over service in the garrison and the additional wages it might provide. He was not alone in doing so.[60]

Despite manifest pressure for pensioners to continue to be "of use" by serving as guards, Lucas's examinations reveal the extent to which the wide-ranging colonial understanding of disability was still in play in post-Revolutionary Massachusetts. In addition to those who suffered from specific wounds, approximately one-fifth of the pensioners argued that they had been more generally "disabled" by sickness, hardship, and general debility born of warfare. Many simply suffered from "old age," were "worn out," or labored under "infirmities." Others were granted disability for complaints—tied to "dis-ease" as much as any discrete disease—from rheumatism, palsy, and rupture. Others suffered from the ravages of diseases common in the earlier pensions, from blindness caused by smallpox, or from epileptic fits. And there were new diseases and conditions that the commissioner encountered as well; Lucas noted that Captain Moses White (age thirty-one) suffered from "what is called lamaptal."[61]

Taken as a whole, the Massachusetts pensioners from the Revolution shared much in common with their colonial predecessors. Despite distrust of some of the invalid veterans, whose reluctance to serve in the Invalid Corps might be attributed to idle habits and even disloyalty, and despite regulations demanding that invalids procure examinations and a range of evidence to substantiate their claims, the pensioners in Revolutionary Massachusetts could count on the same expansive understanding of disability that veterans from the colonial wars had invoked. Old age, discrete disease, general "dis-ease"—all of these conditions, visited upon veterans and ascribed, however vaguely, to their prior service, were understood to be grounds for pension claims.

This was the range of claims the federal government had to confront in the coming years, first in its adjudication of local disputes and later in direct applications made to Congress. The central question became one of determining the degree to which the national government should become involved in addressing local, intimate, and finally indeterminate sufferings that had been so much a part of the protection offered the subjects and citizens of the province and state.

IV. "DECISIVE DISABILITY" AS POLICY

During and after the Revolutionary War, many individual petitioners felt that they had not been treated justly. Some had claims that were dismissed; others did not receive the amount of money they thought commensurate with their disabilities; still others pleaded that while they were unable to gather the evidence necessary to make a persuasive claim, they were deserving nonetheless. What differentiated Revolutionary pensioners from those who preceded them was that they had a new governmental body before whom to lay their appeals, the federal Congress. Like the claimants before colonial and state governments earlier in the century, invalid petitioners to Congress were never overwhelming in number, and those granted pensions were fewer still. As of March 23, 1792, Congress maintained only 1,472 invalid pensioners.[62] But the consideration given to their cases speaks to larger issues about the willingness and capacity of the federal government to meet the needs of its citizens.

Federal oversight of invalid pensions began in the administration of Henry Knox (1750–1806), who served as secretary of war from 1785 to 1794. Knox had made a remarkable ascent into the ranks of the elite and powerful. His father, a ship captain in the West Indies trade, failed at his business when Henry was just six and died six years later. Forced to leave school, twelve-year-old Henry was apprenticed to a bookbinder. After a fortunate marriage in 1771 to Lucy Flucker (1756–1824), from a prominent and wealthy Boston family, Knox was able to open his own bookstore. The Revolution brought further opportunities. Knox joined the militia and became an avid reader on military subjects. During the siege of Boston, Knox impressed Washington with his military knowledge and developed a close friendship with him. Knox rose rapidly through the military command, commissioned as a colonel in the Continental artillery in 1775, later made a brigadier general overseeing the entire Continental artillery, and finally promoted to major general after the victory at Yorktown in 1781.[63]

Like Benjamin Franklin, Knox showed the radical possibilities for self-fashioning in eighteenth-century America. With the proper connections, self-improvement through reading, the cultivation of refined habits, and a good deal of luck, some could bridge the chasm separating commoners from gentlemen. But having risen, Knox, unlike Franklin, was not eager to spread the gospel of progress. As Alan Taylor has aptly observed, Knox aspired to be part of the "natural aristocracy," a benevolent "father of the people," who would come to resent evidence of the social instability that had made his rise possible. Knox's statecraft was, in part, based on his conservative vision of society. He would try to contain the claims that citizens might make on the federal government as a matter of right; the federal government's charge to protect the people might be exercised judiciously in a tightly restricted set of cases that were especially meritorious. But Knox preferred that the pitiable cases brought to Congress be instead addressed in localities, where gentlemen might be better able to exercise their patronage and offer assistance.[64]

During his tenure as secretary of war, Knox struggled with two interrelated problems. First, he had to devise methods that would enable Congress to hear appeals from pensioners dissatisfied with their treatment at the state level without miring the federal government in the intricate politics of state pension relief. Second, Knox was determined to formulate clear and consistent standards that could be applied to soldiers who presented new cases directly to the federal government under the general pension laws of the 1790s.

Both tasks fell under the charge of establishing federal "policy," a word Knox came back to repeatedly in his review of claims. The word carried two meanings in the period. Policy pertained to the conduct of public affairs, establishing the principles advocated by government as "desirable, advantageous, or expedient." But it also bore a private meaning pertaining to personal character, the qualities of prudence, shrewdness, and wisdom that determined one's moral orientation, as in "honesty is the best policy." Both senses of policy were in play as Knox examined the validity of claims. On the one hand, in formulating policy for the federal government, Knox limited government's function as a body that would intervene in and adjudicate controversies percolating at the local and state level. On the other hand, in formulating policy with regard to personal character, Knox significantly shifted the burdens of incapacity from government to the people themselves, who would now be responsible for ameliorating their condition.[65]

The boundaries of Congress's power to adjudicate controversies at the local and state level came up repeatedly in the First Congress. The petition of Ruth Roberts exemplifies the kinds of cases Knox confronted; his report of January 25, 1790, established a precedent that he would refer to in subsequent cases. Roberts had petitioned on behalf of her late husband, Lemuel, a captain of Connecticut's militia in 1776. As Knox represented the petition in his report, Lemuel Roberts had been "attacked with sickness" and obtained a discharge after twenty-three days of service. In the following years, the affliction had not only "prevented his pursuing his customary occupation of a farmer," but "the great length of the disorder compelled him to expend the principal part of his property in ineffectual pursuit of remedies." Connecticut's superior court had refused to put Roberts on the invalid list of the United States, and he had died in 1789 after a fall "occasioned by his infirmities." Left as a poor widow with seven children, Ruth Roberts asked for a pension for her husband from the time of his initial disability until his death.[66]

Knox used the case to argue that the federal government must defer to state decisions, even in the face of apparent suffering, stating that "[t]o suppose that the Congress of the United States, removed at a distance, and from the nature of things acting under more partial information, could equitably reverse the judgments made in respective states, is to suppose that they possess a greater portion of intuition than has been assigned the human race." Congress had been "liberal and honorable" in its conduct by resolving in 1785 to allow states the right to examine and judge who was fit for an invalid pension. By bringing the means of compensation "to the doors of the claimants," Knox argued, "every facility has been offered which could be required of national justice, or national humanity." If after all the gathering of "local information" and the exercise "of all the supposable degrees of local influence," persons like Roberts and her husband had not been relieved, it was evidence of the weakness of their claim. The federal government could offer only sympathy; money and support would have to come from local sources. National humanity and national justice in these instances required deferring to localities.[67]

The report was a remarkable comment on the complex politics of localism in the early republic. A staunch Federalist and supporter of the new national government, Knox nevertheless believed there were domains of local life better left untouched by central power. The moral foundation of monarchical political culture, in which government was the final protector of the people, had enabled appeals of even the very humble to reach the highest level of government for commiseration and relief. But Knox realized that to entangle the federal government in the kinds of local, intimate decisions that were made at the town and state level would be impractical and likely impossible. "If any decision made in the States should be reversed or modified by Congress, unless for powerful and conspicuous reasons," he wrote, "such an inundation of applications would follow as to constrain a new inspection of examination of all the invalids throughout the United States." While some might be overjoyed at the prospect, "it would probably occasion disgust and applications for a greater number," with the result leading to more pleas for relief, more exceptions and reversals, with no final resolution. Cases like Roberts's revealed the limits of national governance. Federalists had promoted the Constitution with the promise that a central government removed from scenes of local prejudice and passion would gain the possibility of wisdom and an honorable disinterest. There was a similar logic in buffering Congress from the details of local life; the famed "filtration" that brought the best men to Congress would also have to screen out the tangled, unsettling, and passionate politics that surrounded misfortune in localities.

Although a Federalist, Knox's vision of local governance was not unlike that of elite Democratic-Republicans of the time.[68] For elite dissenters, such as Massachusetts senator Elbridge Gerry, federalism enabled local men belonging to the "natural aristocracy" to continue to exert their proper influence over local affairs. Knox's deference to "local influence" in the Roberts case shared the same vision; the suffering of the Roberts family was to be addressed in a local economy in which a proper judgment of character and circumstances would lead to benevolence. A national government could never understand fully questions of local desert; a gentleman's "intuition," as Knox implied, could best be exercised not at the national level, but rather in local settings. There, amidst the rituals of conversation and sociability, in interactions that still turned on face-to-face meetings, the moral faculties could best discern merit and worth.[69] One could reach out to sufferers like Ruth Roberts with feeling and wish for her, as Knox did, the "assistance of all humane persons," but that assistance would have to happen in local settings. The sentimental display of feelings was everywhere apparent in the political culture of the new republic—feelings of gratitude for "national characters" like Washington, for example, were a potent means of promoting nationalism. But as a matter of national *policy*, there was a logic to keeping the connection between suffering and commiseration—between humane persons and their assistance—tightly bound within localities.[70]

Regardless of their individual circumstances, the great bulk of petitioners like Ruth Roberts who appealed to the federal government after failing at the state level were summarily rejected; the benefit of the doubt almost always went to local officials. But as Knox anticipated new applications that would come directly to Congress in the coming years, he discerned in the petition of Roberts and others like her a troubling line of argument that would have to be addressed. As he wrote a year after reviewing Roberts's petition, he had seen a "considerable number" of petitions that "state colds, rheumatism, or other disorders, caught ten or fifteen years ago, as causes of a pension." Likewise, there were others "who received flesh wounds as many years past" who felt entitled to a pension. Something would have to be done to break the tenuous connections that pensioners drew between minor ailments in the past and their present distress. Knox understood the problem to be a complex one. For while there could be little doubt about the condition of men of the "highest disability" who were utterly incapable of laboring for their support, he observed that the "grades of disability are several, until they are hardly perceptible." It was this realm of disability, where the detection of incapacity was perplexing and subtle, that Knox feared most. What would keep ill-qualified pension applicants from employing the "influence of humanity" and obtaining certificates of disability from men of "good character" whose sympathies had overwhelmed their reason?[71]

Here was another dangerous dimension of local politics from which Knox hoped to insulate the federal government. What was to be done about the fathers of the people, overly moved by suffering, who might offer compensation to those not fully worthy of it? This sort of question was increasingly also being asked by those advocating changes to poor relief practices that happened "out of doors" of the almshouse and workhouse; the issue became everywhere apparent in the late 1810s. The problem of undeserved relief was particularly complicated with regard to illness. Not only did illness present physical suffering, the spectacle of which could easily overwhelm the rational faculties of the viewer, but it was a condition that begged the question of personal responsibility in a way that accidents and wounds did not. The wound to a soldier on the battlefield had a source that was immediate, knowable, and outside the soldier's control. The sickness visited upon a soldier raised the question of its origins: Was it something that had been lying latent in the soldier's body and only fully manifested in war? Was the illness the result of mental strain and the product of the mind's ability to sicken the body? And sickness raised the question about the invalid's role in prevention and treatment: Had all prudent measures been taken to brace the constitution and restore balance to the body at the earliest signs of dis-ease? Had the invalid pursued an ill-advised course of treatment that had injured his body rather than restoring it to health?

Knox's view of illness as a problem that warranted special attention was evident in other plans he presented to Congress and in his personal correspondence. Asked by Congress to develop criteria for the recruitment of officers to preside over a national army, Knox insisted that recruits be between eighteen and forty-five, at least five feet five inches tall, and healthy. If they were later found to carry any "secret disease" at the time of their enlistment, their associated medical bills would be taken out of their pay. The concern with "secret disease" was likely related to smallpox, which—as we have seen in earlier chapters—was regularly described as being "secretly" brought back by returning soldiers whose symptoms did not suggest the pox at dismissal or even after they arrived home. Inoculation, too, was associated with secrecy because inoculees continued to remain contagious long after they felt well enough to travel about. Considerable effort was devoted to the problem of isolating and policing inoculees, lest they infect the vulnerable, deliberations that Washington and his officers corps were part of in their decision to inoculate the Continental army.[72]

But Knox's concern with "secret disease" also spoke to a broader discussion in the early republic about one's personal responsibility to avoid sickness and to preserve health. True, Knox cultivated a luxurious lifestyle in Philadelphia, where he entertained lavishly and indulged in the kind of culinary excess that so agitated medical reformers of the day, such as William Buchan, who inveighed against both the idle habits of the gentry and the ignorance of the common folk. Yet Knox was also keenly attentive to his health and that of others. A brief consideration here of his medical thought will shed light on his efforts to extricate Congress from responsibility for veterans' illnesses.[73]

Even in the face of terrible loss to disease—he would suffer the deaths of nine of his twelve children—Knox never gave up on therapeutic intervention. During his stay in Philadelphia as secretary of war, he procured an impressive range of medicines for himself and his family, including calomel pills, peppermint water, purging pills, laxative asafetida pills, liquid laudanum, and red bark. He tried diets and exercise, perhaps in response to suggestions that at nearly three hundred pounds he had surpassed a healthy corpulence, but also as a result of his faith in following a balanced regimen to restore health. Medicine, in fact, became one of the means by which he cultivated and maintained sincere friendships, not least with Washington. Hearing that Washington's nephew was dangerously ill, Knox sent off a parcel with tender inquiries and medicine to give the child. Others would receive more direct advice on the rational pursuit of health. David Cobb, appointed brevet brigadier general at the close of the war and later serving two terms in Congress from Massachusetts, had confessed to Knox that his "spirits [were] not good." Knox exhorted, "For God's sake bear up against the devil of Gloom. Put yourself in motion. Visit even me if you can find nothing better. Get Willich, a new author on diet and regimen"—a book that sold itself as "a systematic inquiry into the most rational means of preserving health and prolonging life." "[B]ut above all," Knox concluded, "get—on horseback." Sociability, friendship, and improvement through reason, mental and physical discipline, and learning all pointed to the possibility of preserving health.[74]

But the underside of this faith that the body might be improved and fortified was the sense that improper care or attention could lead to disease. Particularly concerning was the proper regulation of the passions, a lifetime project for those seeking refinement. And here, Knox and others aspiring to gentility found ample room for criticizing enlightened gentle-men and commoners alike. Although the belief in a psychic dimension to somatic illness had deep historical roots, reaching back to the ancients, the idea drew new attention in the early eighteenth century. George Cheyne's influential *The English Malady* (1733) had illuminated the En-glish vulnerability to debility of the nerves and melancholy, an affliction especially acute in the delicate and sensible classes. Commoners, too, might be stricken by the mind's ability to influence the body, though in their case more (it was thought) through indulgence in superstition and a want of a rational degree of self-government.[75]

In response to the yellow fever epidemic that seized the capital city in 1793, stunning Philadelphians and leading to numerous speculations on its origins and proper treatment, Knox and others were prepared to frame the disease as a problem of the mind wreaking havoc upon the body; Knox believed that unwarranted anxieties on the part of common folk had in-flamed the spread of disease. In telling Washington the story of a tailor with a mild case of the fever that need not have been fatal, Knox suggested the man had taken copious amounts of medicine that had only worsened his condition; that, coupled with the curiosity of onlookers, had sealed his dark fate. "[T]he people came into the sick man's room in droves to see the *curious fever*, and he has been so worried, that his life *is* in great danger." Unregulated curiosity here verged on frenzy, feeding disease that might have abated under a properly managed and serene setting, presum-ably in the isolation that the enlightened could seek and the better sort could afford.[76]

For Knox, then, there were ample reasons for being skeptical of veter-ans who claimed that they had been disabled by illnesses suffered in war. He could see many ways in which the invalid might have brought on or worsened a condition that was attributed in pension applications to the hardships of war. Reversing the trend toward broader provision of pensions in colonial and Revolutionary Massachusetts, Knox reported to Congress in 1793 that there needed to be new guidelines for awarding pensions, using a standard he called "decisive disability."

At the heart of decisive disability lay a rigorous social and corporeal ex-amination that would establish the inception, continuance, and intensity of disability as precisely as possible. Congress's act of February 28, 1793, one of several early attempts to regulate invalid pensions under the Con-stitution, laid out the criteria of decisive disability in detail. The veteran was called on to produce a wide range of evidence. As in the past, an applicant needed affidavits from his commanding officer, attending surgeon, or other credible witnesses who could verify the onset of his disability during war. In addition, the applicant would have to secure the testimony of persons who had observed him in his everyday life after the war, witnesses familiar with the "mode of life, employment, labor, or means of support" of the claimant. The law required three "reputable" freeholders from the veteran's place of residence in the two years following his discharge to describe the degree to which he had been disabled by wartime afflictions, and two witnesses to verify the continuance of that disability until the time of application. An in-depth understanding of the claimant in his local context was critical in determining his worthiness of a pension.[77]

Coupled with this social examination was a close inspection of the invalid's body. In its naked innocence, the body presumably signified the nature and extent of its sufferings independent of the potentially misleading stories attached to it by the invalid and others influenced by him. Two physicians were to comment on the degree to which the body was disabled and whether it was plausible that such disability stemmed from war rather than from the ravages of time or some other cause. All evidence was to be examined by the circuit court judge for the district in which the applicant lived and then transferred to the secretary of war, whose office would match applicants' names against muster rolls and add remarks before submitting his report to Congress.[78]

Such stringent requirements proved costly and difficult for prospective pensioners. Laws regulating pensions changed so often that many applicants, especially those who claimed to live "in a remote part of the Country," regularly missed deadlines.[79] The demand for a physical examination proved especially challenging. If previous visits to physicians would not suffice as proof, claimants would have to submit to the expense of yet another inspection.[80] Other requirements could pose difficulties as well. As judges of circuit courts noted, the isolated lifestyle of some desperate veterans made it impossible for them to collect testimony from persons familiar with their local circumstances.[81] Even Revolutionary War officers, who were presumably well-established in their communities, appear to have had troubles. New Englanders had been among the most vocal critics of service pensions for officers, an opinion that appears to have prejudiced some against officers' attempts to secure invalid pensions as well. It was not uncommon for local witnesses, called in to support officers' claims, to deny that these men were truly disabled.[82] The veteran most likely to succeed in his bid for an invalid pension kept abreast of federal laws, could afford an examination, and had the social capital necessary to command witnesses capable of supporting his case. Many others could expect to have their applications denied or found incomplete by Knox's office.

Veterans who based their cases on wartime illnesses must have been especially frustrated. While earlier laws had privileged wounds as a primary cause of wartime disability, they allowed other wartime afflictions like sickness as well: veterans who had been disabled by wartime "wounds or other known cause" were permitted to apply. But in 1793, in an apparent effort to shear claims of ambiguity and the potential for fraud, only "known wounds" were allowed, and claims to disability based on sickness or other afflictions were rejected. The law created the peculiar situation in which two veterans might be similarly disabled, but the one who claimed a wound as the cause of disability would receive a pension and the other who claimed sickness as the cause would be rejected.[83]

The problem is illustrated in striking fashion by certificates that were issued by circuit court judges in 1794 and 1795, compiled and annotated by the secretary of war's office, and submitted to Congress for approval. Arranged in columns that list an applicant's name, disability, recommended pension, and additional remarks by the War Department, the certificates invite comparison. George Airs of Maine was given a pension for the loss of the sight in his right eye due to "the sudden discharge of a cannon to which he was stationed" in 1777. But the War Department denied numerous others who lost the use of an eye as a result of smallpox contracted in the service, such as Stephen Dunham, who served from Connecticut in the Continental army during the same year as Airs. Similarly, Private James Moore, who suffered a "large incurable sore" on the back of his right leg "occasioned by a bruise or wound received in the falling with a barrel of flour," was given a full pension, but the department rejected Sergeant John Charlesworth, who developed an "ulcer in his left knee from disease contracted in the service." Benjamin Fowler, a private from Rhode Island who served during the entire war, stood a good chance of being compensated for one part of his body but not another. The department noted that Fowler's loss of one eye from smallpox fell outside the law, but his criteria left open the possibility of a pension for Fowler's amputated leg, whose cause had not yet been determined.[84] The point is clear: the law created distinctions between bodies that might, to outside observers, have appeared the same.

For invalid pensioners who based their claims on sickness, the secretary of war's strict construction of the law must have been all the more confusing and disappointing because, in the majority of instances, examining physicians considered wartime sickness a legitimate cause of disability. While assessments of the degree of each veteran's disability were by no means uniform, there appears to have been an informal consensus among physicians that disability should be determined by a ranking of incapacitated body parts according to their impact on an individual's capacity to work. In general, one was awarded least for lame or missing toes or fingers, more for hands, feet, eyes, and ears, more still for arms and legs, and the most for crippling back injuries and conditions that affected multiple body parts. What apparently mattered most to physicians was not the narrow cause of a veteran's ailment but the effect of that malady upon his body.[85]

Thus it was perfectly possible for physicians to recommend a full pension to someone like Private David Newton of New Hampshire, who "was overcome by the heat" in retreating from Harlem Heights in 1776 and suffered "universal weakness in all his limbs." Physicians were also willing to consider conditions that, while not permanently incapacitating any part of the body, made it difficult or impossible for petitioners to provide for themselves. Examiners thought Connecticut's Private Samuel Grose worthy of a half pension for recurring epileptic fits "occasioned by hardships" endured at Valley Forge. In a similar vein, examiners recommended that Elijah Morse, a private from New Hampshire, receive a full pension because he had been "deprived . . . of the use of his reason" after wading through the frigid Battenkill River in the fall of 1777 and succumbing to a "nervous inflammatory disorder." In the colonial period, "colds" that had been caught wading through rivers and sleeping on wet ground, and a host of other disorders occasioned by prior stresses on the body that had thrown it out of balance, had been considered just cause for later debility. But while the medical theory and practice of the Revolutionary era would not radically challenge such associations, the imperatives of a federal bureaucracy would.[86]

The War Department noted that none of these men had been wounded, and thus their cases were not "comprehended by the laws." If the department believed such policies were unfair or inconsistent, it made no such comment in its recommendations to Congress. Strict adherence to known wounds as a cause of disability enabled maximum precision in a necessarily complex and messy business. One could never definitively determine if wartime sickness had its origins in civilian life, in a constitution predisposed to debility. But a musket ball that lodged in a soldier's thigh had its own special clarity. Soldiers who had been wounded were regularly able to pinpoint the very day of their disabling affliction, something difficult for those who claimed to have been sickened by the accumulated hardships of war. The fact that physicians could find plausible a veteran's claim to disability based on sickness endured many years in the past did not deter Knox and his successors intent on keeping a tight rein on federal expenditures. The law would create distinctions that medicine and society would not.

When Knox retired in 1794, the ground rules for decisive disability had been established. Congress would only occasionally invite applications from invalids who traced their disability to something other than "known wounds," allowing veterans "disabled by wounds or otherwise" to apply.[87] But such formulations appear to have been used so infrequently that no one was quite sure how to interpret them. In 1816, at the suggestion of the secretary of war, Attorney General Richard Rush issued a special report to clarify the matter. Rush argued for a rather liberal interpretation, maintaining that the serviceman whose constitution was "broken down by rheumatism, or enfeebled by the constant recurrence of fevers, is surely as just an object of this humane stipend at the hands of Government, as he who may have had his arm shattered by a bullet." Yet the peculiar circumstances of sickness would still have to be taken into account. Special scrutiny would have to be applied to men who had lost their health from "careless," "irregular," or "vicious" habits. The uncertain origins and evolution of sickness—its capacity to reach backward in time and across space, its implication in personal habit—continued to lead to perplexing and contentious arguments between claimants and government officials in the coming years.[88]

As of 1816, only 185 officers and 1,572 noncommissioned officers and soldiers from the Revolutionary army received invalid pensions.[89] Veterans in early national America could still point to their injuries and the inability to support themselves and their families as justification for an invalid pension. But without recourse to the range of explanations that their colonial predecessors could turn to in claiming to be disabled from labor, the quest may have seemed too difficult to undertake. When in 1818 Congress finally offered pensions to all in the military who were "in reduced circumstances," a gesture made at a time of budget surpluses and nostalgia for the aged and fading figure of the Revolutionary soldier, more than twenty thousand veterans applied.

Overwhelmed by the volume of applicants, Congress severely limited pensioners two years later with a strict means test that required applicants to document their poverty. From the perspective of federal administrators, the property schedule was a way to rationalize and contain the affective potency of the stories of physical suffering told by colonial pensioners. There were simply too many potential applicants, too many hazy details to sort through and evaluate. Applicants with estates valued below $200 were awarded pensions; those with estates over $400 were denied, no matter the pathetic details they related. Poverty could be objectified and adjudicated in a way physical suffering could not. The law had made it far easier to prove impoverishment than incapacity in the early republic.[90]

V. EPILOGUE

The Revolutionary War Pension Act of 1818 has been recognized as the first entitlement program of the United States and a critical development in what Laura Jensen has called the "early American state." Contrary to earlier major studies of the subject, Jensen argues that federal social provision has a long history that reaches back to the early national period when the federal government developed "programmatic entitlements," benefits directed at groups of Americans deemed "worthy." America was not a welfare state "laggard," as some have charged; rather, social provision was part of federal public policy from the early days of the republic. From the early nineteenth century onward, entitlements for select groups of Americans expanded and, along with them, state institutions emerged to adjudicate and manage claims.[91]

However, as Jensen notes, the selective, "programmatic" conception of entitlement set an early precedent for future entitlements in America, which were never universal but always tied "rights to reasons." Entitlements were limited to specific groups of citizens deemed meritorious and in need of special aid. Further, entitlements for some could come at the cost of others. Most poignantly, in the case of bounties of land that were offered to soldiers in the early national period, Native Americans bore an extreme cost. In awarding land for service, the early American state enlisted entitlements as a means of furthering westward expansion and underwriting America's imperial ambitions.

A focus on invalid pensions over the course of the eighteenth century helps us to see another loss here in the early history of entitlements in America, another possibility that was not pursued. To see that loss, we have to look at several developments that took place over the course of the eighteenth century in Massachusetts.

The monarchical political culture of the colonial world had been remarkably generous in its conception not of entitlement, but of protection, perhaps nowhere more so than in New England. The General Court might hear any number of petitions by persons in distress who were laboring under life's misfortunes and asking that their complaints be "commiserated" with money. The misfortunes of war folded into this general picture while adding something to it. In obliging men to serve and suffer, government incurred a special obligation to attend to their subsequent claims. Over the course of the eighteenth century, both the number and the range of claims by soldiers grew. The rise of the colonial assembly, which tried to enhance its power by hearing and adjudicating claims and offering disbursements, gave political license to what was already common medical understanding: that many years after battles had passed, a soldier's "disease" might be traced to war. Even as the figure of the pensioner in Revolutionary Massachusetts became an emblem of the ancien regime, the assembly continued to consider a range of conditions, from wounds to discrete diseases such as smallpox to the much more amorphous "dis-ease," as legitimate causes for a disability pension.

What was lost with Henry Knox's development of new criteria for "decisive disability" was this expansive sense of the bodily woes for which government was responsible. In addition to the limitations we see with the development of programmatic entitlements beginning in the early national period, we also can see a conceptual limitation to the provision of social welfare that had its roots in the 1790s and the first years of Congress. Over time, disability pensions would offer soldiers who had been sickened by warfare the opportunity to apply to the federal government for relief. But there would continue to be struggles over the degree to which disabilities born of disease could or should be compensated. Well into the twentieth century, the uncertain origins of disease, the unsteadiness of its presentation, and the difficulties of quantifying its exact toll on the stricken would mire veterans and their families, physicians, and pension administrators in confusion and inspire debate.[92]

CHAPTER EIGHT

State Paupers and Patients

In a series of articles in the *Massachusetts Gazette* in the spring and summer of 1788, "Juvenis" offered scathing commentary on vicious and disorderly conduct in Boston and in the republic at large. After indicting gambling, prostitution, idleness, and the want of religion, Juvenis turned to the public disturbance caused by "crazy people" who walked freely in the metropolis. In one unsettling incident, "[a] crazy woman was standing opposite a house in which was a sick person confined in bed, when suddenly she seized a large club, and threw it against the window of the room in which the person was confined; the club passed through the window, and reached the bed on which the person lay." The anecdote served as an extreme example for Juvenis of the disorder that had become commonplace in the city. For the honest, industrious, and sensible, life in Boston was a seemingly unremitting assault on the senses. Even the sickbed, a site that should have commanded tranquility, was vulnerable to the incursions of the street.[1]

That the crazed woman in this case was one of the "state poor"—a person who did not have a legal inhabitancy in any town in Massachusetts and whose care was paid for out of state coffers—raised troubling questions for Juvenis. How could one "scarcely fit to be trusted with their liberty" be wandering Boston's streets? And what failure of government allowed her the freedom to roam? The orientation of public poor relief was intensely localist; towns were only responsible for providing for their legal residents. This case exposed the confusion, and the potential corruption, that attended the care of strangers. As Juvenis reported, when one of Boston's overseers of the poor was questioned in the wake of the incident, he allegedly replied that "as the crazy woman did not belong to the town, he had nothing to do with the matter." Although the woman was both violent and indigent—"not only disordered in her intellects, but poor, in every sense of the word"—the overseer was apparently unmoved. Because towns throughout the commonwealth received money from the state government to care for those with no legal settlement in Massachusetts, the overseer's indifference suggested the possibility of graft. Given the hefty town taxes that Bostonians were paying to care for their own town poor, it was tempting to skim money from the state to lessen outlays required from the town. "It has heretofore been said by some that the town's pay for taking care of the poor of the state, was nearly sufficient to defray the expenses of the almshouse," Juvenis reminded his readers, adding dryly, "it is hoped that no neglect of the town will ever deprive them of that form from which they derive so great a benefit."[2]

We turn in this chapter to the "state pauper," a prominent figure in the province of affliction in late eighteenth-century Massachusetts. The General Court had long provided for sick wanderers with no legal settlement in any town, paying for care through the "province poor" accounts. The accounts, which drew on province coffers, were yet another mark of the capacious provision and precocious development of social welfare in Massachusetts. The province had been among the first of the British North American colonies to adopt such legislation, which complemented the poor law provision by which towns cared for those with legal settlement. Although similar accounts were later adopted by other New England colonies, it appears that there was no comparable program elsewhere in the colonies that was as robust as that found in Massachusetts.[3]

In the wake of the Revolution, the problem of impoverished wanderers with no legal settlement in the state assumed new significance as a regular feature of society and governance. Veterans of the late war, returning Loyalists, free blacks, seamen wandering through the ports, Indians under guardianship, widows, deserted wives, orphans, and a host of foreign nationals—all failed to acquire legal settlement, and when affliction struck, the towns in which they resided turned to the state for aid. Although the state paupers were never significant as a percentage of the overall population—even if one allows for a rough estimate of one thousand state paupers at the turn of the century, the 1800 census records 422,845 persons in Massachusetts, which would make state paupers only about 0.24% of the total population—the costs associated with their care were considerable. The pauper accounts regularly amounted to nearly three times the combined state expenses for militia, sheriffs, coroners, printing, and other miscellaneous costs; next to payments to legislators, the pauper accounts were the largest recurring item on the state's budget, both in raw numbers of claims and in total costs.[4]

The presence in early national Massachusetts of poor persons unconnected to family or town, often ill and incapacitated, repeatedly raised the question of who had the responsibility to provide for those unable to care for themselves. The answer was ultimately ironic. With the "state pauper" system, which became central to poor relief not just in Boston but in towns throughout the state, Massachusetts increasingly relied on state funds to support the poor, involving the state to an unusual degree in the provision of social welfare. But the state pauper program was undertaken not to usher in a new age or enhance the administrative force of the new state, but rather to hold fast to earlier ideals. Indeed, while there were numerous proposals in the Bay State to redesign poor relief on "new principles"— especially to allow entrepreneurial individuals and corporations to attend to the care of strangers—these proposed solutions foundered on the long-held notion that the poor were the responsibility of localities and that the sick among them could not be removed if they lay in an extreme state. But in adhering to the older principles of locality and extremity regarding the afflicted, and in developing its earlier efforts to support the province poor, the Massachusetts legislature expanded the bureaucracy to accommodate the needs of the poor, including the sick and their caregivers.

In the end, the rising expense of tending the state poor, especially the sick and infirm poor, led to cost-cutting measures. In response to a potentially overwhelming number of requests by towns to aid state paupers, the legislature developed uniform standards for town submissions and a uniform schedule for fees and reimbursements for relief. In this scheme, state paupers were treated as members of a class rather than as individuals with differing needs and wants. Once paupers became a class, it became possible to cut benefits across the board; the medical care offered to state paupers would diminish with the declining fortunes of the program as a whole. When charitable institutions for the sick and worthy poor opened, such as Massachusetts General Hospital (which admitted its first patient in 1821), the limited care offered state paupers became these institutions' most potent example of the failure of public entitlement (a topic we will take up in the epilogue).

This chapter begins with an overview of the state pauper system and the unusual narrative form of "pauper certificates," the central piece of evidence required by the General Court. The state pauper program faced many obstacles in the wake of the Revolution, some generated by the persistence of the ideals that had guided arrangements for the "province poor" in the colonial period, ideals that compelled the state government to continue and to extend an expensive program. In the second half of the chapter, we turn to the paupers themselves, whose sickness was implicated in the rise and expense of the pauper accounts; those illnesses frustrated administrative efforts to reform the system. The growth of the state pauper system and the efforts to contain medical costs point to the role of affliction in the development of poor relief, another instance in which the province of affliction threatened to overrun the social and political practices meant to contain it.

I. FROM PROVINCE POOR TO STATE PAUPER: NUMBERS AND THE NEW NARRATIVE OF "FOREIGN SETTLEMENT"

The stranger posed a special threat to New England's "peaceable kingdoms." Outsiders could upset the sometimes fragile consensus that sustained community life. The wanderer who became incapacitated and required immediate assistance might saddle a town with a debt that could take months or even years to be repaid by his or her legal place of settlement; following English precedent, localities (parishes in England, towns in Massachusets) were held responsible for care. Over the course of the seventeenth century, settlement laws were enacted to stave off this possibility. "Foreigners" had to be registered with town authorities and granted permission to live in town. Non-residents were served legal notice (or "warned") that they were not entitled to the benefits of poor relief and could be asked to leave town at will. Laws against vagrancy were passed, "Supressing and Punishing Rogues, Vagabonds, Common Beggars, and other Lewd, Idle and Disorderly Persons" with the lash and confinement in newly constructed houses of correction. Ports were especially vulnerable; in order to prevent the landing of the "poor, vicious and infirm," shipmasters were required to post a bond that the "lame, impotent, or infirm" would not become chargeable to the town. All of these laws directed at the stranger were in place by the beginning of the eighteenth century.[5]

The early settlement laws presumed a world of small-scale, face-to-face interactions, in which the limited numbers of outsiders could be tracked and removed by towns when necessary. The laws proved no match, however, for the outsiders generated by the periodic outbursts of violence and social dislocation that attended colonial conquest, imperial warfare, and the steady integration of Massachusetts into an Atlantic community. In these instances, towns turned in desperation to the General Court for relief. Starting with King Philip's War (1675–76), in which two dozen English towns were badly damaged or destroyed, Massachusetts made special allowance for those wandering unfortunates "forced from their habitations" who found themselves in towns in which they had no legal claim to assistance. The Acadian exiles deported to Massachusetts beginning in 1755, some one thousand impoverished refugees whose homes and farms had been destroyed by the British, also became part of the province poor, although authorities in Massachusetts found it disagreeable to care for a Catholic population unwilling to swear allegiance to the British king. Finally, when soldiers or sailors or other transients passing through towns in Massachusetts became impoverished or incapacitated and made a plausible claim that they had no legal residence in the colony, they, too, became part of the "province poor." Although these outsiders were largely concentrated in Boston, with its close connections to the Atlantic world, strangers also dot the provincial records from outlying towns, as we have seen earlier.[6]

The system of state pauper accounts that emerged in the Revolution built upon colonial precedent. The early stages of the war drove thousands from Charlestown and Boston into the countryside, and the costs for their care, along with sundry other accounts submitted to the General Court, came under the purview in 1780 of a joint standing legislative committee of both houses, which came to be known as the Committee on Accounts. The committee reviewed the claims, made whatever allowances it thought justified, and presented its lists of possible disbursements to the General Court for approval. Towns were then obliged to send someone with a warrant to Boston who would collect the money from the state treasurer and presumably see that it was correctly dispensed. The expenses were numerous, varied, and unwieldy, comprising everything from provision for soldiers to payments to coroners. By 1786 the committee established a standard form, the account roll, in which expenses were listed in categories, the largest of which was given the heading "pauper accounts." Towns were asked to send in lists of the poor in their midst with no legal place of settlement along with bills for their care and (after 1795) certificates documenting each pauper's settlement history.[7]

What had started as a way of providing for the episodic, if profound, dislocations of colonial life became routine, involving state government in town affairs. The pauper accounts presented at each session of the General Court grew steadily from the mid-1730s onward. In the first session in which "rolls" were systematically collected, the Committee on Accounts was asked to pass judgment on 93 accounts with towns and individuals submitting claims; by 1790 the number had grown to 124; by 1800 there were 189 accounts. In the single year of 1798, fully one-third of the towns in Massachusetts submitted accounts (including many that submitted in each legislative session). Large and small towns, old and new, upland and valley, coastal and peripheral, asked for reimbursement for their care of paupers. The eastern towns, particularly the ports in Suffolk and Essex Counties, dominated in numbers of accounts (a problem we will return to below). But, overall, a vast range of places drew on state government.[8]

If the growth in numbers of state paupers was plain to see, those with a keen eye would have detected a subsidiary development: medical bills had grown as well, not only in gross amounts but, more significantly, in proportion to the number of accounts. The published rolls placed at the end of the resolves for each legislative session contain a digest of each town's case, listing names and "types" of persons: "widow," "soldier," "Negro," "Indian," and so forth. In a similar fashion, the digest entries note if costs for board, medical attention, or funeral arrangements (and, less consistently, nursing) were part of the account. While less precise than a tally generated from the manuscript bills themselves, the upward trend in the published digests is revealing. In 1786 (the first year the digests are available), medical bills were included in 20% of the total submissions; in 1790 the proportion had grown to 28%; in 1795 it was 36%; and by 1800 it was 56%. In other words, a little over half of all accounts with the state at the turn of the century contained medical expenses. More and more towns were submitting medical bills in addition to submissions for the reimbursement for room and board. The link between medical care and pauper was becoming not just common but expected.

We will discuss the complicated question of *why* this remarkable development in state governance occurred at length below. But first we will consider the new form of the evidence, itself a major departure in the kinds of information that individuals and towns had to collect to procure funds for the poor. The new requirements focused on what I will call "foreign settlement," on criteria to determine whether the poor had no legal residence anywhere in Massachusetts (and thus were the state's responsibility). As discussed above, New England had long charged each town with caring for its own, those who had acquired legal settlement, documented by birth, marriage, and continuous years of residence without being warned out, or served legal notice that they could be removed. In establishing rules for "foreign settlement," the General Court asked that towns search for precisely the opposite sort of evidence—evidence of *not* belonging. Only by demonstrating that a pauper belonged to no one and no place in Massachusetts could towns expect compensation from the state government. In thousands of applications to the General Court, town after town submitted their bills for "foreign paupers," searching for a narrative of the pauper's dislocation that would satisfy the General Court. Early submiss ons by the towns stressed the pauper's plight and the cumulative burdens that paupers placed on towns, with less attention to documenting that the pauper belonged to no town in Massachusetts. By 1795 the General Court had devised clear rules mandating that each application come with a "certificate" proving that the town in which the pauper resided could turn to no family or place of legal settlement in the state for aid; without valid certificates, claims would be summarily rejected, no matter the degree of suffering of the pauper or townspeople that might be presented.[9]

Consider the development of the evidence in the case of John Demming, a transient soldier living in Sandisfield, Massachusetts, a town of 1,600 in Berkshire County at the far southwest corner of the state.[10] The material on Demming, quoted here at length (with added notations in the manuscript italicized in brackets), was reviewed for the May 1798 legislative session. The Committee on Accounts, consisting of two senators and three representatives, spent twenty-three days wading through this and other cases, the exacting nature of the enterprise earning them that rare reward for committee work, a salary.[11]

> Sandisfield May 15th 1798
> We the Subscribers Selectmen of the Town aforesaid do hereby give information to Your Honours that a Person by the name of John Demming {*who came from state of New york into this Commonwealth about thirty three months past*} being a transient person and unable to Support himself & being in this Town on the twentyeth Day of January 1797 {& *having no relation of sufficient ability or obliged by Law to support him in this Commonwealth*} and being chargable to said Town for cloathing and every other Necessary of Life, Said Deming aforesaid being in a deplorable Situation having been unable to Stand on his feet or help himself for sixteen months past, & his Disorder is such that no person would take him into their house, that the {*Town*} aforesaid was put to the cost of Prepareing a place for his abode for which reasons do exhibit the following Account.

The selectmen signed the certificate and added a summary account below: $158.67 for "boarding cloathing & nursing at two Dollars and thirty three Cents pr. week"; $11.33 for the doctor's bills; and $5.00 for Demming's final days, including funeral charges. They signed again below the account, attesting to its accuracy. Then John Caufield, a selectman and the town representative in the General Court, added a note in diminutive script at the very bottom of the page, affixed to the document two weeks later in

Boston. (One assumes that this was done when Caufield submitted the material to the committee. It is clear, at least, that he was in town for the June session of the court.)

> Said Deming in the Account above mentioned says that he spent some part of his life in the late American war as a soldier & some part in the westindin Islands & some part in Canada and has stroaled through the United States & by the best information was born in the state of Connecticut Town of Norrige.[12]

The Sandisfield selectmen struggled to find the right tone and to emphasize elements of the pauper's story that would warrant attention. Their initial impulse was to write in the mode of the general petition, highlighting the strains that the afflicted placed on community life. Overwhelmed by Demming's "deplorable situation," they had been forced to make special (and costly) provision; his "Disorder" of body, such "that no person would take him into their house," had become their own. Government was asked to restore order through the healing balm of money—a familiar story, presented at all levels of government in Massachusetts throughout the eighteenth century.

For its part, the Committee on Accounts was looking for a different story, and the selectmen's additions in the narrative (italicized and bracketed, above) reflected their unfamiliarity with the new questions put to them. While the selectmen had emphasized a story of community life laboring under affliction, the Committee on Accounts, in its efforts to establish the pauper's credentials as an outsider, had focused on those interjections the selectmen had squeezed between the lines and placed at the margins of their petition. The selectmen's interjection that Demming had come from New York was a good start. But it is likely that when Sandisfield's representative, John Caufield, presented the town's documents to the committee in Boston, he was encouraged to come up with more details. In his note added to the petition, he drew on what must have been an earlier interview with Demming, more detailed but also, perhaps, less reliable; the representative noted that the travelogue he inscribed in the record was largely Demming's, what the soldier "sa[id]." Demming had been born in neighboring Connecticut and wound up in Massachusetts, but in between, if he could be trusted, he had taken an Atlantic odyssey through the West Indies, Canada, and other portions of the United States. Satisfied, the Committee on Accounts accepted the account.

"Foreign settlement" was the key element of these narratives, rendering other personal information secondary, if it was considered at all. The Sandisfield selectmen had been careful to insert (again, as an afterthought) the legal phrase that Demming had "no relation of sufficient ability or obliged by Law to support him" in the commonwealth. No account could expect to pass without such language. The law asked selectmen to determine the pauper's social suffering, less his own physical limitations than the incapacities of those who, through custom or law, were charged with his care. But while the language of social suffering was required, the committee never put it to serious scrutiny. In the case of the poor who were legal inhabitants of a town, considerable effort was often made to identify family members and press them into service, thereby containing a town's poor rates. Not so in the case of the state poor, perhaps because it was assumed that if one was displaced and needing care, traditional social and legal measures had already fallen through. To be without legal settlement was to be socially disabled.

The sharp focus on foreign settlement, stripped of extraneous detail, in the pauper account is clear in the rolls submitted by the state's eastern towns, which dealt with larger numbers of strangers than provincial Sandisfield. In Salem, the roll submitted to the state by the end of the century contained simple entries such as these: "Ruth Austin, born in N. Hampshire came to Salem 2nd January 1798 from Marblehead," or "Jacob Suck, Born in Africa, Came to Salem in 1798 a Crazey Man, reports himself from Virginia." In Boston, the form was leaner still, single-word notations in answer to the following: "Name," "where born," "how long been in this state," "weeks" and "days" at the almshouse.[13] There was no need to get mired in personal stories or to excavate social relations.

In the eyes of the state government, foreign settlement trumped both society and sentiment. The expressive range allowed by the state was circumscribed, placing pauper accounts at variance with other popular genres in the early republic that claimed to represent feeling. The pathetic details of personal narratives, once "published" in petitions before the General Court, now found a ready home in privately published, sensational accounts of disastrous misfortune. But in the pauper accounts, personal and communal sufferings were subordinated to the narrow issue of foreign settlement.[14]

II. THE EVOLUTION OF STATE PAUPER RELIEF

Why did towns turn so eagerly to the state for help? And why did state government take on such a burden? The quick answer lies in the problems of "locality" and "extremity," ubiquitous, as we have seen earlier, in the lives of families, households, and towns. An overriding commitment in Massachusetts to localities taking care of their own, coupled with the shared understanding that very ill people needed special accommodation, led to the growth of the pauper accounts. When ailing "foreign" paupers fell ill or became otherwise incapacitated in towns, poor relief laws offered towns the theoretical possibility of removing the strangers, but sickness argued against removal—it was, as many petitioners put it, simply "not possible." And so the towns turned to the General Court for help, as they had for the "province poor" in the colonial period.

But that answer fails to take into account the considerable obstacles that the state pauper accounts faced in post-Revolutionary Massachusetts. By considering those obstacles, we see the overwhelming force of affliction in driving the growth of the pauper accounts. In this section, we turn to the public discourse concerning paupers and poverty and to the discrimination that free blacks and "aliens," who were major recipients of pauper relief, might confront in Massachusetts. In the following section, we turn to the failed efforts of New Englanders to convince Congress and their fellow states to follow New England's lead in providing for the "foreign" poor. With both of these larger contexts in place, we will return to the paupers themselves and to the place of affliction in bringing their plight to the attention of the General Court. The chapter concludes with an extended consideration of a possible alternative to the pauper accounts that emerged in Massachusetts in the late 1780s and early 1790s: that chartered corporations devoted to the state poor might allow cost savings. Both the call for the reform of the pauper system, and the ultimate rejection of the new proposals drawn up to meet the challenge, were motivated by the particular problems of attending to the sick poor.

Although Massachusetts had been pioneering in its provision for the province poor, little in the social and political climate of early national Massachusetts favored the state government's increasingly deep involvement with poor relief. Despite the gentlemanly commonplace that abject poverty melted the heart and aroused the benevolent affections, the governor and the General Court displayed a notable impatience with the poor, especially the poorest among them, in the wake of the Revolution. The drafting of the new state constitution and the agrarian unrest that culminated in Shays's Rebellion became public occasions for reflection on the failures of character that marked the poor as something less than full citizens. In his address to the Massachusetts State Constitutional Convention in 1780, Governor James Bowdoin offered an unapologetic explanation for what some considered unnecessarily stringent property qualifications for voters. The propertyless consisted of two classes of men: those "who live upon a part of a Paternal estate, who are but just entering into business," and those "whose Idleness of Life and profligacy of manners will forever bar them from acquiring and possessing Property." It was in the interest of the former "to have their right of Voting for a Representative suspended for [a] small space of Time, [rather] than forever hereafter to have their Privileges liable to the control of Men, who will pay less regard to the Rights of Property because they have nothing to lose." Poverty, irresponsibility, and the selfishness that grew out of desperation all folded together.[15]

Despite strenuous opposition to such views, even the most radical voices in the debate over the state constitution and the plight of the Shaysites stopped short of defending the pauper. When Massachusetts sent a draft of its constitution of 1780 to the towns to ratify, forty-two towns, concentrated in the western part of the state, raised objections to the proposed constitution's strict property qualifications for suffrage. Town after town claimed the franchise as a "natural right" of small property owners who would fall short of the proposed requirement for voters. As the town of Petersham put it, "Riches and Dignity Neither makes the Head Wiser nor the Heart Better"; indeed, it was "the overgrown Rich we think most Dangerous to the Liberties of a Free State."[16]

But claims of the worthiness of those with little property were promoted, in part, by differentiating them from groups whose poor judgment, misfortune, and lack of connection to community were construed as personal failings. When Richmond protested that property qualifications were "an infringement on the Natural Rights of the Subject that will exclude many good members of Society," they asked that voters have their character ratified by town officials. Like Belchertown, which wanted to exclude "foreigners" from voting without the unanimous approval of town selectmen, Richmond asked that all voters "obtain Certificates from the Selectmen of the Towns in which they live that they are good members of Society and of sober Life and Conversation. . . ." In its richly detailed consideration of who constituted "a part of the people of the state" entitled to full participation in the polity, Northampton thought it scandalous that ordinary men who paid taxes and might well have "gone for us into the greatest perils, and undergone infinite fatigues in the present war to rescue us from slavery" were to be deprived of full citizenship alongside "villains and African slaves," the most publicly debased persons in the commonwealth.[17]

In like fashion, six years later, when the Shaysites drew on the language of enslavement that had figured so prominently during the imperial crisis, the moral force of their argument consisted in the imperative to avoid the fate of the most powerless and the poorest of the poor. The paper money, in-kind payments, and stay laws that the Shaysites initially demanded were meant to preserve for the honest yeoman the possibility of attaining a competency; without these protections, corrupt and avaricious men in government might bankrupt the farmer, take his property, reduce him to tenancy, and finally bring him into slavery. Yet the Shaysites were not advocating cash outlays for the poor in the manner of the state pauper system. To have done so would have been to invite the pity and scorn visited upon the pauper—a figure at best pitied, at worst debased beyond the boundaries of dignity.[18]

When we consider who did find relief under the state pauper program, the ever-increasing outlays on their behalf seem unlikelier still. To be sure, there were categories of persons on the state pauper rolls considered "worthy" of public relief—the aged, the widow, the soldier, the abandoned wife and mother. Yet many of these paupers were free "negroes" and "alien" immigrants who had been unable to secure legal inhabitancy. While it is perhaps not surprising to find free African Americans or immigrants labeled as dependents under the supervision and discipline of government officials, considerable efforts had been made to keep both groups from access to the public treasury, efforts that were undermined by the pauper accounts.[19]

The end of slavery in Massachusetts was an ambiguous and protracted affair. A final ruling in 1783 in the Walker-Jennison cases held that slavery was incompatible with Article One of the bold Declaration of Rights in Massachusetts' new constitution (1780)—that "all men are born free and equal." Yet as the historian Joanne Melish has observed, kidnappings, extended indentures, and misinformation and confusion about the terms of freedom for former slaves ensured that persons of color moved from outright slavery to "statutory slavery," from slave status to "slavelike" status. There was an advantage here for government officials in extending the bounded, dependent state of ostensibly free persons. The uncertain status of former slaves meant that former masters continued to be held ultimately responsible for them. Legal provisions encouraged the freeing of young, healthy slaves and demanded that masters post bonds and other securities so that the aged and infirm would not be abandoned and become wards of the state. And lest former slaves indulge in "disorderly" and "idle" habits, statutes compelled them to find paid employment or face punishment or removal.[20]

In "An Act for suppressing and punishing Rogues, Vagabonds, common Beggars, and other idle, disorderly and lewd Persons" (1788), a remarkably expansive vision of the range of threats to public order, a special section addressed the problems posed by the "African or Negro" who could not prove citizenship anywhere in the United States. After two months' residence in Massachusetts, such persons could be ordered to leave the state by a Justice of the Peace, or, if they refused, could be confined in a county jail, whipped, and then deported again after a hearing and punishment. The law reinscribed a dependency status upon persons nominally free, whose conduct would be regulated under the vague and contingent definition of vagrancy (a crime that, as Linda Kerber has pointed out, is always in the eye of the beholder), but it also kept the state government from providing the protections traditionally accorded dependents by removing free blacks before they (or anyone on their behalf) could make claims on public treasuries for poor relief.[21]

The state's laws regulating "aliens" and "foreigners" were similarly exclusionary, extending a long history of vigilant concern about incorporating outsiders into town life. Like other states, Massachusetts had room for "good" immigrants, persons granted citizenship after their character and industry were approved by the General Court; between 1782 and 1794, Massachusetts naturalized eighty-seven adults (including returning loyalists) and twenty-one children. But unlike most other states, which were moving to liberalize immigration policies, Massachusetts maintained and considered strengthening its alien property disabilities, which did not allow aliens to hold land in their own names without a special act of the assembly. Given that landholding was a requirement for suffrage, this disability effectively denied aliens the right to vote. The legislature also continued to deny entrance to aliens who might become a public charge, renewing in 1788 earlier statutes (from 1701, 1723, and 1757) that barred entry to the "poor, vicious, and infirm" with no legal settlement in the state.[22]

By the middle of the 1790s, with Federalists in control of Congress, Massachusetts representatives played a significant role in anti-immigrant legislation, notably the extended period of residency required in the Naturalization Acts of 1795 and 1798 and the punitive Alien and Sedition Acts of 1798. From Governor John Hancock's address to the General Court in 1790 pointing to the dangers of "foreign invaders" in a free society, to President John Adams's approval of laws ordering the apprehension, restraint, and removal of "alien enemies," Massachusetts was at the forefront of America's nativist turn in the 1790s—and hardly where one would expect to find the majority of state taxes going to the relief of the foreign-born.[23]

Despite an increasingly intolerant public discourse surrounding poverty, especially the pauper, and strict restrictions on some of the major recipients of state poor relief, the state pauper program grew rapidly in post-revolutionary Massachusetts. Why? To find the answer, we must explore the ways in which the state government came to mediate between the long-standing practice of towns asking for protection from the General Court—for example to address the costs of epidemic or accommodate the province poor—and the federal government's refusal to intervene in matters of social welfare.

III. LOCALITY AND NATION

In the aftermath of the Revolution, amid what David Waldstreicher has called the "geopolitics of celebration," New Englanders touted their own virtues as those of the new nation, conceived as New England writ large.[24] As God's chosen people, New Englanders had been, from the outset, evangelists charged with spreading their "due form of government," both civil and ecclesiastical. But New Englanders also championed their way of life for defensive reasons. In order for the New England way to succeed in the new nation, other states needed to play by their northern neighbors' rules. This can be seen clearly in the efforts of Massachusetts (and other New England states) to amend the Constitution so that Congress could create uniform laws of inhabitancy in all states (an effort that failed) and in the strong objections that Massachusetts representatives voiced to the first national insurance program, an "Act for the Relief of Sick and Disabled Seamen" (1798), which only seemed necessary because other states in the union were not as responsible in taking care of their indigent and their wandering strangers as New Englanders.

The Articles of Confederation had in effect stripped paupers of the right to enjoy the protections of localities outside their own state. "Free citizens" under the Articles were allowed both the "rights and immunities" of the several states, but "paupers, vagabonds, and fugitives from justice" (including runaway slaves) were explicitly denied such rights, including the basic right to enter or leave any state other than their own. While the Articles did not create a uniform law of inhabitancy or regulate settlement laws regarding the poor, they did ensure that state governments would not be obliged to receive and potentially to support the poor from beyond their borders.[25] The Constitution, however, was silent on this matter and left the states vulnerable to the incursions of outsiders, including those who might seek out places with the most generous poor laws. The problem opened Massachusetts to the claims not only of "foreigners" from abroad but also of those traveling from state to state.[26]

Massachusetts was at the forefront of an effort to amend the Constitution to remedy this problem. As in several other large states, the Constitution was subject to vigorous debate in Massachusetts. Federalists were only able to secure ratification by agreeing with Anti-Federalist demands that the Constitution be amended after it went into effect. But when Congress submitted twelve amendments to the states for approval, the Massachusetts Senate and House, both of which largely favored the amendments, failed to give joint approval to any in their deliberations of January and February 1790. In the meantime, a joint committee was formed by the General Court to consider further amendments to the Constitution. The majority of the proposed amendments aimed to restrict Congress's power, both by limiting potential federal overreach in such matters as granting monopolies and by demanding that "the general government exercise no power but what is expressly delegated" (a provision later enacted in Article X of the Bill of Rights). But Massachusetts also asked Congress to extend its powers in one critical way: the third amendment proposed by the committee urged that "Congress have power to establish a uniform rule of inhabitancy or settlement of the poor of the different States throughout the United States." In this area, Massachusetts found that the Constitution left congressional authority too weak and state sovereignty too strong.[27]

The final Bill of Rights, adopted in 1791, included no concession to the request of Massachusetts (and, later, Rhode Island) for uniform laws of settlement for the poor, leaving the commonwealth to devise its own means of attending to the poor arriving from other states and countries. With no help from Congress in regulating inhabitancy, Massachusetts began to use its own poor laws more vigorously, as we shall see below. Seven years later, when Congress finally did enact a measure that had the potential to influence provision for the poor, Massachusetts representatives strongly objected. In the debate over what was finally approved as an "Act for the Relief of Sick and Disabled Seamen" (1798), Massachusetts representatives made it clear that if all of the states in the union had followed their lead in providing for the poor, the federal law would not have been necessary.

The bill proposed deducting 20 cents from each seaman's monthly wages to support the incapacitated at district hospitals in America's ports.

Although the plan had its origins in Boston's Marine Society, which drew on earlier precedents in Elizabethan England and in colonial Virginia and North Carolina, by the time it reached Congress, Massachusetts representatives made a forceful case against it, arguing that the bill suffered from a want of moral imagination in taxing seamen to pay for their own care. The first national insurance program of the United States would be subsidized by the sick themselves, not by Congress.[28]

The opposition to the bill was led by Samuel Sewall, representative to Congress from Marblehead, who had earlier sat on the committee to amend the federal Constitution. A lawyer and later chief justice of the Supreme Court of Massachusetts, Sewall shared with his famous great-grandfather not only the same name but also a commitment to locality, to the necessity of good citizens aiding in the welfare, improvement, and protection of their community. Sewall argued that it was precisely this commitment that was lacking in Massachusetts's neighbors to the south, who stood to benefit from the generous provisions allowed the poor in New England. Never mind that sailors were "a set of men at all times valuable to the United States," an argument made by petitioners to the First Congress from Sewall's Marblehead and other fishing ports in the Bay State, who maintained that fisheries were "nurseries" not only for commercial development of the union but also for the knowledge and skills of the sea that were essential in times of war. Even in the absence of such worthy subjects, concern for the preservation of local society should have prompted his southern compatriots to adopt new ways. In "the part of the Union from whence he came," Sewall scolded, "provision is already made for sick and disabled persons of every description, sailors as well as others, with which every person in the community is charged." With town and first province, then state provision, "[n]either native or foreigner was there sick without care and relief being afforded him." New England's care for the sick poor had been hard earned, requiring town and province and state provision; others should follow such a responsible example.[29]

Southerners in Congress charged that New England seamen often became sick in southern ports and needed attention, thus justifying the tax on them. Like federal pensions for disabled soldiers, the bulk of which went to New Englanders, the bill would be a boon to the northern states; their men would benefit from it. But Sewall responded that if southern states "would provide relief for such unfortunate persons," there would be no need of the tax. As it stood now, New England seamen had to enter the South as if "they go into foreign countries." Sewall's detractors noted dryly that his "federal disposition" as a New Englander seemed in this instance to be waning. But they missed the point. Sewall envisioned the republic as New England writ large, its parts integrated by an expansive localism. The basis of a strong union was for all of the states to adopt the example of New England, which would create a uniformly robust sense of local responsibility for social welfare.[30]

A moral ambiguity underlay Sewall's vision. His generous commitment to providing for those who rightfully belonged in a community was tied to a narrow view of belonging. For all of his celebration of New England's care for "native and foreigner" alike, Sewall's legislative record reveals that he was made uneasy by the stranger. In 1797 he had supported a tax on naturalizations, wanting the country to be an "asylum" but "not wish[ing] to see foreigners our governors"; he had inserted the language in the Naturalization Act of 1798 that extended the length of residence before citizenship could be granted from five to fourteen years; and a month after the debate on disabled seamen, he became a major proponent of the "Alien Friends Act," arguing that deportations of foreigners inimical to the interests of the United States were sanctioned by the Constitution's expansive preamble. The general welfare could best be secured through the careful restriction of outsiders. From the local warning-out system, firmly in place in New England since the early seventeenth century, to Sewall's advocacy of the deportation of foreigners—which might, given Sewall's localist orientation, be thought of as a national warning-out system—New England's communal ethic worked by exclusion as well as inclusion.[31]

Even so, towns throughout Massachusetts seized on the state pauper system in the years after the Revolution and actively provided for "foreigners" in their midst. At the very moment Sewall pressed his case for New England's localist form of care, his own town asked the state government for compensation for two years' worth of board, clothing, and medical expenses for one John Cavender, a "foreigner" born on the island of Jersey. The seaman had been "badly wounded" some twenty-six years earlier after a fall from a masthead and had been "immediately committed to the Poor house," where he had remained ever since. Now, years later, the town of Marblehead noted that the hapless Cavender had no legal place of residence and no one liable to support him. The state government granted the town's request for $186.83 in aid. With his pedigree as an outsider duly certified, the sailor could be absorbed into local society.[32]

Why did Massachusetts towns not simply remove "foreign" paupers? Towns retained the legal right to remove persons who could not claim residency. Instead of exercising this right, why did they instead turn to state government for aid? To answer this question, we need to examine changes in the local laws regulating poor relief as well as the state paupers themselves, their movement across the landscape, and the afflictions that stopped them in their tracks.

IV. SETTLEMENT LAW, MIGRATION, AND THE CLAIMS OF EXTREMITY

Not only did laws relevant to the settlement, support, employment and removal of the poor in eighteenth-century New England change over time, they were complex in their components, defying any simple narrative of their development. Throughout the century, settlement laws generally were meant to accomplish two related goals. On the one hand, they were intended to protect towns from charges associated with care for outsiders. Measures such as physical removal and "warning out" meant that towns could act defensively to safeguard their limited treasuries. On the other hand, the laws were designed to allow some degree of movement throughout the region, which was vital for social visiting, trade, and the procurement of labor. In offering towns certain protections, the settlement laws made it possible for them to allow non-residents entrance without undo worry that outsiders would become a public charge. In theory, at least, the settlement laws enabled towns to hold certain people or entities legally responsible for an outsider's care, whether it was family members, the person who had hired a stranger, or the outsider's town of legal residency. In practice, as we have seen, there were complications; when outsiders suddenly became sick, bills could pile up well in advance of any final determination of responsibility, and in the meantime, caregivers and towns could be left with debts that went unpaid for months and sometimes years.

Compounding this problem, and figuring centrally in the development of the state pauper accounts, was the elaboration of the poor laws themselves. Over the course of the century, legal inhabitancy became more difficult to obtain, in part reflecting the desire of towns to protect themselves from increasing numbers of transients "strolling" through the countryside and the ports. Between 1760 and 1775, some 264 towns were created in New England as the result of migration both to western Massachusetts (and beyond) and to the ports. Some migrants entering towns like Beverly, a port in Essex County, did well enough to rival locals in wealth. But others, with less luck and lesser means, faced new sets of restrictions on settlement by the late 1760s. New laws halted the practice of granting legal settlement to persons based on a certain number of continuous years of residence in a given town, which had been a primary means for poor persons to achieve a legal residency. The elimination of continuous residency as a basis of acquiring legal settlement meant that towns could (again, in theory) essentially rid themselves of men and women of lesser means at will. In the 1780s, however, continuous years of residence again became a means of acquiring legal settlement, and the towns lost some of their power to regulate inhabitancy.[33]

Finally, in 1794, a general revision of the poor laws made a concession to both towns and wanderers alike. Towns were disallowed from removing newcomers for the first three months of their residency, which weakened the towns' ability to regulate who could reside within their borders. But at the same time, other means of obtaining a legal inhabitancy were restricted, increasing the population of persons in Massachusetts without legal settlement in any town. The poor were stymied by increases in the number of continuous years of settlement that were required before legal inhabitancy could be granted, from two years in 1789, to three in 1791, to four in 1792, to five in 1793, and finally to ten in 1794. Free blacks, who were often poor, faced other legal disabilities. As we have seen, vagrancy statutes could force blacks either to perform labor considered suitable to their condition or to face eviction, fines, or imprisonment. Antimiscegenation laws forbade marriages between whites and "any Indian, negro, or mulatto," thus restricting marriage as a means of obtaining settlement. And "aliens" were denied the ability to demonstrate that they had the means to support themselves. The 1794 law on inhabitancy provided "citizens" with a variety of means of proving their financial security, either by pointing to freeholds or personal estates of sufficient worth. Aliens could not use these means of establishing legal inhabitancy nor could they purchase land without special permission from the General Court.[34]

The general difficulty in acquiring legal settlement in eighteenth-century Massachusetts helps to explain the nearly continuous record of migration and physical movement—Atlantic crossings, travel between states, movements between towns—revealed in the pauper accounts.[35] Perhaps only personal history can account for a man who moves six times between Connecticut and Massachusetts in his final years, or someone who jumps from South Carolina clear to the commonwealth. Occasionally testimony gives glimpses of motivations. Robert Jackson, a "Negro man" who fell sick and died in Deerfield in 1797, had come to the town six years earlier. He had been "employed in the Business of boating on [the] Connecticut river," but he had left the river for the fields, deciding to make a go of it "as a common Labourer" before he became terminally ill. More often, there is a record of movement without a story to explain it.[36]

Many paupers had been dislocated by the Revolution. The war created large numbers of refugees. Thousands of Bostonians fleeing the British-held capital were joined by those from Charlestown, whose city was burned during the Battle of Bunker Hill. The General Court had made provision for the displaced, assigning towns in the state a quota of war-born migrants they were required to take in. In the 1790s, the "poor of Charlestown" appeared on the state poor rolls, as did Loyalists. By 1784, one year after the Peace of Paris, Massachusetts's Loyalists were slipping back into society, returning to claim what had not been confiscated. Redcoats "from Burgoyne's army" and former prisoners of war showed up on the rolls. Finally, there were the veterans of the American forces. The fortunate few earned a pension for their "service and suffering," but when the United States took over the pension programs of the states in the early 1790s, as we have seen earlier, the stricter criteria for disability pensions prompted ailing soldiers to turn to state governments for help.[37]

The pauper narratives make visible the difficulties, dangers, and general misfortune that both led to and resulted from migration in the Revolutionary and early national periods. Paupers returned from Maine, Vermont, and New Hampshire to towns like Groton or ports in Essex County; from upstate New York to western Massachusetts and finally, perhaps, to Boston. In the southeastern part of the state, in Bristol County, one finds an assortment of persons whom Ruth Herndon has brought to light, nearly two thousand unfortunates repeatedly warned out from towns in Rhode Island between 1751 and 1800. By the end of the century, some were state paupers living in Massachusetts towns like Attleboro, Rehoboth, and Dartmouth. And Boston—to which we will return later—seemed a magnet for state paupers, pulling them in from all directions.[38]

Illness, both chronic and acute, figures prominently in many of the pauper stories and helps to explain why towns might have been eager to turn to the state government for relief. Towns emphasized the extremity of the paupers, the precariousness of their physical condition, and the great labors that they demanded of town residents. While towns were able to deny state paupers legal inhabitancy, they could not, and evidently would not, ignore persons who were lying in their midst in an extreme condition.

In the great bulk of pauper narratives, there is a point at which the pauper's story of wandering comes to an end, arrested by affliction. For some, acute illnesses clearly stopped them in their tracks. Thomas Mart was "on his way from Canady to Boston" when he was "taken violently ill with fits" in Billerica (in the northeast corner of the state). He "remained extremely ill" for two weeks before continuing on his way. The town called in a doctor, provided "watchers and attenders," and, at Mart's request, paid for his conveyance to Boston. Perhaps with a sense that this account alone might not warrant compensation, the selectmen added: "That said Mart was a foreigner and Frenchman, and totally destitute of any means of support and that he has not any kindred compellable by law of sufficient ability to discharge the aforesaid account."[39] Other cases of similar tempo ended less happily, in death and funeral costs. When such sudden disruption could be tied to foreign settlement, towns could look upward to the state for aid.

More commonly, infirmities of old age, physical disabilities, and mental illness could leave applicants unable to care for themselves. In many instances, selectmen and townsfolk specified that they were caring for the elderly. Danvers wrote that John Woodin had been picked up six weeks earlier, "being a Man 82 Years of Age, sick and helpless, taken up in the Highway very ragged and lousy." He would need "extra nursing." So, too, would "Black Catherine an Indian," who had been "strooling from house to house" in Attleboro. Although the selectmen there confessed that she might belong to nearby Rehoboth—and had even directed the householder with whom she had finally found shelter to compel her to leave (something they discovered was "Impracticable")—they hoped to receive funds quickly. For "she appears to be not less than 80 years of age & for seven weeks past has been very much unwell and stands in need of Nursing, & more than Common Care." Catherine's account also included Hannah Jane, "a very aged Woman," whose settlement history remained elusive; she had married a Frenchman years earlier, and the selectmen had discovered that the two had been warned out of Cumberland, Rhode Island (just south of Attleboro), before 1766. But they had been unable to learn if she was born there, and as they noted in another account, "to certify Exactly, how many Different places she has lived in, or what time they [she and her husband] resided together in Attleborough, it is out of our power."[40]

The elderly poor often suffered from physical disabilities, as less frequently did the younger poor. Boylston, Massachusetts, for example, asked to be reimbursed "For Supporting Topsfield a Negro being a Foreigner— Supposed to be about one hundred years of Age—Blind for many years, and confind to his bed for many months."[41] The terms "blind," "lame," and "cripple" are sprinkled liberally through the accounts without unusual alarm. Both physical disability and age presented "trouble" and helped towns justify extra expense. On occasion, a particularly difficult situation warranted special comment. The selectmen from Hardwick, Massachusetts, noted that John Veal was a "person so Debilitated as to render him allmost incapable of Wearing Mens Apparel or Helping himself which makes it necessary to be with him by Day & by night. . . ." A note was added to further the case: "The with Named John Veal I know him to be a Very old Man and allmost intirely Unable to help himself. . . . I know him to be a very Troblesome Object to Take Care of." A man on the brink of losing his manhood ("almost" but not quite incapable of dressing the part); a man who was, perhaps, slipping from subject to "object"—surely he was worthy of extra compensation. The selectmen let the Committee on Accounts know that they considered prior allotments to be "Inadequate to the Trouble & Expence" they had undertaken.[42]

Finally, states of mental illness, coupled with physical ailments or not, proved incapacitating. Judith Royal in New Gloucester (present-day Maine) was considered "subject to frequent fits of Delirium which incapacitates her from takein Cair of herself. . . ." The selectmen found that "by Reason of Lameness & Lunicy," she was "very troublesom." Andover's John Dunlop, a native of Ireland, was considered "a Cripple and non compis mentis." At the western border of the state, Rachel Galusha's mental anguish was rendered as a frontier tale. She was the daughter of Jacob Galusha, "who appeared to be a foreigner But came from the western part of Connecticut" to western Massachusets prior to Rachel's birth. Rachel was born on an unincorporated plot to the west of Hancock (cementing her state pauper status), but her father, "Being an old Man and very poor went away and abandoned her." The girl "wandered into Williamstown and was found in the woods in a helpless Situation Some time in the Spring of the year 1789 & take[n] care of." Her father had since died, she had no other relatives in the area able to support her, and the selectmen were confident that she would remain in a helpless condition: "[S]he is an Idiot Incapable to Do any thing towards her own Support—and will Doubtless remain So while she Lives." Contests over guardianships in Massachusetts made much of the distinction between the "lunatic," who suffered temporary delirium, and the "idiot," whose insanity was considered permanent. The determination between the two categories in court could tip the balance in deciding whether the disturbed person was allowed to dispose of their own estate. In the world of the state poor, however, "lunatic" and "idiot" were less distinct, both potent tools for ratcheting up the price for the town's "troubles."[43]

The pauper accounts raised the question both of the degree to which the charitable inhabitants of the commonwealth would respond to the plight of strangers and of the degree to which the General Court would reimburse their efforts with cash. By making "foreign settlement" the primary criterion for admitting paupers onto the state rolls, the court begged the question of whether the extent of misfortune itself warranted compensation. If paupers had a legal inhabitancy in Massachusetts or family that could be made to care for them, the General Court would not pay for their care, no matter how dire their circumstances. But if paupers' foreign settlement could be established, the government assumed liability. How much care could be asked for? How much allowed? Having cleared the hurdle of establishing a pauper's foreign settlement, towns and the Committee on Accounts would have to negotiate over bills for care, including those for medical attention. The elaboration of settlement laws ensured that there would be increasing numbers of "non-residents" and "strangers" within the state. Poverty would continue to be closely allied to affliction. What amount of charitable care for the outsider was allowable, what amount excessive?

V. MEDICAL NEGOTIATIONS

From the beginning of the pauper accounts in the 1780s, physicians in Massachusetts appear to have been quite interested in the program. With no hospital in which to receive clinical training, no dominating figure like Benjamin Rush around whom to coalesce, and no coherent medical philosophy, medical practice in the Bay State was subject to considerable negotiation and empirical testing. The state poor, whose care was paid for out of the commonwealth's treasury, represented a unique opportunity for medical practitioners to serve an ailing population, gain experience, and receive reimbursement.

Harvard's Medical School was founded in 1782 and appointed three professors over the next year: John Warren, Chair of Anatomy and Surgery; Benjamin Waterhouse, Professor of the Theory and Practice of Physic; and Aaron Dexter, Professor of Chemistry. Members of the General Court quickly sought to tie the medical school to the almshouse by means of a contract for care of the state paupers. In 1784 the Massachusetts House of Representatives considered a resolve calling for the appointment of a committee to contract with a physician or physicians to tend to the state poor, with "preference to the Professors of Physic, Anatomy and Chemistry . . . at the University [word "Harvard" crossed out] at Cambridge to take care of and provide medicines of the States poor as shall be lodged in the Alms House and work house at Boston." While the resolve did not pass, prominent physicians in Boston were able to secure the yearly contract in support of the state poor. John Warren, for example, served from May 1782 to May 1783. The almshouse was not an ideal environment in which to practice—indeed, complaints about the wretched and riotous condition of the sick there would be one impetus for the eventual creation of Massachusetts General Hospital, which opened its doors in 1821. But until the arrival of the hospital, medical practice at almshouses was a primary means for physicians to acquire clinical experience, train students, and earn an income.[44]

A surviving notebook kept by Dr. Nathaniel Appleton in 1783–84 helps us see the depth and range of medical attention that the state poor could receive. During the year, Appleton made 579 visits to the almshouse to see state paupers, often coming twice a day. In that time he tended 95 patients, 51 men and 44 women, seeing between 4 and 15 per day. He provided "advice & attendance," prescribed and delivered medicines, dressed wounds, ulcers, and abscesses, served as a midwife, and performed occasional operations, amputating toes and legs. The expenses varied considerably, ranging from patients whose treatment cost less than £1 to others whose chronic conditions were quite costly. Sarah Partridge's account over the year amounted to £76 14s. 1d. Ulcers on her neck and knee required dressings, replaced nearly every day, and a steady administration of medicine (which is not specified). At the end of his one-year term, Appleton asked the state for £543 16s. 1d.—a considerable sum.[45]

Facing this large medical account, the Committee on Accounts looked for possible deductions. They struck two persons from Appleton's list (who may have been properly the poor belonging to Boston, not the state's poor) and pared the account further by £163 0s. 6d., a 30% reduction. Appleton was allowed a little over £370. There was no charge of fraud nor any indication that any particular patient's account troubled the committee. After examining the bill, the committee must have had a conversation about what was reasonable. Medical attention was necessary, but the committee guarded against what it considered excessive.

While the committee rarely explained its deductions, in the occasional cases in which it did offer brief comments, we can see what kinds of practices it deemed beyond the bounds of state responsibility. The committee was, in the first place, on the lookout for what might be called therapeutic exuberance. When Dr. Oliver Prescott Jr. submitted extensive bills for "electrilizing" two of Groton's paupers in 1797, the committee cut his charge by a third. The committee considered Prescott's electrical treatment of Molly Kemp to be particularly outrageous. She was a "Strolling Girl" who had come to the town five years earlier and then wandered from "town to town," last residing in neighboring Westford before falling ill in Groton in 1795. The town was allowed twenty weeks of board for the girl at 6s. a week, a standard compensation. But Prescott's care strained credulity. He had started the medical treatments in May, one month before the town began providing Kemp board and nursing, and issued her a steady diet of cathartics. In July the "electrilizing" started, with three sessions that month and an additional charge for transporting the machine. Six sessions followed in August and six more in September before Prescott slowed his pace in November and December. After six more sessions in January, he submitted his bills to the town, for which he received payment in full. The committee went through the bills and noted repeatedly that Prescott was to be deducted "on account of the great Number of Electerilizing." On the final bill, the committee noted simply: "One third deducted on account of the poor woman Liveing Through such opporation."[46]

At the opposite end of the spectrum, the committee confronted the practice of therapeutic nihilism, based on the theory that the body could heal itself without medical intervention. Boston's doctors during the late eighteenth century tended to believe that the heroics of Benjamin Rush were nonsense, that his practice of bleeding frequently and copiously was based more on philosophy than experience. Perhaps this was the frame that Josiah Bartlett (1759–1820) had in mind during his service to the almshouse at Charlestown, Massachusetts, in 1797. As a recording secretary of the Massachusetts Medical Society, a post he held from 1792 to 1796, Bartlett would have been exposed to the idea that some cases called for the physician to step out of the way and allow the body to return to its natural equilibrium.[47] Charlestown's account with the state in 1797 featured four paupers, and Bartlett saw all of them. They were a varied group of men: two had arrived from London and lived in and around Boston for a few years (one as a tallow chandler, the other in an unknown occupation) before being committed to the poorhouse; another, born in Philadelphia, had arrived five years earlier from South Carolina; and lastly a sailor who had been shipwrecked off the northern coast of Maine, at Machias, and had secured passage to Hingham before making his way to Boston and finally Charlestown. Of the four, the bill indicated the immediate need for medical treatment only in the case of the sailor, Ebenezer Hubbert, who had been "much exposed" and "Sissed with the rehumitism" in the aftermath of the wreck.

Bartlett's detailed medical bill presents a therapeutically conservative response to each patient: an occasional purgative or emetic and a steady regimen of visits. After prescribing an emetic for Benjamin Long and visiting with him two times in January 1796, for example, Bartlett visited thirteen more times through February without administering any further medicine. In December he offered Long medicine on six occasions but visited with him sixteen times, twice on several of the days in which medicine was administered. From the committee's perspective, the number of visits relative to the treatment seemed extravagant. They docked the account by one-third, noting that this "considerable" deduction was justified "on acct of the number of visits & few medicines." Their challenge to Bartlett's bill was both medical and financial: treatment normally meant medicines, and visits were costly. Bartlett charged 50 cents a visit, no matter how many times a day he visited (some physicians would charge considerably less, or nothing at all, for subsequent visits on the same day). Bartlett's medicines, which varied in price depending on what was administered, were often half as much as his visits—25 cents or less. When physicians consulted with the elite, they might well take Bartlett's conservative approach, making repeated visits and simply offering advice, sometimes prescribing a special diet or sending patients off on a journey for health, on the theory that one should not rush healing or disrupt the body's natural tendency to restore itself if properly encouraged. But these were indulgences that could not be accorded the state poor. The demands of speed and limited budgets, from the committee's standpoint, argued in favor of drugs.[48]

Towns faced similar if not greater complexities in their relation to the Committee on Accounts. Because many doctors submitted bills directly to town selectmen and expected payment before the town heard back from the committee, selectmen risked losing money when the committee deducted from accounts. Those who boarded and nursed the poor also submitted their chits to the selectmen before final decisions were made.

In the end, towns hedged their bets. They prodded the committee with tales of "trouble," backing their stories with the depositions from doctors and those closest to the case; they continued to send in hefty bills for long-term board and nursing; and they mastered the bureaucratic forms demanded by the state, molding the pauper's story into a narrow issue of foreign settlement.[49]

Towns were on surest footing when they had already documented that a person was one of the state poor. Then, as the pauper aged and became infirm, it was possible to add incremental charges. Westborough, Massachusetts, for example, submitted an account for "taking care" of John Scudmore in 1786, including all charges that had accrued in earlier years. In 1798 the town added "extra nursing and medicines" to its standard claims for yearly board and occasional clothing. Both nursing and doctoring appeared regularly in the following years until Scudmore's death, at which time the town added funeral costs to the bill.[50]

But towns also learned to demonstrate to the committee that they were conscious of costs, making do with less. Franklin, Massachusetts, sent in a certificate with its bill in 1798 showing that it had auctioned off Alexander Read to the lowest bidder. Newburyport wrote of William Dow, "a person subject to epileptic fits, which frequently make him distracted," that "the sums charged for his Board have been the lowest price the overseers of the Poor could have boarded for." The selectmen of Freeport, Maine, somewhat indignantly noted their treatment by the committee the prior year; the town had suffered "a loss" in caring for Thomas Hovey, "an idiot," "for he was a troublesome Person and we have taken the cheapest Method to Support him." Such formulations, couched in the rhetoric of frugality, reflected the pressures that townsfolk might feel in requesting reimbursement for the care of the sick poor.[51]

For both the Committee on Accounts and the physicians and towns who submitted bills, two implicit rules seemed to govern the medical treatment of paupers. First, some degree of medical attention for the poor was necessary and would be approved. Even if deemed extravagant by the committee, medical costs were rarely denied entirely. Both physicians and towns may have tried to exercise restraint in offering medical treatment to paupers, knowing that excessive accounts would be met with disfavor. But all interested parties assumed that medical bills were a natural part of tending to the state poor and that some portion of them, at least, should be paid by the state.

The second assumption was that each medical case had to be decided on its own merits. The condition of each patient, the character of the treating physician, the location of care ("indoors" at an almshouse or "outdoors" in someone's home), the length of treatment, and the particular therapeutic modalities practiced by healers—all of these would be considered on a case-by-case basis. There were simply too many variables in play to make categorical decisions about state provision for medical care, save for cutting it altogether, which not even the severest critics of the state pauper system proposed. In the meantime, the numbers of towns asking to be reimbursed for the medical expenses of "their" state paupers increased ever more rapidly over the course of the eighteenth century.

VI. BOSTON, NEW BRAINTREE, AND THE FAILURE OF THE CORPORATION TO RELIEVE STATE PAUPERS

From the inception of the state pauper accounts in the 1780s until the first deep cuts in the accounts in 1820, an alternative to the pauper system was seriously considered just once. Reformers interested in cutting costs and addressing charges of misconduct at Boston's almshouse, where the largest number of the state poor resided, convinced the General Court that the state poor of that city should be contracted out to individuals or corporations in the commonwealth. Although the plan was finally defeated in 1793, the reform effort—and the larger debates it ignited—is worth close examination because it reveals how the paupers' debilitated physical state necessitated certain solutions to relief and precluded others.

In proposing that "corporations" might be contracted to care for Boston's state poor, reformers were both drawing on a long history of corporations in the commonwealth and tapping into a new development in the political economy of Massachusetts, one that would soon be prominent in the republic at large. The first corporation in Massachusetts was the Bay Colony itself, chartered in 1629. Under the new charter of 1691, the General Court was allowed, with the king's consent, to pass acts of incorporation. By the middle of the eighteenth century, the General Court allowed the incorporation of districts, churches, schools, and other organizations. In the wake of the Revolution, Massachusetts turned to incorporation earlier and more forcefully than any other state, anticipating a move that others would make later in the nineteenth century. The explosion of charitable institutions in post-Revolutionary New England—from about 50 at the time of the Revolution to 1,500 by 1820—was due in no small measure to acts of incorporation.[52]

By the 1790s, when the General Court invited "corporations" to contract with the government for the care of Boston's state poor, a new meaning of corporation was emerging. Incorporation laws were used by the state to sanction private enterprise for the economic development of the commonwealth. Private individuals gathered together and were incorporated for such purposes as building turnpikes and canals, establishing banks, creating insurance companies, and starting manufacturing companies. Government used its power to incorporate for internal improvements; private enterprise was meant to serve a public end.[53]

The "corporations" that made proposals to contract for Boston's state poor were other towns, and, as such, they embodied the older sense of the corporation as an essentially public body deriving its special rights and obligations from the government in whose name it acted on behalf of the public. In small and informal ways, towns in the commonwealth had long made such arrangements with each other—for example, paying for the support of impoverished persons who legally belonged to one town but resided in another where they were receiving public aid. As we have seen above, these arrangements between towns were necessary and convenient.

But in bidding for contracts to take over the responsibility for Boston's state poor, towns were also acting as corporations in the newer sense that the word suggested in the 1790s. Towns were not quite the same as individuals asking to be incorporated for the purposes of private enterprise. But in making proposals inspired by the possibility that they might profit from state contracts awarded to them as corporate bodies, towns were acting according to a new ethics in political economy: in pursuing their own separate interests, corporations might act for the greater good of the commonwealth.

We turn now to an extended legislative history of the plans that towns offered throughout the commonwealth to contract out for the state poor. Those plans, drawing on both older and newer conceptions of incorporation, finally failed in large measure because of intractable problems posed by illness—that caring for the sick in localities was considered the province of the town fathers and townsfolk alike and not outsiders, that it was considered cruel to remove the severely ill to places far afield, and that the new principles advocated by reformers threatened a spare and cruel treatment of the ill in the name of savings. But even as the reformers lost their bid to create a new system to handle the state poor, including the sick among them, the cost-cutting measures they introduced were adopted by the state in later years, adding fuel to an incipient movement to create a general hospital that could be a refuge for the sick and worthy poor who might be spared the ignominy of state provision (a topic taken up in the epilogue).

Boston's almshouse stood at the center of debates over medical care for state paupers in the 1780s and 1790s. There was broad agreement that many of the residents were "infirm," "impotent," "ailing," and "diseased," but the question of what kind of attention they should receive remained contentious.

Beginning in 1787, the General Court appointed committees to review the expenses of the state paupers residing at the almshouse and "consider the expediency of Distributing Said Poor Among the Several Towns in this Commonwealth." In November a committee of five praised the benevolence of the overseers but made it clear that costs could be cut. The committee was of the unanimous opinion that "a very Great Saving might be made to this commonwealth and the Poor as well provided for in sum Country Town," and they assured the court that they had received an offer that promised to care for the paupers at "one forth the Present charge."[54]

The proposal that the committee apparently had in mind had been drawn up by five gentlemen from Essex County, headed by Dr. John Manning, who was both a representative to the General Court from Ipswich and a prominent physician there. Manning and the others claimed that they could relieve "the good people of this Commonwealth from the burdens they are Labouring under" by taking the poor from the almshouse and providing them with "good Accommodations," "Good & wholesom Diet" and "every Necesary both for Sickness & Health" for 9s. per week. Savings would also come from reducing such "other Charges as medicine and attendance," which could be had for "three forth the sume which is Now allowed to the Town of Boston," all of which would reduce the pauper accounts by half. The commonwealth could retain its honor by discharging its duty to provide for the poor in comfort, but the economy and wholesomeness of country care would insure that benevolence for the few would not injure the many.[55]

In 1790, following a report that the Boston almshouse had been charging for residents who were no longer staying at the facility and had placed some residents who were properly the responsibility of the town on the state pauper rolls, a committee of inspection appointed by the General Court recommended that Boston strictly account for each state pauper and document his or her place of birth, age, marriage, and settlement history, requirements that the General Court later asked all towns to follow. Equally important, the committee suggested that it might be best to have the state poor distributed to other towns in the commonwealth, or to individual households within them, who would contract to care for the state poor, "taking them as they are Infirm or Sound old or young in Proportion," which might be done at three-quarters the cost of the present care in Boston. A new committee, including Dr. Manning, who had earlier tried to secure a contract for the state poor, was appointed to find likely applicants.[56]

In the meantime, Boston's selectmen and overseers sent their own set of complaints about the almshouse to the General Court. In a memorial to the court on January 14, 1790, Boston catalogued the difficulties it was under in caring for the poor. The town had incurred extraordinary burdens during the war that had never been adequately reimbursed by the state, and it had been overwhelmed by strangers since its "ports have been open to all nations."[57] Even as it protested that it was not being adequately compensated, the town began its own investigations into the almshouse and, in particular, the problem of tending the sick poor there. In July 1790 the town meeting discussed the possibility of building a hospital in the almshouse yard, but this was rejected as being impossible without "great Injury to the almshouse," which was already situated badly in the town and in need of restoration or removal.[58]

Although the hospital proposal was rejected, the investigation revealed significant challenges facing the almshouse, including a failure to properly attend to the sick poor. The almshouse was too crowded, with as many as three or four hundred residents in the winter months. There was no proper ventilation in the buildings nor was the yard "Spacious enough to Admit of Sufficient walk for the Patients," who were imperiled by the "Noxious" air pouring forth from the pits and vaults that lay too close to the dwelling houses. Most damning was the promiscuous mixing of sick and well, the virtuous and the vice-ridden, which bred disease and fostered moral contagion. "In all infirmaries, poor houses, and hospitals, it is considered an essential provision that separate and detached buildings should be appropriated for the reception and accommodation of such Persons, as are diseased, more especially those whose diseases are infectious," the committee noted. "The Almshouse in Boston, is perhaps the only instance known where Persons of every description and disease are lodged under the same roof and in some instances in the same or Contiguous Apartments, by which means the sick are disturbed, by the Noise of the healthy, and the infirm rendered liable to the Vices and diseases of the diseased, and profligate."[59]

The state paupers were centrally implicated in this morass. Accounting for many of the sick, they were the strangers who could not be warned out and those who freely roamed through Boston, now that the port was open to "all nations." When Boston's committee investigating the conditions of the poor returned its next report at the annual town meeting in March 1791, the sad circumstances of the state poor featured in its assessment. Although the almshouse was unsuitable in general and especially for the sick poor, establishment of an infirmary seemed impossible without further increasing Boston's debt or raising town taxes, neither of which the committee recommended.[60]

Given the troubling reports on the almshouse, the General Court announced in its June 1791 session that it would be accepting proposals from "each and every Corporation within this Commonwealth, who are disposed to contract to support the whole, or any part of the poor of the Commonwealth for ten years. . . ." Most favorable consideration would be given to proposals that "shall in the opinion of the Legislature be most conducive to the interest of the Commonwealth, and the comfort of the said poor." The call for proposals attracted significant interest throughout the state. By February 1792, nine towns, including Boston, had submitted plans for contracting with the commonwealth to tend to state paupers. The proposals came in from Stoughton in Suffolk County; Woburn, Stow, Framingham, and Holliston in Middlesex County; and Fitchburg, Westminster, and New Braintree in Worcester County. With the exception of Boston, the towns all contained under two thousand persons, and the smallest was a village of only eight hundred.[61]

Most of the proposals tried to anticipate the costs the towns would incur in tending to an ailing population, putting safeguards in place to avoid costly medical bills. Many towns sought to make competitive bids that would allow for some flexibility in difficult cases. When the committee chosen by the town of Holliston to contract for the poor offered to take all 173 of Boston's state paupers immediately and keep them for ten years, at 4s. 6d. per week for adults and half as much for children, it tried to ensure that the town would benefit from the healthy and not be weighed down by the costs of the ill. The committee asked to "have [the paupers'] labour," if they could work productively, but it also anticipated charges for the demise of many: 20s. for each adult and 10s. for each child to pay for funeral costs. The town of Framingham offered the lowest bid for boarding the paupers, at 4s. 4d. per week, promising to furnish them with "good & comfortable Houses, firewood, victualling, washing & lodging." But so that it might also "nurse Doctor & furnish all kinds of Hospital Stores," they asked for an additional £100 each year. And it recognized that some could not be moved from Boston due to their debility. Its agents would need "free use of an House situated at West Boston [evidently the "province hospital" used as a pesthouse in epidemics] being the property of the Commonwealth for the term, for the purpose of receiving such of said Poor as cannot be removed from the town of Boston." The town of Stow added to weekly board an extra "one penny per week for every pauper . . . to compensate for such extraordinary necessaries, as may be needful for the sick & other contingencies."[62]

Boston's committee appointed to contract for its own state poor unapologetically submitted the most expensive proposal of the lot, justified, in part, by the costs of the sick poor. The town's proposal required 6s. per week for adults and half as much for children. The charge, the committee suggested, was more than reasonable, given the many poor in the town who lay in dire circumstances. The "additional cost in providing . . . fuel, nursing & medical attendance" for persons who could not be removed, the committee indicated, was not sufficiently considered in other plans. Boston had absorbed such costs in the past as a matter of course, even tending to persons whom the town had the legal right to send elsewhere (to another town in the state, for example), but whose physical condition would not allow it. These long-standing commitments that Boston's overseers had honored in the past should not be jeopardized by "new principles" or wishful thinking.[63]

But when New Braintree offered its own proposal a few weeks after Boston, it won over the General Court with its comprehensive plan, which promised to protect the poor in a decent manner, preserving order and promoting good morals, all at less cost than Boston or any other town had proposed. New Braintree was located in central Massachusetts, furthest west of all of the towns proposing incorporation plans and, with a population of only 939 in 1790, one of the smallest. Situated in the "upland" where residents lived modestly and farming was difficult to conduct profitably, the town knew rural poverty. New Braintree had been part of the Regulation and the only site of bloodshed in Worcester County—two government men sent to the town had been fired on and wounded in February 1787. Like other upcountry townspeople who had participated in the Regulation, the residents of New Braintree had seen in the government's seizure of destitute farmers' property the specter of the ancien regime. Calling on "the people" to do their duty to regulate a government that was supposed to protect them, the town had drawn on the earlier language of the "protection covenant" and applied it to the new practices of republican governance.[64]

Now, in 1792, New Braintree sought a new way of promoting the vision of a well-ordered society. The town promised to support all paupers, regardless of age or sex, at 4s. 6d. per week. This would include "sufficient & comfortable House room, fire wood, meat, drink, cloathing, washing, beds and bedding; and also in case of sickness proper nurses and experienced physicians and medicines." Children would be schooled until they could be bound out as apprentices, and "prudent care should be taken in forming their morals, and in providing masters & mistresses for those who Should become apprentices as should consult their spiritual and temporal interest." The dead would be given "christian burials." All of this, taken together, was more than any other town had promised, and it was consistent with obligations that towns had taken on since the founding—the education of children, the regulation of the labor market, and care for the poor and infirm.[65]

Moreover, the town promised to take responsibility for all of the state paupers in the commonwealth, not only those living in Boston, provided that they did not reside farther away from New Braintree than Boston. Given its location at the center of the state, this would have meant that

New Braintree would have also taken on the state paupers from much of western Massachusets. Towns had long cared for local inhabitants who had no legal settlement in the town on an ad hoc basis, trying to recover costs of care from the afflicted person's place of legal residence within the state, or, if they had no legal residence, from the province and state accounts. But for a corporation to attend to the state poor in large swaths of Massachusetts, special provision needed to be made for the sick and disabled. The town recognized that there were persons too ill or disabled to be removed from Boston, and it promised to make some "suitable accommodations in the town of Boston, or some neighbouring town" until they could be safely taken to New Braintree. In the meantime, New Braintree offered to allow the selectmen of Boston, or of any other place where the state poor were being held until they could be removed, full ability to "visit inspect and superintend" the accommodations.[66]

New Braintree's plan was selected by the General Court's committee and presented to the state legislature, where the senate gave its approval while the house voiced objections. A new committee was appointed to iron out differences in March 1792, and although the bill was eventually approved by both houses, the governor did not sign it before the end of the legislative session, likely swayed by the objections that Boston's representatives had to the plan.

In the meantime, a debate ensued on the house floor in early June 1792, pitting Benjamin Josselyn (representative from New Braintree), Jerathmeel Bowers (of Somerset, in southeastern Massachusetts), and John Gardiner (representative from Pownalborough, in present-day Maine) against two of Boston's most prominent physicians, William Eustis and Charles Jarvis. Both Eustis and Jarvis served as representatives from Boston and had also been on the committee to devise Boston's plan for the state poor. The fight in one sense reflected a geographic division in the state—Boston men against those from the periphery. But the debate on the house floor, continued in a petition to the General Court submitted by Eustis, Jarvis, and other committee members from Boston, more deeply concerned the future envisioned for Boston as part of the public culture of the early republic.[67]

Although Gardiner was a representative from Maine in 1792 (a position he had assumed in 1787), he was a Boston native. After early training in Boston as a lawyer, he was sent for further study to London and Glasgow, where he was influenced by the Scottish Enlightenment. He lived in Wales and the West Indies before resettling in Boston in 1783, moving to Pownalborough three years later. Gardiner argued that while he retained "affectionate regard" for Boston, duty compelled him to recall that Boston's overseers had complained endlessly about their burdens. "Their groans were heard," and now a satisfactory solution had been found. Gardiner then took aim directly at Eustis and Jarvis. Boston's representatives to the General Court had entirely too cozy a relationship to public relief. Gardiner noted that Boston's overseers had allowed £150 to the master of the almshouse and £60 for the attending physician. Jarvis, who along with Eustis had served as almshouse physician, admitted that the salary was actually £100.[68]

Beyond money, however, Gardiner suggested that "humanity compelled him" to urge that the state poor be removed from Boston. If they were sent "to the country, they would draw a pure air, and not the polluted, putrid air of the holes they are often crammed into, in the Boston Alms-House." Gardiner reminded the legislature that in a recent smallpox outbreak, in which Dr. Eustis had tried to inoculate the poor who remained in town, those of means "flew to the country for a change of air, and a restoration of health." He hoped that the "Legislature would not debar the Poor from so great a blessing, but permit them to enjoy this common bounty of Nature, equally with the rich."[69]

In their rebuttal, Eustis and Jarvis drew on an older tradition championing Boston's special obligation, as the "Capital of the Commonwealth," to protect everyone living within the Bay State's borders. In a report written to the General Court, Eustis and Jarvis (along with other members of Boston's committee) reached back to the founding of the Massachusetts Bay Colony. "By laws of the Commonwealth, coeval with almost its settlement, it appears that when poor persons are by special acts of providence, or any other cause deprived of the means of support that it is a duty enjoyned on the Selectmen" to "provide them with the comforts and conveniences of life." The overseers of the poor were chosen annually as men evincing "the virtues of integrity, benevolence and charity," and they could make no "invidious distinction" between the poor of the town and the poor of the commonwealth. They had requested as reimbursements no more than the official allotments for the poor allowed by the state, which had, in any case, been insufficient, particularly during the late war. In fact, the overseers had been compelled to minister to the poor with their own money, placing their concern for their public obligation above their narrow self-interest in matters of the purse.[70]

This spirit of "benevolence and patriotism" differed starkly from the plans to hire out the poor presented by New Braintree, which seemed to Boston's representatives to be based primarily "on the principle of economy." There could be no more vivid display of the danger of operating on this principle than the spectacle of the ailing being removed from Boston in carriages to New Braintree. Surely "transportation by land fifty or sixty miles would be attended with pain distress and danger to the unhappy victims of this measure. . . ." How many months during the year would be "favourable to the removal of Invalids over a rough road?" And those engaged in the transportation would not be the people of New Braintree who had designed the plan but "waggoners and others who may not at all times be guided by principles of tenderness and humanity when it comes in competition with their own interest."[71]

The New Braintree plan threatened Boston's sovereign right to conduct its own affairs and the town fathers' duty to protect members of the town, particularly in cases of affliction. Boston's committee suggested that the illnesses of the state paupers would present insuperable difficulties. New Braintree had acknowledged that some of the sick poor could not be immediately removed. But the "contractors" plan to leave the sick in Boston at some suitable place until they could be transported to New Braintree would in effect "establish hospitals in the Town uncontrouled by the Inhabitants and Selectmen." This breach of town sovereignty, "unprecedented in the Government since the first settling of the country," would surely invite apprehension and complaint. What was to be done, for example, when "disease may prevail and disorders may and probably will arise in such an hospital, where the interference and controul of the Selectmen may be absolutely necessary to preserve the lives and health of the Inhabitants"? It was difficult to imagine even "the smallest district or plantation" allowing such an infringement of local control, never mind the most populous town in the region. The prerogatives of the town fathers to protect all residents—the sick, their caregivers, and the population at large that might be affected by disease, as in the case of smallpox—could not allow contractors residing outside the town to intrude on the authority of local selectmen.[72]

New Braintree's plan raised the specter of an "imperium in imperio," the inevitable conflict that arose when there were two sources of sovereignty where there should have been only one. That tension had animated much of the conflict in the imperial crisis. It had been a rallying cry of dissenters who feared the power of the central government intruding into their lives. And it was now an argument against incorporation. Those in favor of the craze to incorporate in early national Massachusetts could argue for the public benefits of the corporate form, of the ways in which private enterprises could advance a public good. But the afflictions of state paupers resisted such a solution. The very diseases that sent strangers to the almshouse made it unthinkable that they should be removed; to demand removal for those in extremity was simply too inhumane. And so long as they remained in the town of Boston, no outside authority should be authorized to regulate matters that inevitably impinged on public health.[73]

After considerable debate in the General Court, New Braintree's plan was rejected. The vote was extremely close; of the twenty-three votes cast, eleven supported the little town and its efforts to take in Boston's state paupers. New Braintree's advocates in the legislature were outraged, and the town asked for compensation. In anticipation of being awarded the state contract, New Braintree had incurred a "Great cost and Charge . . . in Erecting a large and commodious Building for the . . . accommodation of the said Poor." For this, and for the money spent to send agents from the town to wait on several legislative sessions, the town called for reimbursement, and the General Court agreed.

However, reformers achieved some success in cutting the costs of state poor relief. In the wake of the bidding war over its state paupers, and facing increased pressure to reduce its allotments, Boston agreed to lower its weekly costs for boarding the poor from 6s. a week to 5s., more in keeping with the plans presented by other towns. And Boston was forced to submit to further inspections. On the committee appointed by the General Court to inspect the almshouse were John Gardiner and Benjamin Josslyn (representative from New Braintree), both of whom must have relished the duty. Their tasks included a review of a "full and perfect list" compiled by the master of the almshouse, which would now include, in addition to the name, sex, and age of each inmate, an account of his or her health: "how and when they came into the Alms-House, and if any are sick and infirm, under what disorders they respectively labor & how long they have been confined."[74] The new requirements implied the need for closer supervision of medical care at the almshouse and the possibility that such inspections might save the state money.

In the coming years, the savings on state paupers did not, in fact, come primarily from supervising medical accounts. Medical bills charged by physicians for their care of the state poor, whether submitted by the physicians themselves or by towns and their inhabitants, continued to be negotiated with the Committee on Accounts. While the medical care provided to the indigent at Boston's almshouse continued to be scrutinized by the Committee on Accounts, sometimes with the help of local physicians, there was no concerted campaign to eliminate medical costs altogether, no assumption that somehow the connection between poverty and sickness might be eradicated.

But the scandals and reform efforts that centered on Boston's almshouse did have wide-reaching implications for state paupers throughout the commonwealth, including the sick poor. When Boston agreed to lower its weekly boarding costs for state paupers, in part as a response to other towns who offered to care for paupers more cheaply, it set a precedent. In the coming years, the Committee on Accounts would lower weekly rates allowed to board paupers, first in towns and then throughout the state.

In 1820 the General Court reversed its policy of allowing towns a proportion of the actual costs submitted for state paupers (each case would be vetted), instead setting a maximum rate of one dollar per week for adults and fifty cents per week for children. In the following decade, the General Court reduced allowable costs further, to seven cents per day for persons over age twelve and four cents for those younger. By lowering the allowance for state paupers, the General Court made it difficult for towns in the commonwealth to provide aid to strangers without going into debt themselves. And the reductions directed attention to the physical condition of the ailing state paupers as never before. In 1823 Boston's overseers of the poor defended themselves against charges that they had been too lenient on paupers residing at the almshouse, which critics suggested had become a refuge for the vicious and idle. The overseers were eager to show that the state poor, in particular, were ushered out of the almshouse as soon as possible: "Foreign paupers, unless disabled, have found no liberty to remain: And of the cargoes of poor emigrants that have arrived and found their way to the capital, scarcely a person has remained in the Alms-House after his recovery from sickness."[75] Ailing state paupers were expected to heal as quickly as possible and then leave the almshouse so as not to drain state coffers.

The ailing and extremely ill would still have a place in poor relief. But in the early republic, the sick poor were subjected to special scrutiny. Foreign paupers were the first group of the poor to face the imperative to recover speedily and leave the almshouse. The town poor would follow. For much of the eighteenth century, the sick had been counted among the "worthy" poor, whose condition warranted attendance and accommodation. In the early republic, reformers tried to differentiate further among the poor and to divide the sick into the worthy and unworthy. Who were the truly disabled and who, although ailing, might be made to work? Who warranted charitable assistance, and who could be sent to the almshouse or workhouse? These questions were central to the reformation of the poor laws and the emergence of the first voluntary hospital in New England, topics we will take up in the epilogue.

I. ENDURING PATTERNS IN THE
PROVINCE OF AFFLICTION

Over the course of the eighteenth century, much in the province of affliction remained the same. Each sickness created its own society. Families, households, and towns struggled to accommodate the "body in a state of becoming," rearranging schedules, calling in favors, asking for exceptions and allowances. Illness created an edgy, uneven texture in daily life, a blend of work, striving, and industry, of absence, delay, and excuse. Most fundamentally, illness posed basic questions for which there were no ready answers: Who would be finally responsible for life's misfortunes? How much could be asked of the sick, of their caregivers, and of the public at large? In striving to address these questions, New Englanders were forced to explore, define, and test the boundaries between family and household, household and town, town and province, state and nation.[1]

Their ongoing challenge was that the province of affliction regularly threatened to overrun the metropole of health. The burdens of any given illness often stretched well beyond the stricken, ensuring that suffering was a social affair. In the extreme, in cases of severe illness and in the uneasy knowledge that even an ordinary ailment might escalate into something more threatening, social suffering called forth political accommodations. Sickness became part of the making of New England, shaping society and government.

Family in New England was at once a source of affliction and a potent means to address its consequences. The family life course was affected by illness and other misfortunes. Childhood diseases, youths falling ill and getting injured as they were farmed out to new households in apprenticeships and labor exchanges, young men called to the field of battle or to sea and facing afflictions, young women asked to serve as nurses and to support "new" families or required to remain home to nurse elderly parents—these and more prosaic scenes of malaise forced families to confront sickness as a potentially major obstacle to maintaining a competency. Competency lay at the intersection of a corporeal "luck of the draw" and a family's resilience and resources in the face of those challenges. The intensity and magnitude of illness in family life could separate the competent from the dependent. Families with the financial means and the social credit born of neighborly exchange, deployment of caregivers, and kindnesses stood a far better chance of remaining afloat than the poor, the disconnected, and others on the margins. But everyone faced the specter of dependency in the wake of serious illness.

Poor law provision, which was closely bound to affliction, shaped family life as well. First, the poor law offered a social safety net of sorts for families. While spare and a means of last resort, public provision to care for the poor, supported with taxes and sustained by the imperative of the town to protect its own, ensured that legal inhabitants could claim succor in their time of need. Second, the poor law constructed a particular definition of family by stipulating lines of responsibility that bound family together: the line joining grandparents, parents, and children was deemed primary, and in the absence of a family of whatever constitution being able to care for itself, the law in effect defined filial bonds with mandates concerning financial responsibility. Before poor rates could be applied, each member in the determined line was urged to tend to what the law considered their special burden. That many family members resisted this pressure, claiming their own limited means (and often their own calamities that made taking on additional care impossible), only elaborates the point: the accommodation of illness was a moment to define and test the boundaries of family, and to point to bonds of responsibility, even and especially when none were readily accepted.

Household was an even more heterogeneous and fluid social category than family. And yet it is in the houses of New England, with their changing assemblage of persons of different ages, blood relatives, distant kin, apprentices, hired workers, enslaved laborers, long-term visitors, and an array of neighbors and friends, that the appearance of illness could sharpen the blurred boundary between family and household, especially when visitors or apprentices were stricken.

In the numerous comings and goings in the house, recorded by diarists as a kind of social register, it was not uncommon for a visitor to become sick and need care away from their family of origin. To "fall" sick was an apt metaphor, suggesting a sinking down in a new locale, temporary roots established because of the risk of removal. Extremity commanded that care and accommodation be arranged. The costs would have to be attended to later, worked out informally between host and other parties deemed responsible. When a family like the Parkmans had a daughter or son fall ill abroad, it was ultimately incumbent upon them to arrange retrieval and to negotiate bills with their host. When a stranger passing through was sick enough to preclude removal, the long and difficult process of sorting out bills might involve turning to the town of legal inhabitancy, the selectmen of that town scurrying to find responsible relatives, and the courts, province, and state drawn in by default, as we have seen, if no one could be found.

In times of health the line between children and youths residing in the household as blood kin and those residing as laborers could be blurred, but sickness could sharpen the distinction. In New England's labor market, children and youths were exchanged between households in the name of training and discipline that would finally allow them to participate in a "free" labor market (though one managed by town fathers). A family that took on an apprentice promised good training and care in exchange for productive labor. But what constituted proper care in time of affliction? And at what point did the illness or injury of an apprentice that made it impossible to labor, or to labor well, dissolve the bonds of obligation? There were no hard-and-fast rules, but those persons whose belonging to a household depended on their productive performance within it were vulnerable to removal. The family of origin was called and asked to address the shortfall, but arguments and final resolutions could wind up in court, perhaps to determine whether improper care or abuse had brought on debilitating affliction in the first place, or whether a child or youth had a predisposition toward debility.

In the contests involving enslaved laborers deemed less than fully able, despite sellers' assurances of "soundness" at purchase, sickness embodied the paradox inherent in being both person and productive property. Was an enslaved person's debility the fault of a duplicitous previous owner or slave trader, who had given a false promise of the enslaved person's soundness at sale? Was it the fault of a negligent or abusive current owner, who had caused the enslaved person's illness through improper treatment? Was it the fault of a recalcitrant enslaved person himself or herself, who claimed illness as a pretext for unwillingness to work? Even as families like that of Elizabeth Porter Phelps went to extreme lengths to care for an enslaved laborer considered part of their household, the possibility that a "defective" enslaved worker might be sold marked a sharp boundary between family and household.

Family and household were further shaped—and tested—by town authority during times of epidemic, particularly smallpox. As we have seen, New England's successful regimen of strict quarantine was carried out with a vigilance and compliance that eluded other regions in British North America. That Ashley Bowen's Marblehead could be rocked by the sudden infection of a seventy-nine-year-old matriarch could be viewed as a kind of perverse achievement. The public health strictures that succeeded in protecting enough inhabitants from infection in their youth and beyond ensured that many were vulnerable later in life. But families and households did not necessarily comply peacefully with these strictures nor did towns exert an absolute authority. A more nuanced picture is warranted. For in contagion, the routine ways in which illness was socially accommodated became fuel for further infection. The social gatherings and watching through the night, the visits with food and fuel and medicine, the daily inspections that were dutifully noted in diaries and town records—those on the decline, those on the mend—all ran counter to the basic need to isolate the sick. And social interaction, the stuff of friendship and neighborly goodwill and, indeed, survival, was not easy to stop in its tracks. Town fathers were obliged to board up and mark houses of the infected and police entrance and egress. Members of an infected house might face an excruciating choice of boarding together in place, or removing the ill to a pesthouse, a fate that could be as ignominious as it was deadly. Parents also might need to decide the fate of their children residing in a sick house abroad. Families and households had some agency, but their choices were circumscribed by towns in a time of crisis.

Even as that grim calculus took place, town governance worked to prevent the fraying of community bonds, often disapproving of inoculation campaigns because the inoculated might not adhere to isolation, visiting and carrying on the imperatives of workaday life while they were still contagious. And in the meantime, with infection afoot, fear took hold in social relations, gossip prevailed, and the specter of secrecy and invisible danger loomed. Neighbors demanded that infected beds and other objects remain clear of their property, out of breezeways that might carry infection to the vulnerable, and, most starkly, that the dead be removed in such a way that their infected essence and the risk it carried would not favor one household over another.

The town in the extremity of epidemic, and especially of smallpox, thus exerted authority *and* made accommodations to families and households, demanding individual sacrifices and protecting community members in the service of the public good. To be sure, the town's demands on families and households were met with a host of infractions and a steady register of concerns. And yet New Englanders mustered a compliance that proved impossible to achieve elsewhere in the British colonies. Illness became the occasion for town authority to enact a collective sensibility, a drama in which the excruciating sufferings of the few would not be allowed to threaten the health and well-being of the town.

To this tangle of local claimants and caregivers grappling with the demands of affliction, we need to add the province and state. Sickness in eighteenth-century New England has a place in a larger story about broad patterns of disruption and dislocation coursing through the Atlantic world. War and epidemic stretched the boundaries of family, household, and town responsibility for their own many miles from local society. When sick soldiers were left behind in the wake of expeditionary warfare and needed to be fetched from the theater of battle, when veterans returned and "secretly" infected a town with camp distempers or returned home incapacitated by wounds and debilitating blows to their constitutions, when the Atlantic carrying trade that allowed the region to flourish also meant encounters with the fevers and mysterious maladies carried aboard ships and spread from ports through infected goods or ailing sailors—in these cases and more, as families, households, and towns struggled to care for their own, and define exactly who would be responsible for life's perils, they turned to the province and later the state for help. The petitions that were fielded by the General Court pledged humble allegiance to a government that was expected to protect the people. With heads down and hands out, the suffering and those acting on their behalf filled their petitions with stories of affliction and asked their governors for relief.

A remedy that began in the "catastrophe" of early settlement and colonization became increasingly routine in the eighteenth century. The momentum from the dislocations of the early settlement carried into the eighteenth century and became routinized in petitions to the General Court, an instance of reaching upward and outward when there was nowhere else to go. The petitions reveal just how common extreme and disruptive events could be. For much of the century, a political remedy was sought for extreme social suffering.

At the close of the eighteenth century, government began to push back against these accelerating demands. New Englanders asked the new national government to apply the healing balm of money to the wounds of warfare. The rejection faced by soldiers and those petitioning on their behalf for disability pensions had much to do with a recognition that should such petitions be granted regularly, a flood would be unleashed. Henry Knox's notion of "decisive disability," which challenged illness as a cause of debility, not only invoked local society as the desirable locus of rightful provision, but also pointed to the impossibility of accommodating the stories that were so much a part of New England's past: that the burden of one person's suffering was borne by many; that injuries and misfortunes from long ago might manifest themselves years later. An integrated story of affliction with temporal depth and wide social implication was simply impossible for a national government to comprehend.[2]

At the same time, the province poor accounts that had emerged from the dislocating violence of King Philip's War and subsequent years of warfare entangling New England in the imperial struggle between the British and French ballooned in the wake of the Revolution, leading to restrictions in the state pauper accounts that replaced them. The warning-out system and the increasingly complicated laws restricting inhabitancy became a means of addressing poverty and mobility that resulted in increasing numbers of "strangers" roaming through the state—and rising bills for their care. When care could be accommodated within local society, as it was for legal inhabitants, each town had discretion over allowances, which varied according to the circumstances of the ill and local resources. The new state pauper system, by contrast, elaborated bureaucratic means to standardize rates for anyone in Massachusetts without legal residency. With the move to comprehend paupers as a class, regardless of individual circumstances, it was possible for the state to reduce costs across the board.

By the turn of the century, the care for the sick stranger, the person without legal inhabitancy in Massachusetts, became an emblem of all that was wrong with the poor laws. The state pauper program was the stuff of scandal and disgruntlement, with charges that towns were moving their legal inhabitants to state rolls in order to spare town coffers and complaints that the state was reducing compensation. Finally, in the mixing of the worthy poor and the stranger, critics saw moral corruption and particular dangers facing the sick poor.

We now turn to new arguments and arrangements concerning social welfare around 1820, new ways of grappling with misfortune and frank assessments of the undesirability, if not impossibility, of continuing in an earlier vein. We will examine developments in the accommodation of the sick poor within poor law provision as well as the new medical charities that emerged in the early nineteenth century, including the first voluntary hospital in Boston. All major stories in their own right, we can simply offer a brief view here, enough to see developments that would take hold more firmly later in the century.

II. A NEW WORLD UNFOLDING

At the heart of the change was a reassessment of social suffering, the idea that each sickness implicated not just the stricken, but many people in his or her orbit. The residents of the province of affliction had recognized the power of social suffering and did their best to accommodate its demands: they understood that illnesses from prior years might return and consume sufferers and those around them; that sickness meant not just the loss of labor of the afflicted, but also wrenching changes in the lives of those who needed to labor in their stead; and that in the most dire of situations, governing bodies at all levels might be called on for some degree of relief. These accommodations were not easy, and the strains in sorting out lines of responsibility for affliction became a crucial part of defining the boundaries between family, household, town, province, and state.

The new approaches to the sick poor in the early nineteenth century challenged the ideas and practices of social suffering in two very different ways. Reformers interested in revising poor law practices increasingly placed the blame for sickness and poverty on the sick themselves, who had formerly been considered the worthy poor. Perhaps the sick had been imprudent in husbanding resources for a future time of malaise; more insidiously, perhaps the sick were taking advantage of public generosity. The ill and otherwise afflicted might be made to work off their debts through redemptive labor in the almshouse and workhouse, and institutions might be devised to rationalize care and to limit its costs.

Taking a different tack, champions of new medical charities directed at the sick poor tried to rescue the worthy sick from the indignities of poor law provision, which was becoming increasingly punitive and spare. Charities like the dispensary could allow persons and families otherwise supporting a competency to receive free medicines without the shame of public discovery. Female charitable societies could offer basic articles of food, clothing, and other means of aiding the sick, removing the sting of want from the sick poor and other sufferers and offering modest comforts in its place. And the hospital could offer succor and the promise of cure to those with laudable ambition, persons who had left home in search of new opportunities, but who found themselves bereft of the social connections necessary to sustain themselves in affliction. Medical charities aimed to use the new power of association to enhance aid where traditional social and political means had failed, and in so doing, to offer, particularly in the case of the hospital, an institutional means to shore up worthy individuals.

Despite such innovations, the obstinate challenges of the province of affliction persisted into the new age. The force of illness overwhelmed newly devised plans. The seriously sick could not be made to work, much less moved easily to new institutions, whether to the workhouse or the hospital. Extreme cases resisted easy solutions. And the costs of care endured as a vexing problem for poor relief and medical charities alike. The poor law accommodation of the sick swelled the public outlays to such an extent that draconian cuts were called for, subjecting poor law reformers to charges of cruelty. Medical charities, in the meantime, offered aid but, given their limited means, only to a select few.

What emerged in the early nineteenth century were new ways of framing old and seemingly intractable problems. However, one sees most clearly how the force of affliction resisted ready solution, generating problems that would endure well into the nineteenth century and beyond.

III. NEW APPROACHES TO THE SICK POOR AND POOR LAW PROVISION: THE QUINCY REPORT

In a remarkably ambitious and influential investigation into the poor laws of Massachusetts (undertaken at the behest of the General Court in 1820 and published a year later), a committee chaired by Josiah Quincy III sought to quantify a "pernicious," "palpable," and "increasing" threat that needed to be addressed by the legislature. The report was based on questionnaires sent to all towns in the commonwealth asking about the numbers on poor relief, what accommodations had been made, and what costs had been associated with care. Although the total returned fell short of Quincy's aims—162 towns sent in responses, just over half the towns in the state—he was impressed with the "intelligence, precision, and zeal" that the complying towns had demonstrated. While a complete report would have to await additional responses, Quincy suggested that what he had on hand was more than enough to make summary comments and recommendations, if not detailed plans for revising pauper provision throughout the state. The legislature agreed and ordered the report to be widely reprinted, with copies to be given to local overseers of the poor and selectmen, who were in charge of poor relief in each town. And in the meantime, beginning in March, the newspapers published digests of the report's central findings.[3]

The findings were unsettling. Judging from expenditures on state paupers alone—cash payments by the state to aid persons with no legal settlement in Massachusetts—the rise in poor relief had been substantial and alarming. Between 1801 and 1820, the cash outlays from the public treasury had risen from $28,000 to $72,000, well more than doubling in two decades. Even in England, where the "evils of pauperism" were considered "desperate and malignant in their nature," it had taken three decades to witness such increases. While care for paupers might present overwhelming fiscal challenges, it was the malignancy of *pauperism* that posed a more serious threat to the society, economy, and governance in the new republic. The ultimate threat was moral contagion, that the habits of the pauper would infect the industrious and lead to the dissolution of a free society.[4]

In one sense, the report rehashed long-standing critiques of poor relief in New England. The poor laws, as we have seen, had been subject to scrutiny and revision over the course of the eighteenth century, and Boston alone had undertaken several inquiries into expenses and potential fraud at its almshouse. While the report drew on English authors who pointed to the poor laws themselves as an important cause of poverty, it might as well have cited homegrown critics to bolster its case. The criticisms that poor relief removed the incentive to work, that misguided charity encouraged bad habits, and that vice itself would lead to poverty—these were commonplaces in the discourse on poverty. The belief that moderation and prudent self-regard, the hallmarks of a temperate lifestyle, were critical to well-being could be found in everything from private correspondence to advice freely doled out in conduct guides and the columns of the public prints.

What distinguished the Quincy Report was the cumulative effect of seeing, for the first time, just how sharply poor relief costs were rising throughout the state and just how many towns had experimented with new modes of relieving the poor in recent years, especially in the construction of almshouses to shelter the poor and farms on which the poor were set to work. Both the costs of poor relief and the rise of the almshouse had important implications for the understanding of bodily misfortune, including illness, as a major cause of poverty. In a world in which poor relief was divided between the "worthy" and "unworthy" poor, sickness had commonly exempted the poor from accusations of moral failing; the afflicted had been reduced to dependency through no fault of their own. The Quincy Report pointed to a new ambivalence regarding the sick poor.

At the heart of the matter, Quincy maintained, was the difficulty of discerning the worthiness of recipients of relief, a problem that pointed to the ambiguities of the "body in a state of becoming." Eighteenth-century folk knew that they lived in a perilous and contingent world. One might be healthy today but stricken tomorrow; one might be called upon to mind the sick or fill in for those who tended them; one understood that alongside the workaday world of muscle, movement, and industry, there was one of absence, excuse, and delay fueled by affliction. Quincy's genius lay in his probing and synthetic discussion of the social and corporeal vagaries that the eighteenth-century world had accommodated—sometimes with uneasiness, always with sacrifice, and finally with a sense that a world of perils demanded no less. He argued that such a world must be understood in all of its complexity so that a new response to it might be devised.

Poor relief rested on a convenient fiction that sharply distinguished between the "impotent" and "able" poor, those "incapable of work, through old age, infancy, sickness or corporeal debility" and those "capable of work, of some nature, or other; but differing in the degree of their capacity, and in the kind of work, of which they are capable." While the rhetoric of poor relief turned on this crisp division, the boundary, so easily delineated on paper, was quite difficult to police in practice. There was extreme "difficulty of discriminating between the able poor and the impotent poor and of apportioning the degree of public provision to the degree of actual impotency." To determine *actual* impotency meant a careful unpacking of social, physical, and mental capacities that varied among individuals and might well change over time.[5]

The problem, Quincy explained, lay in the "shades of difference between, the pauper, who, through impotency, can do absolutely nothing, and the pauper, who is able to do something, but that, very little." For even within what would seem to be such a narrow divide—between those utterly unable to help themselves and those able to work in some degree for their sustenance—lay subtle distinctions that could not be comprehended in law and "removed by any legislative provision." Along the chain linking those able to help themselves in some degree and the totally impotent lay "so many circumstances of age, sex, previous habits, muscular, or mental, strength," that "society is absolutely incapable to fix any standard, or to prescribe any rule, by which the claim of right to the benefit of the public provision shall absolutely be determined." No two individuals were alike in capacity, it seemed. Even if one could think, in the abstract, of the different capacities of the sexes, a distinction that had grown sharper in public rhetoric since the Revolution, other categories of difference blurred the distinction: one's personal history, one's peculiar habits, and the changes that inevitably resulted from the effects of age upon one's body made the consideration of capacity to work an exceedingly difficult one.[6]

That those considerations had been "entrusted to men in good, generally in easy, circumstances" exacerbated the problem. Overseers of the poor were surely men of good character and benevolent disposition, "guided by sentiments of pity and compassion" that made it impossible for them to refuse relief to those in want. But such charity had ill effects, inadvertently encouraging "habits of idleness, dissipation, and extravagance among the class, which labor." As overseers became overwhelmed by tender feelings of sympathy and the exacting labor to "ascertain the exact merit of each applicant," aid flowed indiscriminately, sometimes being "excessive" and at other times "misplaced." The poor themselves soon came to think of their relief "as a right" and something that "they calculate upon . . . as an income." And with that calculation, they lost in proportion to their degree of relief "just pride of independence, so honorable to man, in every condition," a fatal source of corruption in the republic.[7]

The report presented abstracts from towns across Massachusetts in support of these claims, praising the salutary role of almshouses that had the character of "Work Houses, or Houses of Industry, in which work is provided for every degree or ability in the pauper. . . ."[8] Town after town reported that the prospect of sending a family member to the almshouse, as opposed to offering them "out relief" in their homes or those of relatives or caregivers, was enough to keep many from asking for alms. For those who were sent to the almshouse, work proportionate to their abilities could be found, and all the while, the poor contributed to the upkeep of the property. Towns without almshouses aspired to build them as soon as possible.

Even the vexing question of medical care seemed to be addressed by almshouse discipline. As Andover reported, "In many cases where the Overseers have allowed those who have had strong aversions to going to the Poor House" to remain on out relief, the town had "been under the necessity of paying large sums for doctors' bills, nursing, &c. which would not have accrued, had they been at the Alms house." The town happily reported that their poorhouse, with eighty acres of land, allowed for men to labor on the farm and women to be "employed in spinning, weaving, making clothes for the family, taking care of the sick, &c."[9]

Heath, a town of some 1,122 souls in the northwest part of the state, argued that a move away from out relief and toward the poorhouse would provoke just the sort of culture shift necessary to contain medical costs. The compulsory nature of the poor law ensured that "every man knows that as soon as he or his friends become unable or unwilling to support themselves," an application to the overseers of the poor would have legal backing. And so, "a man who makes application on behalf of a sickly or aged relative, claims the privilege of taking care of him" at home, all the while "charging at pleasure, for every item of trouble and expense." The respondents from Heath argued that while the honest poor should be well provided for, they considered that "the greater part of those who are supported by towns, become poor through idleness, extravagance and intemperance." And when sickness inevitably followed from their poverty, the town was obliged to pay the wages of sin. "[W]hen disabled by sickness or old age, a subsistence, as abundant as they even wished, takes away every inducement to lay up something for a rainy day; such ought to be immediately sent to the Poor House. . . ." Heath lamented that such institutions were lacking in many towns. And to add insult to injury, the poor laws benefited the ports, where transients wandered and accepted low-paying work. When "disabled by disease, they become a charge upon the towns [where] they are settled, instead of deriving their support from those who had the benefit of their labor." A grand revision of the poor laws requiring towns where the sick fell ill to pay their bills would remedy the injustice. In the meantime, Heath championed the establishment of more poorhouses across the state, as part of a larger reform in manners that would ameliorate the costs of illness.[10]

But despite these new and seemingly promising developments, the returns in the Quincy Report also revealed problems that had long beset eighteenth-century New Englanders in the province of affliction. The costs of caring for the sick continued to loom large, even in the almshouse setting. In answer to challenges by inland towns like Heath, port cities pleaded that they, too, were affected by the unremunerated costs of the transient ill. Chief among the complaints was that the sick poor might avail themselves of almshouse care and then abscond; in effect, like an enslaved person who might "steal themselves" by running away, the sick could consume healing resources—medicine, nursing, shelter—and then leave. As Charlestown reported, its "proximity to the Navy Yard, Marine Hospital, State Prison, &c.," ensured a steady supply of state paupers who frequented the almshouse and workhouse, "some insane, some distracted, some blind and maimed, and some with broken limbs, who cost us from 3 to 5 dollars per week to restore them." These "foreigners" over whom "we have no control," freely "rove from town to town, to avoid labor, that but few of them who can procure the means of vicious indulgence, continue any longer with us than to be recovered from disease, when they seize the first opportunity to abscond. . . ."[11] But the problem was not confined to the ports. Lanesborough, in western Massachusetts, opined that "Overseers ought to be authorized to bind out to hard labor, in all cases, Paupers who have obtained their health, to pay the expenses incurred by the town. Instances have happened, where healthy persons have been committed to the gaol, and taken the poor man's oath, and the town have been obliged to support them in prison, and when out, the town has no remedy but to sue for the expense, and recommit them, which is no remedy at all."[12]

Taken as a whole, the Quincy Report suggested that the answer to these difficulties consisted in greater discipline of the poor and an increased ability to exact labor in exchange for care—in short, a restoration of order that would have the idle, who now included the sick, pay in wages of redemptive labor and self-sacrifice.

But critics of poor reform made it plain that such goals were fraught with difficulties, particularly regarding care for the ill and ailing. The sharpest rebuttal came from Boston's overseers of the poor. In the wake of the Quincy Report, a report issued in 1823 by the city council of Boston charged Boston's overseers of the poor with dereliction of duty: by providing generously to the poor, they showed blatant disregard for the cost to the public. More importantly, the overseers demonstrated an unwillingness to cull from the almshouse all those able poor who might be sent to a newly built House of Industry in South Boston.

In a long refutation of the charges, the overseers defended themselves in the familiar terms of the province of affliction, pointing to the difficulty in distinguishing the able from the disabled and diseased. An inspection had suggested that there were at the almshouse "78 sick, 77 children, and 9 maniacs and idiots," which left a balance of 155 "able-bodied poor."[13] But on closer inspection, the overseers noted that many of the so-called able-bodied were "old and decrepid individuals, of worn out constitutions," along with those who worked as carpenters, nurses, and servants to help keep the institution afloat. "[T]he line between the 'able bodied' poor and the infirm, was not so plainly marked as had been imagined . . . there were gradations between health and strength on the one hand; and disease and imbecility on the other, so that it would in many instances be difficult to tell whether an individual more properly belonged to one class or another."[14] For their part, many of the poor under scrutiny in the almshouse voted with their feet and refused to be removed to the House of Industry.

Where the Quincy Report had indicted overseers for overindulgence of the poor, positing a future in which every condition would find its institutional match and the requisite discipline to contribute to the commonwealth, the overseers' response reflected a social imagination rooted in eighteenth-century life, one that conceived of out relief as a means of preserving the honor of the industrious who had fallen. Was it really warranted to "withhold relief, or compel to receive it in the Alms-House, the family of an industrious mechanic, or laborer, who, by any temporary sickness or casualty, was thrown upon the wife and helpless children for support"? That "relief granted to the individual extends[,] in most cases, to whole families" heightened the stakes of charity. Social suffering could be alleviated by benevolent and judiciously allocated relief, without the need to inflict unnecessary pain, the *"dread* of absolute want," and injury to ambition and reputation.[15]

Critics of the almshouse solution to affliction queried the fate of the worthy poor, particularly the sick, within the almshouse regime. That question had arisen in the late eighteenth century and continued after the building in 1801, at Leverett Street in Boston's West End, of a grand new almshouse, designed by the prominent Boston architect Charles Bulfinch and considered "second only to the State House among the buildings of Federal Boston."[16]

Within just a few years, the problems that had plagued earlier almshouses recurred.[17] Reflecting on his recent experience as physician to the almshouse in 1805, James Jackson drafted a lengthy critique. With insufficient space for the sick in the almshouse, they could not be gathered in the fresh air and properly attended to; without suitable nursing staff, patients were compelled to care for their neighbors; the budget for food was restrictive; and the physician's meager salary coupled with his responsibility for supplying medicines to the patients pushed him toward compromising his professionalism. Must the physician "not be greetly tempted, when he can do it with safety, to deprive the sick & miserable of the means of relief that his own family can be better supplied with bread? Will not his own necessities make him insensible to the calls of others, whose moral characters perhaps render them in his view of little importance to society?" In straitened circumstances, the beleaguered physician might confound the sick poor with the vicious poor.[18]

Jackson saw hope for physician and patient alike in a new order. In addition to the worthy infirm, the insane, and the vicious poor, he had detected a new class at the almshouse, one that was outpacing the others: those who could support themselves in ordinary circumstances but had been reduced to dependency in sickness. These persons, of whom he had seen several hundred, would have bright futures if they could be treated quickly and expertly. Without care, however, their residence in the almshouse would familiarize them with "the idea of dependence" and acquaint them with those "who have perhaps been more indiscreet, more debauched than themselves." Proper treatment could rescue these persons from such moral debility and restore them to society.[19]

Despite the logic that had fueled the proliferation of almshouses across the state—growing numbers of poor, the attraction of lower costs of care, and the possibility of redemption and reform through work—the institution had, according to Jackson, turned into a breeding place of corruption, as dangerous to the inhabitants as to the physician who might lose his moral bearings.[20] Within five years, Jackson was successfully making the case for the first voluntary hospital in New England. Chartered in 1811, Massachusetts General Hospital admitted its first patients a decade later. Hospital care was designed to address what a threadbare system of public entitlements could not, by providing the compassionate care to the sick poor that society, at its core, required. Other medical charities took aim at the same problem. Comfort and care could be accompanied not only by the removal of dreaded want, but also by an opportunity and impetus for healthy living; and in an age of honest but poor wage earners living away from home—apprentices, mechanics, domestics, and other laborers—aid with medical expenses could encourage industry and ambition and provide the support that would have come from family, town, and state in the eighteenth century.

IV. NEW APPROACHES TO THE SICK POOR: THE GROWTH OF MEDICAL CHARITIES AND THE MASSACHUSETTS GENERAL HOSPITAL

After a period of relatively slow growth compared to other colonies, charitable and humanitarian societies proliferated in post-Revolutionary New England. As Gordon Wood has observed, "In the decade following 1787, New Englanders formed 112 charitable societies; between 1798 and 1807, 158 more; and between 1808 and 1817, 1,101" were created.[21] Republican reform addressed many elements of society and politics, including education, marriage, crime and punishment, and the spread of the gospel. The plight of the sick, and especially the sick poor, became a focus of this reforming zeal, with many new institutions arising in Massachusetts in the first decades of the nineteenth century.

By the time of the Quincy Report (1821), multiple medical charities in Massachusetts sought to help the sick poor of upstanding moral character, whose particular circumstances would, absent aid, threaten them with the almshouse and the moral and physical dangers therein. With a

$5 annual subscription, members of the Boston Dispensary (founded in 1796) could recommend two worthy clients who would receive free medical care, including a visit with a physician (either at the client's residence or at a clinic) and medicines. Aid also came from all-female associations that joined together on a range of projects in the early republic, including those dedicated to assisting the sick poor.

Finally, there was Massachusetts General Hospital (MGH), which opened its doors in 1821 and could be spied from the West Boston Bridge along with the Harvard Medical School (which moved from Cambridge to Boston in 1810). MGH arose at a juncture in early nineteenth-century New England at which a voluntary, charitable hospital, separate from care provided under compulsory poor laws, was deemed essential. The extended campaign for the hospital (and a parallel campaign for an insane asylum) reveals new concerns about the limitations of local society in providing for its own, new anxieties about the problems created by what might in other contexts be considered laudable ambition, and finally a hope that the new institution, as both a place and a governing metaphor, might secure the region, and the region's capital, Boston, its rightful place in a new economic age.[22]

The decade-long case for the hospital was made in private correspondence, in circular letters passed to influential citizens, in newspapers columns, and in a series of pamphlets. Leading the initial charge were John C. Warren and James Jackson, who were to become, respectively, the first surgeon and physician at the hospital. After its incorporation in 1811, they were joined by the Trustees of the hospital, a varied group of New England merchants, manufacturers, legislators, and inveterate reformers, including Josiah Quincy III, whose critique of the commonwealth's provision for the poor coincided with his advocacy for the new hospital.

Jackson and Warren's first address to the public in 1810 promoted the hospital as the answer to several significant problems painfully familiar to anyone living in the province of affliction. While those with means might well provide for themselves in a time of misfortune, the burdens of illness could become overwhelming. Warren and Jackson maintained that even the idle deserved care as a Christian duty. But the force of affliction threatened many more: those suffering from "protracted disease," including insanity, which devastated the ill and overwhelmed their families with the burden of care; those with "good and industrious habits," the mechanic and journeyman early in a career, whose savings would evaporate with serious illness; the domestic sidelined in sickness, forced to lodge "in the most remote corner of the house, in a room without a fireplace," even as the mistress charged with care of the household would face "unusual labours which are thrown on her at a time perhaps when she is least fitted to perform them"; women "unable to provide for their own welfare and safety" during childbirth and lying in; and those struck by an "extraordinary disease" calling for special expertise or by an accident in need of immediate attention.[23]

While current medical charities were surely useful, advocates for the hospital made plain that they fell short in key ways. As the MGH Trustees argued in an address to the public in 1813, the hospital was "designed for cases which neither the Dispensary, nor private benevolence can touch, much less alleviate."[24] In the long campaign to see the hospital funded, boosters paid tribute to other forms of charitable care in the commonwealth while also painting a vivid portrait of the deficiencies that made a hospital a necessity.

According to Jackson and Warren, the Boston Dispensary was to be applauded for the relief it gave "to hundreds every year." Both knew the institution well and had derived medical experience from their tenure there. Jackson had served as a district physician, visiting with the sick for two years before resigning, and Warren served as a consulting physician for six years, starting in 1809.[25] Part of the dispensary's attraction was that it provided care discreetly to the worthy poor. Its advertising pamphlets made the case that "the sick, without being pained by a separation from their families, may be attended and relieved in their own houses," avoiding the indignities of the almshouse: "Those who have seen better days may be comforted without being humiliated: And all the poor receive the benefits of a charity the more refined, as it is the more secret."[26] The dispensary was conceived as a necessary adjunct to family care, preserving the competency of the respectable and protecting the worthy poor from the taint of pauperism.

But the strength of the Boston Dispensary was also its weakness. It was explicitly designed to be a low-cost alternative to care that might be found elsewhere; as its champions noted, dispensary care allowed for the sick to "be assisted at a less expense to the public than in an hospital."[27] While patients might receive the care of a physician and requisite medicines, they were not allowed nursing, something that concerned critics and advocates alike. Moreover, the discreet provision that allowed individuals and families to continue to live at home while under care meant that the material conditions of domestic life, particularly for the poor, could be problematic.[28]

As Jackson and Warren observed in critiquing the Boston Dispensary and other charities, "there are many others among the poor, who have, if we may so express it, the form of the necessaries of life, without the substance." The poor lived on spare diets, in crowded boardinghouses, in garrets and cellars. If they fell ill, they might be threatened with eviction. The patriarch, even if allowed to remain in his "miserable habitation," was "harassed with the idea of his accumulating rent, which must be paid out of his future labours. In this wretched situation, the sick man is destitute of all of those common conveniences, without which most of us would consider it impossible to live, even in health."[29]

The champions of the hospital could look to female societies dedicated to the relief of the sick and suffering to provide just this sort of material comfort. Like the Boston Dispensary, female societies for the relief of the sick often partnered with local physicians, paying for medicines if physicians would provide patients free visits. By also offering comforts such as clothing, bedding, and food, the female societies could supply necessities that a charity like the dispensary could not. For example, the Female Humane Society of Cambridge (FHSC; 1814) and its partner, the Cambridge Humane Society (dedicated to relieving poverty and to resuscitating drowning victims), and the Watertown Female Society for the Relief of the Indigent Sick (WFS; 1816), affiliated with the town's First Parish Church, endeavored to pay for medicine and physician's visits, as well as loaning or donating a range of needed articles. By paying an annual fee or working for the society, subscribers had the privilege of recommending the deserving sick for aid. The female societies offered charity meant to take the sting of want from the harsh material circumstances faced by the sick poor.

It was expensive to provide substantial material aid. Given the high costs of care and the fear that those unworthy of aid might drain coffers, groups like the WFS and the FHSC initially restricted their reach. Both agreed to tend only to members of their respective towns. The FHSC also curtailed outlays for any family "which has a man at its head, who is able to work, and may find employment if he conducts himself with propriety," and for "any female who has real estate, money at interest, expensive articles of furniture, or plate. . . ." Charity was coupled with a normative vision of society: the prudential management of funds called for the exclusion of the profligate man who impoverished his family, and cautioned against assisting those of means who might support themselves.

Within a few years, however, with relatively few applications for aid, both female charitable societies broadened their mission, providing a variety of measures to ease suffering in their towns. The WFS dropped the word "indigent" after its first year and offered to help a broader array of afflicted townspeople. The FHSC went further, addressing the failure of the wage economy to support the needs of workers. Its president made the case, noting that "the hour of sickness is the time of greatest distress with the indigent, but is not the only [time] that they feel the gripping hand of poverty." The wages of day laborers were "at best but a slender pittance for the support of a family . . . and generally least in that season of the year when most is wanted to make a family comfortable. . . . And the case of the female who has nothing but the labour of her hands to support herself and family with, still more deplorable, because her wages are smaller."[30]

Unlike the Boston Dispensary, which solely provided physician's visits and medicines, the two female societies offered a wide variety of items to ensure greater comfort and cleanliness. The Cambridge society provided not only medicine but "groceries," wood in the winter, and a remarkable range of clothing loaned or given—petticoats, cotton gowns, loose gowns, waistcoats, chemise, hose, and robes for infants, children, and adults, and diapers—as well as wine (though always with the concern that not too much be distributed), brandy, cider, sugar, tea, coffee, oatmeal, rice, raisins, nutmeg; and other articles that might help restore the body to balance such as castor oil, arrow root, sago, beeswax, and herbal medicines (senna, chamomile flowers, and rhubarb). Equally impressive was the variety of articles on loan: mattresses, pillows and pillowcases, sheets, quilts, blankets, caps, and easy chairs. The society insisted that all loaned materials be "perfectly cleansed" by the borrower on their return.[31] The Watertown society generated a similar (if larger) set of materials after agreeing to provide for all the sick in the town. The WFS also partnered with the selectmen of the town to have several "public bathing tubs" committed to the WFS's charge, which the selectmen agreed to, provided "their object in rendering benefit to the Sick will be strictly preserved. . . ."[32]

Taken as a whole, the aspirations and practices of the female societies illustrate several new developments in the province of affliction which would take hold more firmly later in the nineteenth century. The emphasis that both societies placed on regimes for comfort and cleanliness reflects a middle-class concern with health that was taking shape in the early nineteenth century. Guidance on these means of improvement might be found in everything from domestic manuals to advice proffered in correspondence and polite conversation.[33] The matriarch of the middle-class household was charged with promoting refined manners and supervising increasingly exacting regimes of cleanliness in the house, its furnishings, and especially its members' clothing. She was also tasked with ensuring the bodily comfort and health of residents. We see both imperatives at work in the loans of pillows, blankets, and garments that might ease bodily suffering during illness, and in the insistence that loaned articles be returned clean and ready for reuse.[34]

Because of the connection between health and cleanliness, the female societies participated in new public health efforts throughout turn-of-the-century New England. Expanding on earlier town efforts and prompted by yellow fever epidemics, local and state officials worked to regulate "nuisances" and "filth." Such developments would lead to increased intervention by the state government in public and private life in the name of protecting "the people's welfare." While full coercive powers given to boards of health would follow much later in the century, the WFS's supervision of the Watertown public tubs illustrates the kind of informal partnerships that brought women's societies into the civic sphere, with the preservation of health as their area of expertise.[35]

Health and its relationship to cleanliness offered female societies an opportunity not only to redress the spare and harsh living conditions of the working poor struck by affliction, but also to remake households in the image of the middle class. As the Cambridge society reported in 1829, they had helped the sick and infirm through the provision of groceries and articles of clothing, but in addition, "some small sums have been expended in order to render the apartments of the sick, more clean & healthful." One sees the early glimmerings in such efforts of the broad-scale assault on filth that informed the later sanitarian movement, the inspections of city slums and their poor by John Griscom, and the late nineteenth-century discourse and practices that waged war on "the germ" in the household. In the meantime, with comfort in view, the female societies could offer the accoutrements of care, supplementing the spare lives of the sick with clothing, bedding, special furniture, food, wood, and limited medicine.[36]

While the female societies were ambitious in their efforts, their meeting minutes reveal that they encountered significant obstacles, in particular limited finances due to the difficulty in recruiting and retaining paying members. The societies would have to make compromises, reluctantly turning to the state and its state pauper program, for example, to fund those who were otherwise deemed worthy.[37] And they would have to choose between the support of acute cases and the ongoing chronic care necessary to meet the needs of the aging in their midst. A single, intractable case could deplete charitable funds.[38]

The champions of the hospital pointed to limitations of piecemeal charitable efforts. Only the hospital could offer the expertise, material resources, and overall capacity to match the magnitude of problems that had arisen in the province of affliction: the insufficiency of wages to cover overwhelming medical costs, the spare material conditions of the poor, the social isolation of sufferers in the metropolis. The hospital would offer the best medical and surgical aid with expert nursing and a built environment that was clean, orderly, and properly ventilated, a world apart from the hovels that the sick poor might inhabit or the disarray of the almshouse. And with patients gathered from all parts of the state, physicians and surgeons would derive new medical knowledge based on clinical experience, which would ultimately benefit everyone in the commonwealth and beyond.

Such grand ambitions would need to be matched by a massive fundraising effort, and the hospital and asylum for the insane benefited from a new and potent amalgam of legislative allowances and business enterprise devoted to the project. The General Court's granting of a public charter to the hospital (1811) had been followed by the donation of the Province House, which could be rented or sold; state prison laborers were enlisted to cut stone for the grand edifice, designed by Charles Bulfinch; and, two years after it opened its doors, the hospital was given a percentage of the profits of the Massachusetts Hospital Life Insurance Company (1823), which became the largest financial institution in New England. In his address at the laying of the cornerstone of the hospital in 1818, Josiah Quincy praised the "liberality" of his fellow citizens and the "munificence" of the legislature. Taking nothing for granted, he and the other Trustees, who had been assiduously fundraising for some eight years, would redouble their efforts and "commence their institution upon a scale and on a system coinciding less with the immediate state of funds, than with the anticipated exigencies of society. . . ."[39]

Essential to this endeavor was the campaign of the Trustees and others to secure voluntary contributions from citizens throughout the commonwealth, who were asked to see the hospital not just as a place serving a locality, the metropole of Boston. Citizens were challenged to rethink the locus of collective responsibility for social welfare itself. In the long quest to secure voluntary contributions, residents of the Bay State were asked to reconceive their long-standing means of accommodating affliction. The key to supporting the worthy poor would not be town or state taxes but voluntary contributions to a corporation charged with serving the commonwealth as a whole.

The immediate attentions claimed by the sick in extremity had meant throughout the eighteenth century that local society was first to absorb costs. That burden had been met, sometimes silently, sometimes with grinding conflicts over who within localities would be responsible for life's misfortunes. Was it the individual, family, or household? Was it the town in which the ill became indisposed or the town of origin? Was it, in the case of the larger calamities of war and epidemic, and the later wanderings of those without legal settlement in the commonwealth, the responsibility of the province and state to reimburse locals? New Englanders had done their best to accommodate life in a community of peril. As they did so, the social suffering generated by illness became the occasion for the definition and maintenance of building blocks of society and politics throughout the eighteenth century.

The hospital asked for a different social and political imagination. Critical not only to its financial success but also to its vitality as a new institution was that citizens see the hospital as a charitable and finally philanthropic enterprise that was essential to their lives, wherever they resided. That persons in towns across the commonwealth, even New England as a whole, should embrace a hospital in Boston required, first, that everyone recognize the increasingly powerful gravitational force exerted by the metropolis. Necessity, opportunity, and ambition had driven the extraordinary growth of Boston after the Revolution. After losing population during the Revolution, the city had grown from 15,500 in 1774 to 43,298 in 1820.[40] Many of the Boston Associates themselves, who comprised the great bulk of hospital Trustees, had migrated to Boston in search of new opportunities, seeking an escape from the social and financial confines of their rural towns. They were joined by many others with lesser means, persons on the make who were especially vulnerable in times of illness.

As the Trustees noted in 1814, they were especially concerned about those "who resort to the metropolis, from remote parts of the Commonwealth, in the capacity of labourers, of mechanics, of sailors, or servants, or teamsters. Such persons are often seized with sickness, in taverns and boarding houses; and fall victims to the neglect, the ignorance, or the indifference of those, with whom they are occasionally inmates; and to whom they are generally unknown." "What town, in the Commonwealth," they asked, "has not some of its inhabitants, every year, exposed to the hazard of accident, or disease, in their occasional intercourse with the metropolis?" Far from being a hospital for Bostonians, the new institution would be, "in its character, a State establishment."[41]

The fundraising drive asked Massachusetts residents to envision themselves as owing their first affiliation to the commonwealth as a whole rather than their particular town. True, they might have a personal interest in an institution that tended to town residents who fell sick in the city (and whose medical bills would be the responsibility of their town of legal settlement), but the hospital campaigners asked, like the Good Samaritan, for a broader sense of who constituted one's neighbor in a time of suffering. In short, residents were asked to go beyond personal, local acts of charity to embrace a more wide-ranging and impersonal philanthropy.[42]

In an 1816 letter soliciting hospital subscriptions from coastal towns, the Boston merchant, investor, and philanthropist Thomas Handasyd Perkins noted that the hospital and asylum for the insane "extend only to those extraordinary incidents which multiply the miseries of human life, & which neither private benevolence, nor the common public institutions can diminish or remedy." At stake in addition to those extreme cases, however, was the Christian duty to think beyond local interests and embrace a larger community in peril. "The Citizens of this Town," Perkins contended, "have therefore no interest which is not common to all the fellow Citizens, no obligation or Duty which is not equally enjoined on all Christians, unless Gentlemen, it should be contended, that Charity is a Duty which is attached only to proximity, & that the distress which is removed from us a few miles is not entitled to our Sympathy."[43] In times of "calamities," such as fires and epidemics, town residents had been forthcoming; now was the time to press further. The hospital would not supplant public outlays for the poor nor private acts of charity, but if liberal donors were to provide sufficient funding, the hospital and asylum could alleviate and even remove "Evils to which our common brethren, may be exposed."[44]

In printed circulars and private letters sent between 1816 and 1818, the Trustees personally reached out to prominent citizens in towns across the commonwealth and asked them to help gather subscriptions of amounts they deemed commensurate with the capabilities of each town. The campaign as a whole was a grand success. As many historians have noted, following the lead of the hospital's first historian and avid booster, Nathaniel Bowditch, the average size of donations to the hospital as of 1843 was around $110, and three-quarters of the gifts were less than $100. While the majority of funds came from larger donations, including a spectacular gift of $20,000 from the Phillips family, there was no doubt that people of lesser means contributed with enthusiasm.[45]

Clear failures in the fundraising campaign, however, reflected the enduring limitations of the earlier province of affliction. In letters to the Trustees in the wake of their solicitations, towns, particularly in central and western Massachusetts, revealed their hesitation to support the hospital. Several towns, having received the appeal in August, noted it was an unfavorable time of year for contributions. As Daniel Waldo of Worcester noted, "money is scarce at this season of the year[;] people in the Country seldom have any." From one of the leading families in the county, Waldo contributed a generous $200, and he suggested another campaign later in the fall might be more successful. But others were less sanguine. Thomas Kitteredge from Andover noted that the hospital was just one of a "multiplicity of subscriptions" circulating through town "for various charitable purposes," and that between "the heavy Taxes for four of five years past and the embarrassed state of the times, I judge very little, if any thing is to be expected from this town." Asa Packard, writing from the Second Parish in Marlborough, enclosed $90, noting, "In a small society, so distant from the capital, and where little surplus property is found, this collection, I hope, will not be thought indecent." But other towns made the subtle case that perhaps the request for donations itself was misdirected, if not futile. The Fitchburg town meeting, for example, had been read the entire plea for funds, "and explanations were made in an earnestness to dispose the People to contribute the small proportion assigned them in a most noble, useful and honourable Charity—but all without effect." As the town clerk in Holden reported, the prior day's town meeting had been unsuccessful: "there was not any person appeared Disposed to contribute any thing— they thought it would not be of much Use to this Town so far Distant from the Capital." Bolton's respondent could not fathom how contributions could be forthcoming. There were, he claimed, "only three wealthy men here," but they had large families "each with nine or ten Children—they probably expend their income, & neither family has a Servant!" Despite the worthy cause, "I see what small incomes" they "obtain from their hard labor—& I think their Children ought to have it."[46]

The scarcity of money; the burden of local and state taxes, which, after all, supported both social welfare for legal residents and town dwellers without settlement; the din of other requests in a society proliferating with new charitable enterprises; the underlying sense that the hospital, however worthy, would not benefit those remote from Boston—all of these concerns spoke to the ongoing challenges facing town residents. The burdens of affliction in the eighteenth century had stretched upward and outward, from family and household, backed by what Barry Levy calls the "town state" and its poor law provision, to the General Court. But appeals for relief had been in the service of helping make whole the sick and their providers, who of necessity bore the immediate costs of affliction in *local* settings where the sick fell ill.[47]

The hospital offered to step into the place of local provision by plucking the sick out of local society and healing them in an institution set apart from it. But for that system to work, the hospital would have to be something that was readily accessed by locals. As an abstract institution, the hospital was a transcendent answer to the burdens that illness placed on local society, a way of knitting together a new community of peril whose diffusion was animated by the ambitions and necessities of a new economic and cultural order. But as a physical artifact existing in a single place, the hospital was seen as too remote to be of use to the many who would continue to confront extremity in their towns. It was too difficult to imagine, much less afford, removing the afflicted—too dangerous for the sick, the costs of transport and a protracted stay at the institution too high.

Underlying these manifest material concerns was a latent barrier to restructuring the priorities and affiliations of local society: even if particular patients might herald from towns in the hinterland, the hospital as a whole would be comprised by strangers—anonymous, disconnected, removed from a lived familiarity that might evoke fellow feeling. In a letter authored by "The Massachusetts General Hospital" published in the *Columbian Centinel* in 1817, the boosters of the hospital asked readers to reconceive of sufferers everywhere as "family" in search of a "home." The hospital was personified as a worthy woman in desperate need of gathering her ailing family. "TO MY COUNTY FRIENDS," began the letter; it was with pride and humility that so many benefactors had contributed toward "building me a house, and providing an income to support me and my poor distrest and sick family, which is already large and every year increasing; a family which is now scattered about, and suffering neglect, and pain, and distress, for want of a common home, where they might be comfortably nursed, and their disorders skillfully attended."[48] The piece evoked a harmonious image that at once promoted the home as a place of family nurture and belied the ideological work that was bringing a new conception of family, home, and work into being. The new middle-class "home" was designed as a haven for family, a sanctuary for the fine feelings of the sensible and refined, a place of cleanliness, comfort, virtuous and cheerful industry, and expert nurture presided over by the matriarch. The unremunerated work of home life, set apart from the wage market where the male breadwinner was to secure his family's maintenance, was obscured by the pastoral narrative of home.[49]

The hospital, its boosters could claim, was to be a new kind of home populated by a family of strangers. Over the course of the eighteenth century, the residents of Massachusetts had worked through the numerous complications of caring for the sick poor in local settings, backed by the complementarity of the poor law, "town state," and province and state support. The hospital offered an alternative to care in local settings, bringing to the fore a new complementarity of impersonal markets, large-scale philanthropy, and, in short order, the new financial practices of corporations such as the Massachusetts Hospital Life Insurance Company (MHLIC). The company was chartered by the General Court to serve the public good. Behind the scenes, however, the company was soon making enormous profits for its shareholders, investing the fortunes of many of the Boston Associates who served as trustees for MGH, and calling in interest payments of farmers in western Massachusetts according to strict reimbursement schedules, with lawsuits threatened if they were late.[50] But the imagery of the hospital as home might quiet such unrest, its boosters could hope. The hospital could stand as a new kind of institution knitting together society. Strangers as family, hospital as home—such framing imaginatively brought the dislocations of a new era into a new domestic fold.[51]

Six months after the Massachusetts General Hospital opened its doors in September 1821, the Trustees and chief physician and surgeon, James Jackson and John C. Warren, published an account for hospital subscribers and the public at large. It was, on the whole, a highly favorable report. Jackson noted that "obstinate diseases have yielded more readily than I have commonly found them to do in private practice." He pointed with pride, for example, to two patients admitted with bronchitis, a female who had lost her voice and was "discharged well within six days" and a male whose "disease had assumed a most unfavorable character, so that at first I nearly despaired of his recovery." The patient had originally been seen by a "respectable Physician" outside of the hospital, his condition considered "desperate." But after being admitted to the hospital, he was out of danger within just two days, and by six days nearly well. Jackson observed that the "great amendment in this case was produced by the removal of the patient from a small chamber in a filthy boarding house to the pure air and clean apartments of the Hospital." The carefully controlled environment of the hospital was central to recovery. Warren was similarly optimistic, noting that through bone setting, surgery for strictures of the urethra and rectum, and treatments applied to rashes, inflammations, ulcers, and frozen limbs, he had allowed many patients to resume their occupations.[52]

Despite the successes underscored by Warren and Jackson, their record with patients also illuminates structural failures rooted in the earlier province of affliction. Jackson noted that the hospital would necessarily see "a great proportion of grave, aggravated and protracted diseases," sufferers whose ailments had been "increased by the want of care arising from poverty and negligence." Patients came to the hospital too late to be helped. And even if patients' symptoms diminished at the hospital, they would have to return to the squalid living conditions deemed to be the seedbed of disease. The hospital could not address the intemperance, the filth, and the riot outside its doors. It might offer the sick poor care that would stand in for the ministrations of family and town, connections lost to them in their moving across the countryside, driven by ambition or necessity. But in the end, patients would have to return to their own quarters.[53]

The creation of the hospital pointed to the best that a new world of associations and medical philanthropy might offer—that strangers might be helped, that the ambitious who had left their home towns would not be left to languish in the absence of social connections, that with a carefully regulated environment and expert medical care, the worthy sick might be restored to society. But the hospital would be forced to confront familiar and troubling issues. Campaigns to fund free beds for the poor were only partially successful. A strict discipline in separating classes of sufferers began to fray in the absence of adequate finances. Despite the herculean effort to get the hospital up and running, the institution was soon subject to challenges reminiscent of charges made against the almshouse, that it was a hothouse that promiscuously mixed the worthy and morally depraved, a place that one might go as a last resort, a place of danger rather than respite. The hospital would reach its ascendancy decades later, when the province of affliction would be a distant memory.[54]

⌘

Some historical problems hover above time. Concerns about the social and political consequences of sickness remain as vital today as they were in early New England. Two aspects of the particular responses to illness in the province of affliction described in the preceding chapters may have lessons for historians and present-day citizens alike.

First, the command that illness could exert over daily life in early New England points to the centrality of interdependency in social and political relations. A portrait of everyday life with sickness at its center suggests that we temper a narrative that would have early Americans advancing steadily through the acquisition of land that was more readily available than in Europe, or through the procurement of goods in an emerging consumer culture, or though the mastery of codes of refinement as a way to social advancement.[55] Alongside these dynamic means of improvement and competition lay the force of affliction, illuminating the fragility of autonomy, individualism, and advancement in the period. Each sickness in early New England created its own web of interdependent social relations that enabled survival but also could set off an enduring struggle to determine who would be finally responsible for misfortunes. Stricken individuals, families, households, towns, provinces, and states became entangled in the process, as sufferers and those around them reached out for help—to neighbors, townsfolk, and finally their governing officials who might offer protection.

Second, that we can talk so readily about illness in this period reflects just how easily and often eighteenth-century New Englanders themselves broached the topic. Sickness is everywhere apparent in the documents of early New England—in letters and diaries, in the public prints, in the records of governing bodies at all levels. The references were often fleeting and vague, leaving one to wonder what ailed the sufferers and perhaps to skim over numerous and generic complaints. But early New Englanders were insistent in recording the presence of illness as a central problem in their lives. And in doing so, they registered how pervasive illness was, how many lives it touched, and how deeply it was implicated in daily affairs. They saw the problems it caused, the sacrifices it demanded, and the need to monitor its presence insistently and openly.

We need not romanticize this world. The costs of the province of affliction could be considerable, and it is not surprising to find that tensions could abound. Family squabbles over who should care for elderly parents, or disputes between towns insisting bills belonged elsewhere, could find their way into court. And later critics charged that the care afforded the sick poor could be so spare as to be cruel. But it is hard to view our founding generations without admiration for their forthright attempts to accommodate the problem of sickness in their society. They faced issues all too familiar to us—the unexpected dislocations of acute disease; the enormous financial and social costs of caring for the chronically ill—and they did so squarely and resolutely. They understood the province of affliction in daily life, and they did not trivialize its hold on everyday affairs.[56]

ACKNOWLEDGMENTS

In these pages, I claim that each sickness in eighteenth-century New England created its own society. The same might be said all the more of this book. Over the long course of writing, I have been extremely fortunate to have had the help and encouragement of numerous people and institutions.

Several short-term fellowships allowed me to launch the project. I am enormously grateful for the support of the American Antiquarian Society, the Massachusetts Historical Society, the John Nicholas Brown Center, and Countway Library. The Charlotte W. Newcombe Foundation and the Omohundro Institute of Early American History and Culture generously funded long-term fellowships that were crucial in reworking the manuscript. Oregon State University has been extremely supportive over the years, with research fellowships at the Center for the Humanities and an early sabbatical leave supported by Paul Farber, chair of the Department of History, who has been an irrepressible enthusiast and champion since my arrival on a wet weekend visit many years ago. More recently, I was awarded a sabbatical leave from a long-term administrative position, supported by the dean of the College of Liberal Arts, Larry Rodgers, with great appreciation. I extend my heartfelt thanks to all of these institutions and persons for their encouragement and assistance.

I want to thank archivists at a range of institutions who made it such a pleasure to conduct research and to be part of a community of scholars, including the wonderful staffs at the American Antiquarian Society, the Massachusetts Historical Society, the Countway Library, the Massachusetts State Archives, the Peabody Essex Museum, the Massachusetts General Hospital, the Schlesinger Library, the Porter-Phelps-Huntington House Museum (and the Porter Phelps Huntington Foundation that sustains it), the Amherst College Archives and Special Collections, and the Rhode Island Historical Society. I offer my sincere thanks as well to the staffs at libraries and town halls throughout Massachusetts, including those in Lincoln, Brookline, Westborough, and Marblehead, who went above and beyond duty to let me consult archival materials in reading rooms, vaults, and basements. Ross W. Beales Jr. and Ruth Herndon were extraordinarily generous in sharing transcriptions of their archival efforts. I hope they feel that I have put their material to good use.

I've benefited enormously from presenting portions of this work at a variety of venues. Thanks are due to the Columbia Seminar on Early American History and Culture, the John Nicholas Brown Center, the Boston Area Seminar in Early American History, the Rocky Mountain Seminar, the Center for the Humanities at Oregon State University, the Early Modern Studies Institute and the Huntington Library, the Society for Historians of the Early Republic, the Society for Disabilities Studies, the OIEAHC Colloquium and Annual Meeting, the Pacific Northwest Meeting of Early Americanists, and the history departments at New York University, Dartmouth College, and Bates College.

Over the years, many colleagues have read drafts of chapters and larger sections of my work. I would like to thank David Armitage, Elizabeth Blackmar, David Rosner, and Herbert Sloan for their close reading of an early draft. Richard Bushman deserves special thanks. His economy and grace in writing, creativity in teaching, and generosity in spirit have set an example that I can only hope to follow in my own work. His thought is everywhere evident in the pages within. Thanks to Fred Anderson, Carol Berkin, Pat Berman, Daniel Blackie, Kathleen Brown, Eliza Byard, Joyce Chaplin, Elaine Crane, Nicole Eustace, Cori Field, Mike Flamm, Tami Friedman, Christopher Front, Walter Hickel, Erik Hinderaker, the late Thea K. Hunter, Anne Kornhauser, Catherine Kudlick, Peter Mancall, Lou Masur, Michael Meranze, Phil Morgan, John Murrin, Alice Nash, Jennifer Pulsipher, Adam Rothman, Thad Russell, Robert Blair St. George, Michael Sappol, Bob Scott, Robyn Spencer, Alden Vaughan, Douglas Winiarski, the late Al Young, and Michael Zakim for conversation and commentary.

My stay at the Omohundro Institute was animated by the incredible number of early Americanists who took an interest in my work. For reading early drafts, my thanks to Chris Grasso, Paul Mapp, Karin Wulf, Martin Brückner, Ann Gross, Bob Gross, Ron Hoffman, and Cary Carson. The late Rhys Isaac helped me frame unwieldy material over lunches, walks, and at jazz venues. Fredrika Teute saw the early promise of the work and spent many afternoons helping me think through implications; I appreciate her encouragement over the years. Readers for the Omohundro Institute—Laurel Ulrich, the late Roy Porter, Barry Levy, Nina Dayton, and Mark Peterson—offered sharp and discerning comments. Paul Mapp, my co-fellow, made daily life stimulating and occasionally hilarious. I'm quite grateful to Paul for his work as interim editor, a role he took on with great insight, judiciousness, and good humor. I miss Ron Hoffman, most especially his wry smile and his surprising and mischievous generosity with my young daughter, who pined for the secret treats that he kept in his filing cabinet. Thanks to Ron, Sally Mason, and Beverly Smith for making my family feel at home. Thanks to Kim Foley for help with a database and to Becky Wrenn for creative birthday cakes and companionship. I'm so pleased that Becky was able to design a map for the book.

At Oregon State, I've been fortunate to be surrounded by superb colleagues, creative scholars and mensches all. My thanks to the following people for taking the time to talk about the project, to read my work, and to offer valuable feedback: Mina Carson, Marisa Chappell, George Estreich, Paul Farber, Gary Ferngren, Jake Hamblin, Mo Healy, Bill Husband, Jon Katz, Paul Kopperman, Chris Nichols, Bob Nye, Mary Jo Nye, Lisa Sarasohn, Stacey Smith, and Nicole von Germeten. Jeff Sklansky has been an especially close friend who has gone above and beyond in every domain, offering much-needed encouragement and extremely thoughtful and incisive readings of both individual chapters and the entire manuscript. I have had the good fortune to receive the encouragement and aid of many students over the years, both through the stimulation of teaching and through the efforts of several admirably resourceful and enthusiastic researchers: Raul Burriel, Jenna Proctor, Mikaela Schamp, Jason Sharples, and Harrison Schreiber.

It has been an enormous pleasure to have found a home for this book at the University of Chicago's American Beginnings series. I thank series editors Edward Gray, Stephen Mihm, and Mark Peterson for their interest and encouragement. Mark has offered his wise counsel, penetrating critiques, and stimulating exchange since I met him as a college student. It is a happy development to have him as an editor, and the manuscript has benefited immeasurably from his unfailing ability to point to its larger significance. I want to thank Mary Woolsey for her last-minute heroics in line editing; her work has surely made the book much stronger and livelier. Tim Mennel has been a model of efficiency, unruffled by any query, it would seem. Erin DeWitt copyedited the manuscript with a keen eye and good humor. I could not be more pleased and impressed with the entire team at the University of Chicago Press.

Portions of chapter 2 appeared in "Illness in the 'Social Credit' and 'Money' Economies of Eighteenth-Century New England," in *Medicine and the Market in England and Its Colonies, c. 1450–c. 1850*, ed. Mark S. R. Jenner and Patrick Wallis (New York: Palgrave Macmillan, 2007), 175–95. My thanks to the publisher for permission to reprint material from that volume. I thank the libraries and archives noted above for permission to quote from their rich materials.

My family has lived with this project for more years than I care to remember. For their patience, encouragement, and abiding love, I thank Ethan Mutschler, Levi Mutschler, Maureen O'Reilly, Deborah Mutschler, and Peter Murad. My children, Manya and Sam, have grown up with the project, been of good cheer when I stayed late at the office, and, more than anything, have inspired me with their creativity, humor, deep thought, hard work, razzing, and love. It will be a good thing for us to have the book on the shelf. I thank their mom, Sue Aldine, for all of her support and sacrifice over the years.

Erica Prince danced into my life six years ago and has brought me great joy, adventure, beauty, and love—and piano playing, hikes, a stunning garden, vivid tapestries, and tours of houses, landscapes, and ocean fronts. I am a fortunate fellow to share my life with her.

The book is dedicated to the memory of my parents, Phyllis and Louis Mutschler. They always encouraged my curiosity, appreciated my quirks, and offered an extraordinary amount of support for this project and every other that I undertook. I miss them dearly. But I take some solace in knowing that they are a part of this work, and that they would have been so pleased to see it come to completion.

INTRODUCTION

1. *The Diary of Elizabeth Drinker*, ed. Elaine Forman Crane (Boston: Northeastern University Press, 1991), 1: 226. Drinker dated the entry "Augt. 20 or 21" and added to the entry over time, penning an update on Henry's condition on September 6. Drinker often commented on the heat in the city in the late summer, including a note a week before Henry became ill that it was "very hot" (August 14, 1777). That the heat continued into the following week is conjecture on my part. For a genealogy of the Drinker family, see *Diary of Elizabeth Drinker*, 1: lxxi–lxxiv and 157 for Henry's birth. For worms and children, see Lucinda McCray Beier, *Sufferers and Healers: The Experience of Illness in Seventeenth-Century England* (London: Routledge, 1987), 189–90. For a suggestive treatment that explores the theme of the "precariousness of life," including the many illnesses of Drinker's children, see Helena M. Wall, "'My Constant Attension on My Sick Child': The Fragility of Family Life in the World of Elizabeth Drinker," in *Children in Colonial America*, ed. James Marten (New York: New York University Press, 2007), ch. 9.

2. For the full course of Henry's illness, see *Diary of Elizabeth Drinker*, 1: 226–49. Quotes from September 9, 15, 28, and October 26.

3. See, for example, Elaine Forman Crane, "'I Have Suffer'd Much Today': The Defining Force of Pain in Early America," in *Through a Glass Darkly: Reflections on Personal Identity in Early America*, ed. Ronald Hoffman, Mechal Sobel, and Fredrika J. Teute (Chapel Hill: University of North Carolina Press, 1997), 370–403.

4. John Winthrop, "A Model of Christian Charity," reprinted in *Early American Writings*, ed. Carla Mulford (New York: Oxford, 2002), 238–45. Stephen Foster provides an excellent overview of affliction in seventeenth-century New England, chiefly in the context of poverty and poor relief, and suggests that the ideas surrounding affliction carried into the eighteenth century. See Foster, *Their Solitary Way: The Puritan Social Ethic in the First Century of Settlement in New England* (New Haven, CT: Yale University Press, 1971), 127–52, comment on eighteenth century, 132n13.

5. On New England as atypical, see Jack P. Greene, *Pursuits of Happiness: The*

Social Development of Early Modern British Colonies and the Formation of American Culture (Chapel Hill: University of North Carolina Press, 1988). On New England in the Atlantic world, recent studies of Boston have been especially important: Mark Peterson, *The City-State of Boston: The Rise and Fall of an Atlantic Power, 1630–1865* (Princeton, NJ: Princeton University Press, 2019), and Jane Kamensky, *A Revolution in Color: The World of John Singleton Copley* (New York: Norton, 2016). On New England's precocious regulation of public life, including poor laws and taxation, see Robin L. Einhorn, *American Taxation, American Slavery* (Chicago: University of Chicago Press, 2006), ch. 2, which argues that sophistication in its tax regime did not mean its tax laws were progressive; Barry Levy, *Town Born: The Political Economy of New England from Its Founding to the Revolution* (2009; repr., Philadelphia: University of Pennsylvania Press, 2011), ch. 1; Cornelia H. Dayton and Sharon V. Salinger, *Robert Love's Warnings: Searching for Strangers in Colonial Boston* (Philadelphia: University of Pennsylvania Press, 2014), 44–46, 49–50, 53–54. On public health, see note 7, below.

My focus on New England has two significant limitations. First, I do not treat Native Americans at any length. This is because there is already excellent work that has been done to recover native medical practices and, especially, the ways in which the afflictions of Indians became part of provincial governance in New England. On the former, see, for example, the recent work of Kelly Wisecup, *Medical Encounters: Knowledge and Identity in Early American Literatures* (Boston: University of Massachusetts Press, 2013). On the latter, see Daniel R. Mandell, *Beyond the Frontier: Indians in Eighteenth-Century Massachusetts* (Lincoln: University of Nebraska Press, 1996), chs. 4–5, who ties the social and financial costs of illness to Indians' loss of land. Second, I do not focus on church charity or the church as an institution. Here, again, there has already been significant work on clergymen and connections to healing, the charitable work of churches, and the strengths and weaknesses of churches throughout the eighteenth century. The material is so rich that it would have warranted another book project to break new ground. See, for example, Patricia Ann Watson, *The Angelical Conjunction: The Preacher-Physicians of Colonial New England* (Knoxville: University of Tennessee Press, 1991), and Douglas L. Winiarski, *Darkness Falls on the Land of Light: Experiencing Religious Awakenings in Eighteenth-Century New England* (Chapel Hill: University of North Carolina Press, 2017).

6. R. A. Kashanipour, "Contagious Connections: Recent Approaches to the History of Medicine in Early America," *William and Mary Quarterly* 73 (January 2016): 141–59, is a thoughtful overview. This note and the three that follow can only gesture toward a few of the pertinent works. John M. Murrin, "Beneficiaries of Catastrophe: The English Colonies in America," in *The New American History*, ed. Eric Foner (Philadelphia: Temple University Press, 1990), 3–23; William H. McNeill, *Plagues and Peoples* (Garden City, NY: Anchor Press, 1976); Jared Diamond, *Guns, Germs, and Steel: The Fates of Human Societies* (New York: Norton, 1999); Alfred Crosby, "Virgin Soil Epidemics as a Factor in the Aboriginal Depopulation in America," *William and Mary Quarterly* 33 (April 1976), 289–99; and David S. Jones, "Virgin Soils Revisited," *William and Mary Quarterly* 60 (October 2003), 703–42. Gerald N. Grob's *The Deadly Truth: A History of Disease in America* (Cambridge, MA: Harvard University Press, 2002) synthesizes

much of work on morbidity and mortality in North America and the United States, from conquest through the twentieth century.

7. On public health in New England, see John Duffy, *Epidemics in Colonial America* (Baton Rouge: Louisiana State University Press, 1953); John Blake, *Public Health in the Town of Boston, 1630–1822* (Cambridge, MA: Harvard University Press, 1959); Barbara Gutman Rosenkrantz, *Public Health and the State: Changing Views in Massachusetts, 1842–1936* (Cambridge, MA: Harvard University Press, 1972); and Andrew Wehrman, "The Siege of 'Castle Pox': A Medical Revolution in Marblehead, Massachusetts, 1764–1777," *New England Quarterly* 82 (September 2009): 385–429. Other helpful works on public health include Charles Rosenberg, *The Cholera Years: The United States in 1832, 1849, and 1866* (Chicago: University of Chicago Press, 1962); Simon Finger, *The Contagious City: The Politics of Public Health in Early Philadelphia* (Ithaca, NY: Cornell University Press, 2012), which offers a recent effort to integrate public health concerns into the larger constellation of politics in colonial and Revolutionary Philadelphia; and William J. Novak, *The People's Welfare: Law and Regulation in Nineteenth-Century America* (Chapel Hill: University of North Carolina Press, 1996), ch. 6. Jeanne E. Abrams, *Revolutionary Medicine: The Founding Fathers and Mothers in Sickness and in Health* (New York: New York University Press, 2013), has argued that the Founders' intimate experience with sickness and death in their families helps explain their concern for public health measures deemed necessary to support the health of the people.

8. A substantial body of work focuses primarily on New England. On therapeutics, healing, and the medical marketplace in New England, see J Worth Estes, *Hall Jackson and the Purple Foxglove: Medical Practice and Research in Revolutionary America, 1760–1820* (Hanover, NH: University Press of New England, 1979); Philip Cash, Eric H. Christianson, and J. Worth Estes, eds., *Medicine in Colonial Massachusetts, 1620–1820*, vol. 57 of *Collections* (Boston: Colonial Society of Massachusetts, 1980); Eric Howard Christianson, "The Colonial Surgeon's Rise to Prominence: Dr. Silvester Gardiner (1707–1786) and the Practice of Lithotomy in New England," *The New England Historical and Genealogical Register* 136 (April 1982): 104–14; and Christianson, "The Emergence of Medical Communities in Massachusetts, 1700–1794: The Demographic Factors," *Bulletin of the History of Medicine* 54, no. 1 (Spring 1980): 64–77; Ronald L. Numbers, ed., *Medicine in the New World: New Spain, New France, and New England* (Knoxville: University of Tennessee Press, 1987); Norman Gevitz, "'Pray Let the Medicines Be Good': The New England Apothecary in the Seventeenth and Early Eighteenth Centuries," *Pharmacy in History* 41, no. 3 (1999): 87–101; Peter Benes, ed., *Medicine and Healing*, vol. 15 of *Annual Proceedings of the Dublin Seminar for New England Folklife* (Boston: Boston University, 1990); Watson, *The Angelical Conjunction*; Laurel Thatcher Ulrich, *A Midwife's Tale: The Life of Martha Ballard, Based on Her Diary, 1785–1812* (1990; repr., New York: Vintage, 1991); Rebecca J. Tannenbaum, *The Healer's Calling: Women and Medicine in Early New England* (Ithaca, NY: Cornell University Press, 2002); Ben Mutschler, "Illness in the 'Social Credit' and 'Money' Economies of Eighteenth-Century New England," in *Medicine and the Market in England and Its Colonies, c. 1450–c. 1850*, ed. Mark S. R. Jenner and Patrick Wallis (New York: Palgrave

Macmillan, 2007); and Catherine L. Thompson, *Patient Expectations: How Economics, Religion, and Malpractice Shaped Therapeutics in Early America* (Amherst: University of Massachusetts Press, 2015).

9. Beier, *Sufferers and Healers*; Roy Porter and Dorothy Porter, *In Sickness and in Health: The British Experience, 1650–1850* (1988; repr., New York: Basil Blackwell, 1989); Dorothy Porter and Roy Porter, *Patient's Progress: Doctors and Doctoring in Eighteenth-Century England* (Cambridge: Polity Press, 1989); Mary Lindemann, *Health and Healing in Eighteenth-Century Germany* (Baltimore: Johns Hopkins University Press, 1996); Mary E. Fissell, *Patients, Power, and the Poor in Eighteenth-Century Bristol* (Cambridge: Cambridge University Press, 1991); and Sheila M. Rothman, *Living in the Shadow of Death: Tuberculosis and the Social Experience of Illness in American History* (New York: Basic Books, 1994). Several recent biographies of persons in eighteenth- and early nineteenth-century New England integrate sickness and caregiving into their larger narratives: Robert E. Shalhope, *A Tale of New England: The Diaries of Hiram Harwood, Vermont Farmer, 1810–1838* (Baltimore: Johns Hopkins University Press, 2003), ch. 9; Megan Marshall, *The Peabody Sisters: Three Women Who Ignited American Romanticism* (Boston: Houghton Mifflin, 2006), ch. 18; Marla R. Miller, *Rebecca Dickinson: Independence for a New England Woman* (Boulder, CO: Westview Press, 2014); and Jill Lepore, *Book of Ages: The Life and Opinions of Jane Franklin* (New York: Vintage, 2013).

10. Christopher Clark, "The Household Economy, Market Exchange and the Rise of Capitalism in the Connecticut Valley, 1800–1860," *Journal of Social History* 13 (Winter 1979): 169–89; Richard L. Bushman, "Family Security in the Transition from Farm to City, 1750–1850," *Journal of Family History* (Fall 1981): 238–56; Daniel Vickers, "Competency and Competition: Economic Culture in Early America," *William and Mary Quarterly* 47 (January 1990): 3–29; Virginia DeJohn Anderson, *New England's Generation: The Great Migration and the Formation of Society and Culture in the Seventeenth Century* (Cambridge: Cambridge University Press, 1991).

11. Gordon S. Wood, *The Radicalism of the American Revolution* (New York: Knopf, 1992), chs. 1–5; Richard L. Bushman, *King and People in Provincial Massachusetts* (1985; repr., Chapel Hill: University of North Carolina Press, 1992), ch. 2.

12. Wood, *Radicalism*; T. H. Breen, *The Marketplace of Revolution: How Consumer Politics Shaped American Independence* (Oxford: Oxford University Press, 2004); Rhys Isaac, *Landon Carter's Uneasy Kingdom: Revolution and Rebellion on a Virginia Plantation* (New York: Oxford University Press, 2004); Jay Fliegelman, *Prodigals and Pilgrims: The American Revolution against Patriarchal Authority* (Cambridge: Cambridge University Press, 1982).

13. Toby L. Ditz, "The New Men's History and the Peculiar Absence of Gendered Power: Some Remedies from Early American Gender History," *Gender and History* 16 (2004): 1–35, highlights men's "access" to women. For an overview of dependency and its connection to social welfare, see Nancy Fraser and Linda Gordon, "A Genealogy of Dependency: Tracing a Keyword of the U.S. Welfare State," *Signs* 19 (Winter 1994): 309–36. In contrast to Carole Shammas, *A History of Household Government in America* (Charlottesville: University of Virginia Press, 2002), and Christopher Tomlins, *Freedom Bound: Law, Labor, and Civic Identity in Colonizing English America, 1580–1865*

(Cambridge: Cambridge University Press, 2010), who argue that the power of household heads increased steadily through the colonial and Revolutionary periods into the antebellum era, Kristen Sword, "Wayward Wives, Runaway Slaves, and the Limits of Patriarchal Authority in Early America" (PhD diss., Harvard University, 2002), stresses the liabilities of the patriarch.

14. Wood, *Radicalism*, chs. 13–18; Joyce Appleby, *Inheriting the Revolution: The First Generation of Americans* (Cambridge, MA: Belknap Press of Harvard University Press, 2000); François Furstenberg, "Beyond Freedom and Slavery: Autonomy, Virtue, and Resistance in Early American Political Discourse," *Journal of American History* 89 (March 2003): 1295–330; James Kloppenberg, "The Virtues of Liberalism: Christianity, Republicanism, and Ethics in Early American Political Discourse," *Journal of American History* 74 (June 1987): 9–33; Lynn Hunt, *Inventing Human Rights: A History* (New York: Norton, 2007); J. M. Opal, *Beyond the Farm: National Ambitions in Rural New England* (Philadelphia: University of Pennsylvania Press, 2008); Susan E. Klepp, *Revolutionary Conceptions: Women, Fertility, and Family Limitation in America, 1760–1820* (Chapel Hill: University of North Carolina Press, 2009); Richard Bell, *We Shall Be No More: Suicide and Self-Government in the Newly United States* (Cambridge, MA: Harvard University Press, 2012).

15. The literature on disability is vast and growing rapidly. I can only touch on a few of the works that have been most helpful. Martha C. Nussbaum, *Frontiers of Justice: Disability, Nationality, and Species Membership* (Cambridge, MA: Harvard University Press, 2007), uses a "capabilities approach" to explore questions of justice, exploring the broad social, political, cultural, and economic contexts that make each of us capable. Rosemarie Garland-Thompson, "Disability Studies: A Field Emerged," *American Quarterly* 65 (December 2013): 915–26, and Catherine J. Kudlick, "Disability History: Why We Need Another 'Other,'" *American Historical Review* 108 (June 2003): 763–93, are helpful historiographical and conceptual overviews. Several historically informed collections convey a range of perspectives: Paul K. Longmore and Lauri Umansky, eds., *The New Disability History: American Perspectives* (New York: New York University Press, 2001); Susan Burch and Michael Rembis, eds., *Disability Histories* (Urbana: University of Illinois Press, 2014); and Sari Altschuler and Cristobal Silva, eds., "Early American Disability Studies," a special issue of *Early American Literature* 52, no. 1 (2017). Kim E. Nielsen, *A Disability History of the United States* (Boston: Beacon Press, 2012), synthesizes much of the recent literature. Cornelia H. Dayton, "'The Oddest Man That I Ever Saw': Assessing Cognitive Disability on Eighteenth-Century Cape Cod," *Journal of Social History* 49, no. 1 (Fall 2015): 77–99, explores the question of mental competency as it was comprehended in law and in an eighteenth-century community. Dayton is at work on a study of madness in pre-asylum New England. Given her ongoing research and other influential work on the topic, such as Mary Ann Jimenez, *The Changing Faces of Madness: Early American Attitudes and Treatment of the Insane* (Hanover, NH: University Press of New England, 1987), I treat the topic lightly here. References to disability and war can be found in chapter 7, below.

16. E.g., Barbara Duden, *The Woman Beneath the Skin: A Doctor's Patients in Eighteenth-Century Germany* (1991; repr., Cambridge, MA: Harvard University Press, 1998).

17. On the ways of life in England's cultural provinces, see John Clive and Bernard Bailyn, "England's Cultural Provinces: Scotland and America," *William and Mary Quarterly* 11 (April 1954): 200–213; and Bernard Bailyn, *To Begin the World Anew: The Genius and Ambiguities of the American Founders* (New York: Vintage, 2003), ch. 1. I am indebted to Mark A. Peterson for his suggestion that illness can be thought of as provincial in this sense.

18. Susan Sontag, *Illness as Metaphor* and *AIDS and Its Metaphors* (New York: Doubleday, 1989), 3.

19. Ulrich, *A Midwife's Tale*, 170, finds in the case of Martha Ballard's midwifery practice, "one maternal death for every 198 living births." Ballard lost no mothers in nearly a thousand deliveries and only five patients in their lying-in period. On childhood mortality, see note 23, below.

20. On New England and health, see Mary J. Dobson, "Mortality Gradients and Disease Exchanges: Comparisons from Old England and Colonial America," *Society for the Social History of Medicine* (1989): 259–97; Dobson, "From Old England to New England: Changing Patterns of Mortality," Research Paper 38, School of Geography, University of Oxford (1987), 5–64; and Richard H. Steckel, "Nutritional Status in the Colonial American Economy," *William and Mary Quarterly* 56 (January 1999): 31–52. On the sickness and early death of sailors, see Daniel Vickers with Vince Walsh, *Young Men and the Sea: Yankee Seafarers in the Age of Sail* (New Haven, CT: Yale University Press, 2005). The authors suggest that among locally born sailors in Salem, Massachusetts, "three in ten never reached the age of thirty" (111).

21. See James C. Riley, *Sickness, Recovery and Death: A History and Forecast of Ill Health* (London: Macmillan Press, 1989); Riley, "Measuring Morbidity and Mortality," in *The Cambridge World History of Human Disease*, ed. Kenneth F. Kiple (Cambridge: Cambridge University Press, 1993), 230–38; and Riley, "Disease without Death: New Sources for a History of Sickness," *Journal of Interdisciplinary History* 17 (Winter 1987): 537–63. In the latter, Riley broaches the difficulty in calculating morbidity rates and probes the relation between sickness and the social consequences of sickness, a formulation that is consonant with my approach. The distinction between falling sick and being sick is Riley's.

22. Charles E. Rosenberg, "The Therapeutic Revolution: Medicine, Meaning, and Social Change in Nineteenth-Century America," in *The Therapeutic Revolution: Essays in the Social History of American Medicine*, ed. Morris J. Vogel and Charles E. Rosenberg (Philadelphia: University of Pennsylvania Press, 1979), 5.

23. Maris A. Vinovskis, "Angels' Heads and Weeping Willows: Death in Early America," reprinted in his *Studies in American Historical Demography* (New York: Academic Press, 1979), 286, 297; Daniel Scott Smith and J. David Hacker, "Cultural Demography: New England Deaths and the Puritan Perception of Risk," *Journal of Interdisciplinary History* 26 (Winter 1996): 367–92. For an anguishing account of one eighteenth-century New England mother's spiritual attempt to more deeply understand the sickness and death of her son, see Catherine A. Brekus, *Sarah Osborne's World: The Rise of Evangelical Christianity in Early America* (New Haven, CT: Yale University Press, 2013), ch. 5.

24. Robert H. Wiebe, *The Opening of American Society: From the Adoption of the

Constitution to the Eve of Disunion (New York: Knopf, 1984); D. W. Meinig, *Atlantic America, 1492–1800*, vol. 1 of *The Shaping of America: A Geographical Perspective on 500 Years of History* (New Haven, CT: Yale University Press, 1986); Martin Brückner, *The Geographic Revolution in Early America: Maps, Literacy, and National Identity* (Chapel Hill: University of North Carolina Press, 2006).

25. Winthrop, "A Model of Christian Charity," 239–41.

26. Levy, *Town Born*, ch. 3, emphasizes the protective and finally coercive force of the town in issuing warnings. By sharply circumscribing the benefits of poor relief to town residents, a viable safety net was established for town insiders, in the event they needed provision. For the phrase "town state," 290–91. Dayton and Salinger's *Robert Love's Warnings* complicates this view. They depict a two-tiered poor law regime in Boston in which warning did not necessarily mean removal, and in which Bostonians devised a remarkable new accommodation for strangers belonging to no town in the province, who would be placed on a province poor account (I carry this story forward in chapter 8). Paul Slack's *The Impact of Plague in Tudor and Stuart England* (London: Routledge, 1985) and *Poverty and Policy in Tudor and Stuart England* (London: Longman, 1988) provide antecedents in public health and poor law. For comparison of New England and other regions, see Duffy, *Epidemics in Colonial America*, ch. 2, and Whitfield J. Bell Jr., "Medicine in Boston and Philadelphia: Comparisons and Contrasts, 1750–1820," in *Medicine in Colonial Massachusetts*, ed. Cash, Christianson, and Estes, 159–83.

27. On the "protection covenant" that bound together the king and people, and the replication of exchanges of protection for allegiance that linked superiors and subordinates, see Bushman, *King and People.*

28. On petitions in the colonial period, see Bushman, *King and People*, 46–54, and David D. Hall, *A Reforming People: Puritanism and the Transformation of Public Life in New England* (Chapel Hill: University of North Carolina, 2011), 87–92. On petitions to the First Congress, see William C. diGiacomantonio, "Petitioners and Their Grievances: A View from the First Federal Congress," and Jeffrey L. Pasley, "Private Access and Public Power: Gentility and Lobbying in the Early Congress," in *The House and Senate in the 1790s: Petitioning, Lobbying, and Institutional Development*, ed. Kenneth R. Bowling and Donald R. Kennon (Athens Ohio University Press, 2002), 29–56, 57–99.

29. Allan M. Brandt, "From Analysis to Advocacy: Crossing Boundaries as a Historian of Health Policy," in *Locating Medical History: The Stories and Their Meanings*, ed. Frank Huisman and John Harley Warner (Baltimore: Johns Hopkins University Press, 2004), 460–84, offers some useful suggestions in this regard for a "policy-relevant" history.

30. Darrett B. Rutman, "Assessing the Little Communities of Early America," *William and Mary Quarterly* 43 (April 1986): 168–69.

31. The Massachusetts State Constitution (1780) was explicit in its provisions regarding the health of representatives. Health was not considered a positive right, but the constitution made plain that it was not to be endangered as a result of public service. Chapter II, section I, Article V, of the state constitution provided that "in case of any infectious distemper prevailing in the place where the said court is next at any

time to convene, or any other cause happening, whereby danger may arise to the health or lives of the members from their attendance, he [the governor] may direct the session to be held at some other most convenient place within the State." The first comprehensive declaration of health as a human right that I know of resides in Article 25 of the Universal Declaration of Human Rights (1948) of the United Nations: "Everyone has the right to a standard of living adequate for the health and well-being of himself and of his family, including food, clothing, housing, and medical care and necessary social services, and the right to security in the event of unemployment, sickness, disability, widowhood, old age, or other lack of livelihood in circumstances beyond his control." On the contemporary battle to conceive of health as a human right, see Paul Farmer, *Pathologies of Power: Health, Human Rights, and the New War on the Poor* (Berkeley: University of California Press, 2005).

32. Laura Jensen, *Patriots, Settlers, and the Origins of American Social Policy* (Cambridge: Cambridge University Press, 2003).

CHAPTER ONE

1. The Diary of Ebenezer Parkman, Parkman Family Papers, American Antiquarian Society, Worcester, Massachusetts, October 17–18, 1769. The printed portions of Parkman's diary can be found in *The Diary of Ebenezer Parkman, 1703–1782: First Part, Three Volumes in One, 1719–1755*, ed. Francis G. Walett (Worcester: American Antiquarian Society, 1974), and *The Diary of Rev. Ebenezer Parkman, of Westborough, Mass.*, ed. Harriette M. Forbes (Westborough Historical Society, 1899). Unpublished portions of the diary can be found at the American Antiquarian Society, Worcester, Massachusetts, and the Massachusetts Historical Society, Boston, Massachusetts. I am extremely grateful to Ross W. Beales, Jr., for allowing me to consult his transcriptions of the diary. Beales has now placed a transcription of the entire diary online as part of the Ebenezer Parkman Project: http://diary.ebenezerparkman.org/about-this-project/. References below will be to the transcriptions by Beales and given by date in the body of the chapter. Brief biographies of the two men can be found in Clifford K. Shipton, *New England Life in the 18th Century: Representative Biographies from "Sibley's Harvard Graduates"* (Cambridge: Belknap Press of Harvard University Press, 1963), 182–98 (Parkman), and C. Kenyon Shipton and J. Langdon Sibley, *Sibley's Harvard Graduates* (Boston: Massachusetts Historical Society, 1942), vol. 6: 428–32 (Barrett).

2. Catherine L. Thompson, *Patient Expectations: How Economics, Religion, and Malpractice Shaped Therapeutics in Early America* (Amherst: University of Massachusetts Press, 2015), ch. 1, offers a recent overview of therapeutics, including bleeding (which she argues was moderate), in early New England.

3. Patricia Ann Watson, *The Angelical Conjunction: The Preacher-Physicians of Colonial New England* (Knoxville: University of Tennessee Press, 1991).

4. Eric H. Christianson, "The Emergence of Medical Communities in Massachusetts, 1700–1794: The Demographic Factors," *Bulletin of the History of Medicine* 54, no. 1 (Spring 1980): 66; Rebecca J. Tannenbaum, *The Healer's Calling: Women and Medicine in Early New England* (Ithaca, NY: Cornell University Press, 2002), 9, 140; Laurel Thatcher Ulrich, *A Midwife's Tale: The Life of Martha Ballard, Based on Her*

Diary, 1785–1812 (1990; repr., New York: Vintage, 1991), 56; Parkman diary, December 7, 1758. The family regularly saw Dr. Chase, Dr. Crosby, and Dr. Willis. Dr. Hawes was the first town physician in Westborough, arriving from Wrentham in 1764.

5. Charles E. Rosenberg, "Medical Text and Social Context: Explaining William Buchan's *Domestic Medicine*," *Bulletin of the History of Medicine* 57 (Spring 1983): 22–42; *Every Man his own Doctor: or, The Poor Planter's Physician*, 3rd ed. (Williamsburg, VA, 1736), 18, 44–46, 53; John Wesley, *Primitive Physick; or, An easy and natural method of curing most diseases*, 12th ed. (Philadelphia, 1764), 23–24; William Buchan, *Domestic Medicine*, 11th ed. (London, 1790), ch. 33.

6. On reading the exteriors of the sick, see Mary E. Fissell, *Patients, Power, and the Poor in Eighteenth-Century Bristol* (Cambridge: Cambridge University Press, 1991), 29–33. Parkman diary: July 31, 1760; April 1, 1746.

7. Anne Bradstreet, "To My Dear Children," in *The Works of Anne Bradstreet*, ed. Jeannine Hensley (Cambridge, MA: Harvard University Press, 1967), 241–42; Cotton Mather, *The Angel of Bethesda*, ed. Gordon W. Jones (Barre, MA: American Antiquarian Society, 1972). Mather completed the volume in 1724, but it was not published until the twentieth century.

8. *The Diary of Ralph Josselin, 1616–1683*, ed. Alan MacFarlane (Oxford: Oxford University Press, 1976), 146–47; David D. Hall, *Worlds of Wonder, Days of Judgment: Popular Religious Belief in Early New England* (Cambridge, MA: Harvard University Press, 1989), ch. 5; Robert Blair St. George, *Conversing by Signs: Poetics of Implication in Colonial New England* (Chapel Hill: University of North Carolina Press, 1998).

9. The record of God's mercies begins on April 15, 1729. On affliction in the diary, see Rose Ann Lockwood, "Birth, Illness, and Death in 18th-Century New England," *Journal of Social History* 12 (Fall 1978): 111–28; Ross W. Beales Jr., "The Smiles and Frowns of Providence," in *Wonders of the Invisible World: 1600–1900: Annual Proceedings of the Dublin Seminar for New England Folklife, 1992*, ed. Peter Benes (Boston: Boston University, 1995), 86–96; Erik R. Seeman, "'She Died Like Good Old Jacob': Deathbed Scenes and Inversions of Power in New England, 1675–1775," *Proceedings of the American Antiquarian Society* 104 (1995): 285–314; Douglas L. Winiarski, *Darkness Falls on the Land of Light: Experiencing Religious Awakenings in Eighteenth-Century New England* (Chapel Hill: University of North Carolina Press, 2017), Kindle ed., locs. 1308–480 (in "The Loud Calls of Divine Providence").

10. Parkman diary, November 28, 1770.

11. Charles E. Rosenberg, "The Therapeutic Revolution: Medicine, Meaning, and Social Change in Nineteenth-Century America," in *The Therapeutic Revolution: Essays in the Social History of American Medicine*, ed. Morris J. Vogel and Charles E. Rosenberg (Philadelphia: University of Pennsylvania Press, 1979), 5.

12. *Diary of Elizabeth Porter Phelps*, October 18, 1769 (cited hereafter as EPP diary). The diary is dated most consistently on Sundays, but in listing the days of the week within entries, it is possible, in many cases, to determine a more exact date. Extensive excerpts of the diary can be found in Thomas Eliot Andrews, ed., "The Diary of Elizabeth (Porter) Phelps, 1763–1805," *New England Historical and Genealogical Register* (hereafter *NEHGR*), 118 (1964): 3–30, 108–27, 217–36, 297–308; 119 (1965): 43–59, 127–40, 205–23, 289–307; 120 (1966): 57–63, 123–35, 203–14, 293–304; 121 (1967): 57–69, 95–100,

296–303; 122 (1968): 62–70, 115–23, 220–27, 302–9. A list compiled by Phelps of "Births and Deaths in Hadley from 1794–1816" is published in *NEHGR* 123 (1969): 16–32. On the architecture and layout of Forty Acres, including the process of "rustification" that tried to turn provincial wood into the appearance of grand stone, see Elizabeth Pendergast Carlisle, *Earthbound and Heavenbent: Elizabeth Porter Phelps and Life at Forty Acres (1747–1817)* (New York: Scribner, 2004), 12–13, and James Lincoln Huntington, *Forty Acres: The Story of the Bishop Huntington House* (New York: Hastings House, 1949), 5.

13. Marla R. Miller, *The Needle's Eye: Women and Work in the Age of Revolution* (Amherst: University of Massachusetts Press, 2006), 124; Sylvester Judd, *History of Hadley* (Springfield, MA: H. R. Huntting and Co., 1905), 423–24; EPP diary, July 2, 1769, and August 20, 1769.

14. Judd, *History of Hadley*, 381–82. Marla Miller argues that quilting is commonly, and mistakenly, conceived as a classless activity. The intricate embroidery on quilts, the leisure time to execute them, and the money to pay laborers to procure materials and run a household in the absence of quilters were all markers of class. Miller, *The Needle's Eye*, ch. 3.

15. A. Roger Ekirch, *At Day's Close: Night in Times Past* (New York: Norton, 2005), chs. 1–2 (night perils), 114 (watching); Allan Greer, ed., *The Jesuit Relations: Natives and Missionaries in Seventeenth-Century North America* (Boston: Bedford/ St. Martin's, 2000), 72–78.

16. Among other resources, the Porters owned slaves and could send them off to tend others, as they had a year earlier, when the wife of a slave owned by Colonel Patridge in town had given birth. See EPP diary, October 4, 1768, and Carlisle, *Earthbound and Heavenbent*, 62.

17. EPP diary, October 22, 1769.

18. Edward Jarvis, *Traditions and Reminiscences of Concord, Massachusetts, 1779–1878*, ed. Sarah Chapin with an introduction by Robert A. Gross (Amherst: University of Massachusetts Press, 1993), introduction, ch. 1; Robert A. Gross's foreword to the Francis H. Underwood classic, *Quabbin: The Story of a Small Town with Outlooks on Puritan Life* (Amherst, MA: Northeastern University Press, 1986).

19. On nursing and the negotiations surrounding women's wages in antebellum New England, see Karen V. Hansen, *A Very Social Time: Crafting Community in Antebellum New England* (Berkeley: University of California Press, 1994), 95–98. Rebecca Dickinson—whose diary from 1787 to 1802 records her life as a gown maker, stay maker, and tailoress working in Hampshire County (and not infrequently at Forty Acres)—offers us a rare glimpse into the world of the single woman and the special pressures she might face in her own illnesses and in having to tend others. See Marla R. Miller, "'My Part Alone': The World of Rebecca Dickinson, 1787–1802," *New England Quarterly* 71 (September 1998): 358, 363–64, and Miller, *Rebecca Dickinson: Independence for a New England Woman* (Boulder, CO: Westview Press, 2014), 77, 102–9, 121–23, 134–43, 165–69.

20. *Twenty-Third Report of the Record Commissioners: Selectmen's Minutes, 1769–1775* (Boston, 1893), 23: 41 (for the meeting on October 18), 32, 36–38 (for other involvement with the Tuckermans). The record of the smallpox outbreak runs through-

out the volume. The Haithi Trust has a convenient listing of all volumes within this 39-volume series of Boston Records: https://catalog.hathitrust.org/Record/012294051. I will be using both Boston Town Records (hereafter BTR) and Boston Selectmen's Records (hereafter BSR) from these volumes, and I will cite the shortened title provided in the Haithi record for the first use and an acronym for subsequent use.

21. John B. Blake, *Public Health in the Town of Boston, 1630–1822* (Cambridge, MA: Harvard University Press, 1959), 32–35, 109–10. Barry Levy stresses the political achievement of such isolation, part of a larger effort to protect the labor markets of the port city. Levy, *Town Born: The Political Economy of New England from Its Founding to the Revolution* (2009; repr., Philadelphia: University of Pennsylvania Press, 2011), 7–8.

22. Gary B. Nash, *The Urban Crucible: The Northern Seaports and the Origins of the American Revolution* (Cambridge, MA: Harvard University Press, 1979), chs. 9–12; Blake, *Public Health in the Town of Boston*, 247–49; Cornelia H. Dayton and Sharon V. Salinger, *Robert Love's Warnings: Searching for Strangers in Colonial Boston* (Philadelphia: University of Pennsylvania Press, 2014), chs. 5, 8, 9.

23. Blake, *Public Health in the Town of Boston*, 35, 79.

24. For the origins of quarantine at Spectacle and Rainsford Islands, see Blake, *Public Health in the Town of Boston*, 35, 79.

25. John M. Murrin, "Beneficiaries of Catastrophe: The English Colonies in America," in *The New American History*, ed. Eric Foner (Philadelphia: Temple University Press, 1990); Alfred Crosby, "Virgin Soil Epidemics as a Factor in the Aboriginal Depopulation in America," *William and Mary Quarterly* 33 (April 1976): 289–99; David S. Jones, "Virgin Soils Revisited," *William and Mary Quarterly* 60 (October 2003): 703–42; John Duffy, *Epidemics in Colonial America* (Baton Rouge: Louisiana State University Press, 1953), ch. 3; Mary J. Dobson, "Mortality Gradients and Disease Exchanges: Comparisons from Old England and Colonial America," *Society for the Social History of Medicine* (1989): 259–97; Dobson, "From Old England to New England: Changing Patterns of Mortality," Research Paper 38, School of Geography, University of Oxford (1987), 5–64.

26. *The Journals of Ashley Bowen (1728–1813) of Marblehead*, 2 vols., ed. Philip Chadwick Foster Smith, Publications of the Colonial Society of Massachusetts, vols. 44 and 45 of *Collections* (Boston: Colonial Society of Massachusetts, 1973), 1: 142 (1764), 197 (1769).

27. Charles E. Rosenberg, *The Cholera Years· The United States in 1832, 1849, and 1866* (1962; repr., Chicago: University of Chicago Press, 1987), ch. 11; John Duffy, *The Sanitarians: A History of American Public Health* (Urbana: University of Illinois Press, 1990); Barbara Gutman Rosenkrantz, *Public Health and the State: Changing Views in Massachusetts, 1842–1936* (Cambridge, MA: Harvard University Press, 1972); William J. Novak, *The People's Welfare: Law and Regulation in Nineteenth-Century America* (Chapel Hill: University of North Carolina Press, 1996), ch. 6.

28. Carole Shammas, *A History of Household Government in America* (Charlottesville: University of Virginia Press, 2002); Christopher Tomlins, *Freedom Bound: Law, Labor, and Civic Identity in Colonizing English America, 1580–1865* (Cambridge: Cambridge University Press, 2010).

29. John Demos, *A Little Commonwealth: Family Life in Plymouth Colony* (Oxford: Oxford University Press, 1970); David H. Flaherty, *Privacy in Colonial New England, 1630–1776* (Charlottesville: University Press of Virginia, 1972); Levy, *Town Born*; Novak, *The People's Welfare*, ch. 6.

30. The selectmen issued three public notices on the case of the Tuckermans alone: *Boston Evening-Post*, September 4, 1769; *Boston Gazette*, September 25, 1769; *Boston Evening-Post*, October 9, 1769.

31. Conrad Edick Wright, *The Transformation of Charity in Postrevolutionary New England* (Boston: Northeastern University Press, 1992), 36.

32. *Boston, MA: Marriages, 1700–1809*, AmericanAncestors.org (online database; New England Historic Genealogical Society, 2006), 2: 376; *Massachusetts Officers in the French and Indian Wars, 1748–1763*, 360, in *Colonial Soldiers and Officers in New England, 1620–1775*, AmericanAncestors.org (online database; New England Historic Genealogical Society, 2013); Robert Francis Seybolt, *The Town Officials of Colonial Boston, 1634–1775* (Cambridge, MA: Harvard University Press, 1939), 256, 286; Annie Haven Thwing, *Inhabitants and Estates of the Town of Boston, 1630–1800*, and *The Crooked and Narrow Streets of Boston, 1630–1822* (CD-ROM database, New England Historic Genealogical Society and Massachusetts Historical Society, 2001), refcodes #42547, #58605; #50154; *NEHGR* 140 (1986): 284; *Republican Gazetteer*, October 27, 1802; Benjamin L. Carp, "Fire of Liberty: Firefighters, Urban Voluntary Culture, and the Revolutionary Movement," *William and Mary Quarterly* 58 (October 2001): 781–818; Fred Anderson, *A People's Army: Massachusetts Soldiers and Society in the Seven Years' War* (Chapel Hill: University of North Carolina Press, 1984), 38–39.

33. See note 32.

34. *Boston News-Letter*, September 7, 1769.

35. *Boston Town Records, 1758–69* (1886), 16: 298–301 (on town meeting; hereafter BTR). On Bernard and the evolving crisis in 1769, see Bernard Bailyn, *The Ordeal of Thomas Hutchinson* (Cambridge, MA: Belknap Press of Harvard University Press, 1974), 127–55.

36. There have been many accounts of Boston in this period. For an early overview of the imperial crisis in Boston, see G. B. Warden, *Boston: 1689–1776* (Boston: Little Brown, 1970), chs. 8–15. For a recent account of the imperial crisis that offers an intimate portrait of Phillis Wheatley and the losses inherent in that Atlantic rupture, see Mark Peterson, *The City-State of Boston: The Rise and Fall of an Atlantic Power, 1630–1865* (Princeton, NJ: Princeton University Press, 2019), ch. 6. On "Hillsborough paint," see Bailyn, *Thomas Hutchinson*, 135.

37. BTR, 16: 299–300.

38. On laws of concealment, see *The Acts and Resolves, Public and Private, of the Province of the Massachusetts Bay*, 21 vols. (Boston: Wright and Potter Printing, 1869–1922) 2: 621–22 and 3: 35–37. On Mackey, see BSR, 23: 19.

39. BTR, 16: 273–77.

40. BTR, 16: 275.

41. BTR, 16: 275; Gary B. Nash, "The Failure of Female Factory Labor in Colonial Boston," *Labor History* 20 (1970): 169–70; Adam Jay Hirsch, *The Rise of the Peniten-*

tiary: Prisons and Punishment in Early America (New Haven, CT: Yale University Press, 1992).

42. BSR, 23: 3; BTR, 16: 275 (overall numbers at almshouse); Boston Overseers of the Poor Records, 1733–1925, reel 8, box 9, folder 1, Massachusetts Historical Society, Boston, MA (summary list of admissions, discharges, and deaths in 1768–69); Eric Nellis and Anne Decker Cecere, eds., *The Eighteenth-Century Records of the Boston Overseers of the Poor*, vol. 69 of *Collections* (Boston: Colonial Society of Massachusetts, 2007), 629 (birth of boy on February 12), 639 (death of Zerviah and son), 638–40 (running tally of deaths in 1769). The death rate in October was somewhat less than trends over a longer period. Nellis and Cecere have counted 1,836 total almshouse admissions and 424 deaths between 1758 and 1774 (60), or a 23% mortality rate.

43. Boston Overseers of the Poor Records, reel 8, box 9, folder 2. A letter "p" is placed next to the names of those on province account. But not all persons on the province charge are designated in this way. Zerviah Smith, for example, has no "p" next to her name, but is listed as being on province charge in the record of deaths in the house. The total of 37 persons is likely an undercount.

44. Dayton and Salinger, *Robert Love's Warnings*, 50.

45. BSR, 23: 11, 18. Dayton and Salinger, *Robert Love's Warnings*, 50, note that in fiscal year 1769–70, "the treasurer divided £171 between the almshouse keeper and the institution's physician for special ministrations to these inmates."

46. BTR 16: 275; Boston Overseers of the Poor Records, reel 1, box 1, folder 2. See February 5, 1752, for the first mention of Lasenby, and March 1, 1769, for the latest payment to Lasenby recorded in the file.

47. Nash, "Failure of Female Factory Labor"; Laurel Thatcher Ulrich, "Sheep in the Parlor, Wheels on the Common: Pastoralism and Poverty in Eighteenth-Century Boston," in *Inequality in America*, ed. Carla Gardina Pestana and Sharon V. Salinger (Hanover, NH: University Press of New England, 1999), 182–200; and Ulrich, *The Age of Homespun: Objects and Stories in the Creation of an American Myth* (New York: Knopf, 2001), 157–66.

48. *The Diaries of George Washington*, vol. 2, ed. Donald Jackson (Charlottesville: University Press of Virginia, 1976), 188 (on fox hunting), 92 (on Robert Fairfax); *The Writings of George Washington*, vol. 2, ed. John C. Fitzpatrick (Washington, DC: US Government Printing Office, 1931), 528 (on Boucher). *Journals of Ashley Bowen*, 1: 198, 220, 224. John Demos finds that the dead of winter, while food from harvest was still plentiful and not spoiling in the summer heat, tended to be the healthiest time in New England. Demos, *Circles and Lines: The Shape of Life in Early America* (Cambridge, MA: Harvard University Press, 2004), 14.

49. Demos, *Circles and Lines*.

CHAPTER TWO

1. Alice Morse Earle, *Home Life in Colonial Days* (1898; repr., Lee, MA: Berkshire House, 1993), 388, 391.

2. Richard Lyman Bushman, "Markets and Composite Farms in Early America," *William and Mary Quarterly* 55 (1998): 351–74.

3. Paul Starr, *The Social Transformation of American Medicine: The Rise of a Sovereign Profession and the Making of a Vast Industry* (New York: Basic Books, 1982), 22.

4. Emily K. Abel, *Hearts of Wisdom: American Women Caring for Kin, 1850–1940* (Cambridge, MA: Harvard University Press, 2000); Abel, "'Man, Woman, and Chore Boy': Transformations in the Antagonistic Demands of Work and Care on Women in the Nineteenth and Twentieth Centuries," *Milbank Quarterly* 73 (1995): 187–211; Abel, "A 'Terrible and Exhausting' Struggle: Family Caregiving During the Transformation of Medicine," *Journal of the History of Medicine* 50 (1995): 478–506.

5. Margaret Pelling, *The Common Lot: Sickness, Medical Occupations and the Urban Poor in Early Modern England* (London: Longman, 1998); Peregrine Horden, "Household Care and Informal Networks: Comparisons and Continuities from Antiquity to the Present," and Sandra Cavallo, "Family Obligations and Inequalities in Access to Care in Northern Italy, Seventeenth to Eighteenth Centuries," in *The Locus of Care: Families, Communities, Institutions and the Provision of Welfare since Antiquity*, ed. Peregrine Horden and Richard Smith (Oxon, UK: Routledge, 1998), chs. 1, 3.

6. See introduction, above, note 8, for a list of representative works. Catherine L. Thompson, *Patient Expectations: How Economics, Religion, and Malpractice Shaped Therapeutics in Early America* (Amherst: University of Massachusetts Press, 2015), chs. 2, 3, argues that while exchange in goods, labor, and services continued to be common in rural New England through the middle of the nineteenth century, urban areas, and especially Boston, witnessed a change to a predominantly cash economy to execute medical debts. Patients with means to pay were able to take advantage of a robust medical marketplace and were promiscuous in their selection of healers. The respectable poor increasingly found themselves pushed toward new institutions of care, such as the dispensary and hospital, and those in severe want were relegated to almshouses. I return to the rise of new institutions of care that emerged in the nineteenth century in the epilogue.

7. Craig Muldrew, *The Economy of Obligation: The Culture of Credit and Social Relations in Early Modern England* (New York: Palgrave Macmillan, 1998); Karen V. Hansen, *A Very Social Time: Crafting Community in Antebellum New England* (Berkeley: University of California Press, 1994), ch. 4; Laurel Thatcher Ulrich, *A Midwife's Tale: The Life of Martha Ballard, Based on Her Diary, 1785–1812* (1990; repr., New York: Vintage, 1991), 72–101, which argues that the work and exchange activities of men and women were in many cases separate, in others overlapping, and in the end complementary.

8. Craig Muldrew, "'Hard Food for Midas': Cash and Its Social Value in Early Modern England," *Past and Present* 170 (2001): 78–120. On "complex barter," see Michael Merrill and Sean Wilentz, eds., *The Key of Liberty: The Life and Democratic Writings of William Manning, "A Laborer," 1747–1814* (Cambridge, MA: Harvard University Press, 1993), 12; on money economy, see Richard L. Bushman, *From Puritan to Yankee: Character and the Social Order in Connecticut, 1690–1765* (Cambridge, MA: Harvard University Press, 1967), chs. 7–9.

9. Muldrew's insights in "'Hard Food for Midas'" on the difficulties that the marginal had in procuring credit in early modern England are helpful here.

10. Dorothy Porter and Roy Porter, *Patient's Progress: Doctors and Doctoring in Eighteenth-Century England* (Cambridge: Polity Press, 1989).

11. Bettye Hobbs Pruitt, "Agriculture and Society in the Towns of Massachusetts, 1771: A Statistical Analysis" (PhD diss., Boston University, 1975). Daniel Vickers argues that interdependent relations between family farms was actually rising during the eighteenth century in Essex County, Massachusetts. Vickers, *Farmers and Fishermen: Two Centuries of Work in Essex County, Massachusetts, 1630–1850* (Chapel Hill: University of North Carolina Press, 1994), ch. 5.

12. Initial writing on the warning-out system emphasized the cruelty of the practice and the special attention directed at the poor: see Douglas Lamar Jones, "The Strolling Poor: Transiency in Eighteenth-Century Massachusetts," *Journal of Social History* 8 (1975): 28–54, and Jones, "The Transformation of the Law of Poverty in Eighteenth-Century Massachusetts," in *Law in Colonial Massachusetts, 1630–1800,* ed. Daniel R. Coquillette, vol. 62 of *Collections* (Boston: Colonial Society of Massachusetts, 1984), 153–90; and Ruth Wallis Herndon, *Unwelcome Americans: Living on the Margin in Early New England* (Philadelphia: University of Pennsylvania Press, 2001). More recently, Barry Levy has argued that the political economy of New England towns should be seen as necessary adaptations to the New World and on the vanguard of social provision, including the provision of education, regulation of labor markets, and social accommodation of the poor. Barry Levy, *Town Born: The Political Economy of New England from Its Founding to the Revolution* (2009; repr., Philadelphia: University of Pennsylvania Press, 2011). Cornelia H. Dayton and Sharon V. Salinger, *Robert Love's Warnings: Searching for Strangers in Colonial Boston* (Philadelphia: University of Pennsylvania Press, 2014), also argue that Boston's poor relief was generous, and they add that it was built on a two-tiered system, one directed toward those with residency in Massachusetts and the other, the province poor accounts, directed toward the many "strangers" (non-residents) and "sojourners" who moved most often from other areas of New England. The discussion of the province poor runs throughout the narrative. See 49 and 197n23 for the original law (1701) that was targeted at those who fell ill at sea and arrived in the port; in short order, it was broadened to accommodate sick strangers not "belonging to any town or place within the province. . . ."

13. Margaret Ellen Newell, *From Dependency to Independence: Economic Revolution in Colonial New England* (Ithaca, NY: Cornell University Press, 1998), chs. 6–11; Jeffrey Sklansky, *Sovereign of the Market: The Money Question in Early America* (Chicago: University of Chicago Press, 2017), chs. 1–2.

14. Westborough's population was 1,110 in 1765 and hovered around 900 for the last quarter of the century. Heman Packard DeForest and Edward Craig Bates, *The History of Westborough, Massachusetts* (Westborough, 1891), part 2, 345. The original Parkman diaries are held by the American Antiquarian Society and the Massachusetts Historical Society. Ross W. Beales Jr. has now placed a transcription of the entire diary online as part of the Ebenezer Parkman Project: http://diary.ebenezerparkman.org/about-this -project/. References below will be to the transcriptions by Beales (cited as Parkman diary) and given by date in the body of the chapter. Parkman's first entry is in 1719, but the steady record keeping begins in 1723.

15. On the stages of recovery after childbirth, see Ross W. Beales Jr., "Nursing and Weaning in an Eighteenth-Century New England Household," in *Families and Children: Annual Proceedings of the Dublin Seminar for New England Folklife, 1985*, ed. Peter Benes (Boston: Boston University, 1987), 52 (and n. 13); Ulrich, *A Midwife's Tale*, 183–90.

16. There is no explicit record of the arrangement with the maid. Judith Rocke was eventually hired as a maid and arrived at the parsonage on December 6, 1739. On female workers in the Parkman household, see Ross W. Beales Jr., "'Slavish' and Other Female Work in the Parkman Household, Westborough, Massachusetts, 1724–1782," in *House and Home: Annual Proceedings of the Dublin Seminar for New England Folklife, 1988*, ed. Peter Benes (Boston: Boston University, 1990), 48–57.

The wage work of nursing was open to a range of practitioners, and sometimes African Americans (both free and enslaved) were hired for this work: Dayton and Salinger, *Robert Love's Warnings*, loc. 2365; Jared Ross Hardesty, *Unfreedom: Slavery and Dependence in Eighteenth-Century Boston* (New York: New York University Press, 2016), Kindle edition, loc. 2372.

17. Massachusetts Archives Collection, vol. 105: 156–57, November 30, 1738, Massachusetts State Archives, Boston, MA (cited hereafter as MAC).

18. Dayton and Salinger, *Robert Love's Warnings*, locs. 960, 1036, point to extensive spending on the province poor at midcentury.

19. Steven King, "'Stop This Overwhelming Torment of Destiny': Negotiating Financial Aid at Times of Sickness under the English Old Poor Law, 1800–1840," *Bulletin of the History of Medicine* 79 (2005): 228–60.

20. Jonathan Leavitt, *A Summary of the Laws of Massachusetts Relative to the Settlement, Support, Employment and Removal of Paupers* (Greenfield, 1810); Jones, "The Transformation of the Law of Poverty in Eighteenth-Century Massachusetts"; Douglas Lamar Jones, "Charity, Medical Charity, and Dependency in Eighteenth-Century Essex County, Massachusetts," in *Medicine in Colonial Massachusetts*, ed. Cash, Christianson, and Estes. See also the account book of Ebenezer Roby, 1749–1772 (Countway Library of Medicine, Boston, MA), who ranged through Middlesex County; and physicians' accounts with the Boston overseers, Boston Overseers of the Poor Records, 1733–1925, reel 1, box 1, folder 2, Massachusetts Historical Society, Boston, MA. Eric Nellis and Anne Decker Cecere, *The Eighteenth-Century Records of the Boston Overseers of the Poor* vol. 69 of *Collections* (Boston: Colonial Society of Massachusetts, 2007), 65–66, discuss the almshouse physicians.

21. This argument runs through Levy, *Town Poor*, ch. 3, which focuses on local inhabitants of the town, and Dayton and Salinger, *Robert Love's Warnings*, which emphasizes, in addition to the town poor, the significant cash outlays that were devoted to the province poor. See above, note 18.

22. David Thomas Konig, ed., *Plymouth Court Records, 1686–1859* (Wilmington, MA: Michael Glazier, 1978), 3: 398, 401, Petition of Thomas Stockbridge, General Sessions, 1748–1781 (hard-copy volumes in this series cited hereafter as *PCR*, followed volume, page number at the bottom of the page, petitioners and litigants, and court). The *Plymouth County, MA: Plymouth Court Records, 1686–1859* (CD-ROM; Boston:

New England Historic Genealogical Society, 2002) have also been placed online and can be viewed with a subscription to NEHGR. Citations to the online materials have a different volume- and page-numbering system than the hard-copy volumes. These materials will be cited below as "Online *PCR*," followed by volume, page, and petition-ers or litigants. On being sick and lame as cause for contested tax abatements, see the varied responses in Online *PCR*, 2: 130, 141, 152, 158, Petitions of Ephraim Norcut, General Sessions; *PCR* 3: 250, Petition of George Barrow, General Sessions, 1748–1781; *PCR* 3: 278, Petition of Thomas Mansfield, General Sessions, 1748–1781; and *PCR* 3: 385, Petition of Benjamin Bates et al., General Sessions, 1748–1781.

23. Online *PCR*, 2: 161–62, Petition of Samuel Kempton, General Sessions, March 1740/41.

24. *PCR*, 3: 243, Warrant to David Stockbridge et al. on petition of Robert Bradford et al. regarding Ruth Drew, General Sessions, 1748–1781.

25. *Wenham Town Records, 1730–1775* (Wenham, MA, 1940), 246–47. Wenham ranked in the seventh decile in an assessment of the stock in trade, supply of specie, and money lent at interest in all Massachusetts towns in 1784. See the calculations of Van Beck Hall in his "Appendices to *Politics without Parties: Massachusetts, 1780–1791*" (Pittsburgh, 1972), A-11, A-37. (On deposit at the Hillman Library, University of Pittsburgh.)

26. *PCR*, 3: 231, Petition of Nicholas Shaw, General Sessions, 1748–1781.

27. Online *PCR*, 3: 53, 137, 140, Petition of Gideon Bradford et al., General Sessions. This sort of protracted process is evident in the long list of letters, written monthly by Boston's Overseers, to towns across the state. Boston Overseers of the Poor Records, "Daily Memorandum Book, 1 January 1816–31 December 1824," reel 12, box 14, folder 5, Massachusetts Historical Society, Boston, MA.

28. *Selectmen's Minutes, 1742/3–1753* (Boston, 1887), e.g., 17: 37.

29. For the initial law, see *The Colonial Laws of Massachusetts* (Boston, 1887), 238. For variations on the Massachusetts law providing for the province poor, see Laurel Daen's compilation of county, province, and state poor law provision regarding strangers without legal settlement that could be found in other New England colo-nies and states: "'To Board & Nurse a Stranger': Poverty, Disability, and Community in Eighteenth-Century Massachusetts," *Journal of Social History* (2020): 20n4. On Acadians, see John Mack Faragher, *A Great and Noble Scheme: The Tragic Story of the Expulsion of the French Acadians from Their American Homeland* (New York: Norton, 2005), 373–75, 378–80; town petitions, found in MAC, vols. 23–24; Dayton and Salinger, *Robert Love's Warnings*, locs. 1041–42, 1703, 2950, 3026–88.

CHAPTER THREE

1. Daniel Vickers, "Competency and Competition: Economic Culture in Early America," *William and Mary Quarterly* 47 (January 1990): 3; Richard L. Bushman, "Family Security in the Transition from Farm to City, 1750–1850," *Journal of Family History* (Fall 1981): 240. See also Christopher Clark, "The Household Economy, Market Exchange and the Rise of Capitalism in the Connecticut Valley, 1800–1860," *Journal*

of Social History 13 (Winter 1979): 169–89; Virginia DeJohn Anderson, *New England's Generation: The Great Migration and the Formation of Society and Culture in the Seventeenth Century* (Cambridge: Cambridge University Press, 1991), 123, 141–76; and Sarah F. McMahon, "A Comfortable Subsistence: The Changing Composition of Diet in Rural New England, 1620–1849," *William and Mary Quarterly* 42 (January 1985): 26–65.

2. Julie Hardwick, Sarah M. S. Pearsall, and Karin Wulf, "Introduction: Centering Families in Atlantic Histories," *William and Mary Quarterly* 70 (April 2013): 205–24, offer an overview of recent studies of family and household in an Atlantic context, part of a special issue of the journal devoted to the topic. Taken together, the essays stress the social, political, legal, economic, commercial, cultural, metaphorical, and ideological contexts that constituted family and household in the early modern Atlantic. In exploring the "life course" of illness in family life, I understand family to be always under construction, with different versions of family called into being in moments of affliction. In illness, one sees the elaboration of the spatial dimensions of family life, along with temporal reach that severe illness of family members could exact many years later.

3. Estimates vary on the numbers of live births a woman in her childbearing years could expect to deliver. John Demos calculates an average of 9.3 children born to families in Plymouth's third generation; Catherine M. Scholten suggests that "six to eight pregnancies were typical" of the colonial period; and David Flaherty finds that the average total number of persons in families projected in the Massachusetts census of 1764 was a little less than six. To complicate matters, a census must be read as a snapshot at a particular point in a family life cycle—it is not an actual count of the total number of children belonging to a household head. And, as was true in the case of the Parkmans, remarriage could add considerably to the total number of children in a family. Whatever the actual numbers one arrives at, a family of sixteen must be seen as quite substantial. John Demos, *A Little Commonwealth: Family Life in Plymouth Colony* (Oxford: Oxford University Press, 1970), 192; Catherine M. Scholten, "'On the Importance of the Obstetrick Art': Changing Customs of Childbirth in America, 1760 to 1825," in *Women and Health in America: Historical Readings*, ed. Judith Walzer Leavitt (Madison: University of Wisconsin Press, 1984), 142; David H. Flaherty, *Privacy in Colonial New England, 1630–1776* (Charlottesville: University Press of Virginia, 1967), 46–55. The original Ebenezer Parkman diaries may be found at the American Antiquarian Society, Worcester, MA, and the Massachusetts Historical Society, Boston, MA. Ross W. Beales Jr. has now placed a transcription of the entire diary online as part of the Ebenezer Parkman Project: http://diary.ebenezerparkman.org/about-this-project/. References in the chapter will be to the transcriptions by Beales and given by date. The website contains a helpful genealogical table that lists the births, marriages, and deaths of each of the Parkman children: http://diary.ebenezerparkman.org/diary-themes-people/#Children.

4. Laurel Thatcher Ulrich, *A Midwife's Tale: The Life of Martha Ballard, Based on Her Diary, 1785–1812* (1990; repr., New York: Vintage, 1991), 186–87; Christopher M. Jedrey, *The World of John Cleaveland: Family and Community in Eighteenth-Century New England* (New York: Norton, 1979), 70; Daniel Scott Smith and J. David Hacker, "Cultural Demography: New England Deaths and the Puritan Perception of Risk," *Journal of Interdisciplinary History* 26 (Winter 1996): 372. Smith and Hacker suggest

that 11.2 years may be "closer to the mark" than earlier calculations based on the first American life table, from which a median of 18.1 can be derived. The latter figure is based on statistics from the late eighteenth century in well-established communities in which lower fertility and increased longevity probably pulled the figure upward. On the age of the Parkman children at death, see table 1.

5. Ernest Caulfield, "Some Common Diseases of Colonial Children," in *Transactions, 1942–1946*, vol. 35 of *Publications of the Colonial Society of Massachusetts* (Boston: Colonial Society of Massachusetts, 1951), 4–65. The spectrum might run from the mumps, which were considered a nuisance but not lethal, to the throat distemper, which killed thousands of children in New England in the 1730s and 1740s and inspired numerous sermons and accounts of remarkable deaths. See note 9, below.

6. The year 1736 does not appear on the Ebenezer Parkman Project website. Readers can find the original diary for this year at the American Antiquarian Society, Worcester, MA. I have consulted the microfilmed originals for this year and compared them with a transcription that Ross W. Beales Jr. has generously provided me.

7. Even after his remarriage in 1737, Parkman continued to mark the anniversary of the occasion with somber reflection. Ross W. Beales Jr., "A Minister's Bereavement and Remarriage: Ebenezer Parkman of Westborough, Massachusetts," *History of the Family* 17 (2012): 397–406.

8. Mary died early the next morning. Parkman diary: January 29, 1736.

9. Ernest Caulfield, "A History of the Terrible Epidemic, Vulgarly Called the Throat Distemper, as It Occurred in His Majesty's New England Colonies Between 1735 and 1740," *Yale Journal of Biology and Medicine* 11, no. 3 (January 1939): 219–72; John Duffy, *Epidemics in Colonial America* (Baton Rouge: Louisiana State University Press, 1953), ch. 3; Douglas L. Winiarski, *Darkness Falls on the Land of Light: Experiencing Religious Awakenings in Eighteenth-Century New England* (Chapel Hill: University of North Carolina Press, 2017), 59–62, 68, 70, 75, 82, 106, 122, 508, 511–12.

10. Parkman's frustration at Deborah Ward's absence gave way to concern when the horse she had borrowed returned to Parkman's neighbor and kinsman without her (October 31, 1736). One wonders about the incident. Some thought the throat distemper contagious. Was Ward fleeing the scene? Why had she left on a Thursday (October 28, 1736), at least a day before an acceptable time for a weekend visit occasionally allowed hired help? It seems possible that after going through the intensive process of caring for Ebenezer Jr., Deborah Ward did not want to do the same when young Thomas Parkman became ill. Ward herself had been quite ill during the year and left the family in August before returning again on September 25. Perhaps another string of illness was more than she felt able to undertake.

11. On August 31, 1736, Parkman wrote: "Hannah under great Discouragement at the Thought of 4 Children to have the Care and Government of. Person—Country Life—Westborough—Ministerial Life—no objection—but the first mentioned Article insuperable *as yet. . . .*"

12. Ross W. Beales Jr., "In Search of the Historical Child: Miniature Adulthood and Youth in Colonial New England," *American Quarterly* 27 (1975): 379–98.

13. Steven C. Bullock and Sheila McIntyre, "The Handsome Tokens of a Funeral:

Glove-Giving and the Large Funeral in Eighteenth-Century New England," *William and Mary Quarterly* 69 (April 2012): 305–46.

14. Thomas had been ill for a week at Concord before Parkman sent son Ebenezer to fetch him on February 7, 1750, returning with Thomas to Westborough the next day. Thomas stayed at the parsonage until February 28. This absence might explain why the twelve-month contract that should have ended around September 19, 1750, appears to have finally finished on October 12, 1750. Thomas returned from Concord to Westborough on September 20, but he stayed for only a week before he resumed work in Concord. When Thomas returned to the parsonage for good on October 12, Parkman was filled with gratitude that his son had finally completed the agreement: "Towards evening came home my Son Thomas from Mr. Goold of Concord. . . . I thank God my son has been carry'd out, through the Agreement and that no Evil has fallen upon us to Grieve us."

15. Jack Larkin, *The Reshaping of Everyday Life, 1790–1840* (New York: Harper Perennial, 1988), ch. 5; Patricia Cline Cohen, "Safety and Danger: Women on American Public Transport, 1750–1850," in *Gendered Domains: Rethinking Public and Private in Women's History*, ed. Dorothy O. Helly and Susan M. Reverby (Ithaca, NY: Cornell University Press, 1992), ch. 6.

16. See Parkman's 1742 diary entries for October 26; November 2, 4, 23, 26, 30; and December 1, 4, 14. It is unclear whether Molly was ill until she was retrieved, or whether Parkman left her at the Marlborough parsonage until it was convenient to fetch her. Ebenezer Jr. had also been charged with fetching a doctor in Marlborough for Parkman, who was suffering from rheumatic pains.

17. It is possible that the entry did not mean that Molly kept house, but that she was confined to the house. The final portion of the entry reads: "Lodged at Sister Bettys. Molly had been long laid up with a Severe ague and Still Kept House" (November 30, 1742).

18. The account book contains sporadic entries for the years 1766 to 1782, and in many instances it is not clear what debts Parkman is discharging. As it happens, the account book offers an entry that clearly coincides with the incident involving Suse: "Jan. 26 1768 To Rev. Mr. Eb[eneze]r Morse for his Care of Suse. £6.15.6." In other cases, such as Parkman's reckoning for the boarding costs of his daughter Sarah, who stayed with Captain Clark for a month while she sought the help of a doctor in Hopkinton, there is no entry in the account book to match the transaction. See the diary for October 1, 1766. The account book can be found in Parkman Family Papers, Octavo volumes, American Antiquarian Society, Worcester, MA.

19. Ross W. Beales Jr., "The Reverend Ebenezer Parkman's Farm Workers, Westborough, Massachusetts, 1726–1782," *Proceedings of the American Antiquarian Society* 99 (1989): 121–49, provides a detailed discussion of the mechanics of this process.

20. Twitchell denied the minister on July 21 and again August 5, though he had worked on July 10 and 12. Perhaps he felt that his earlier efforts had discharged the debt. The possibility of confusion and contest here speaks to the ambiguities inherent in placing a price on work in a barter economy. Parkman regularly complained that he had a difficult time receiving his rates, either in cash or in work in lieu of it.

21. Parkman summarized the matter nicely in his diary the following spring when writing about Billy's work on the farm: "It is to my great Comfort that Billy is able to do So well for me as he does, since it is so exceeding Difficult for me to get Help" (April 27, 1756). An able-bodied son saved time and money.

22. *The Diary of Rev. Ebenezer Parkman, of Westborough, Mass.*, ed. Harriette M. Forbes (Westborough, MA: Westborough Historical Society, 1899), 83–89. It is also possible that Mrs. Crosby, who left the following day, was merely cleaning her quarters.

23. Clifford K. Shipton, *New England Life in the Eighteenth Century: Representative Biographies from "Sibley's Harvard Graduates"* (Cambridge, MA: Harvard University Press, 1963), 196.

24. Bernard Bailyn, *The Peopling of British North America: An Introduction* (1986; repr., New York: Vintage, 1988), 52; Richard L. Bushman, *From Puritan to Yankee: Character and the Social Order in Connecticut, 1690–1765* (Cambridge, MA: Harvard University Press, 1967), esp. chs. 3–6; James A. Henretta, "The Morphology of New England Society in the Colonial Period," in *The Origins of American Capitalism: Collected Essays* (Boston: Northeastern University Press, 1991), ch. 1; D. W. Meinig, *Atlantic America, 1492–1800*, vol. 1 of *The Shaping of America: A Geographical Perspective on 500 Years of History* (New Haven, CT: Yale University Press, 1986), 91–109; Douglas Lamar Jones, "The Strolling Poor: Transiency in Eighteenth-Century Massachusetts," *Journal of Social History* 8 (1975): 28–54; Richard L. Bushman, *Joseph Smith and the Beginnings of Mormonism* (Urbana: University of Illinois Press, 1984), which follows the Smith family and its trek into greater New England and beyond.

25. For a consideration of the importance of the life cycle in its relation to the Parkman family's need to hire domestic and farm help, see Ross W. Beales Jr., "'Slavish' and Other Female Work in the Parkman Household, Westborough, Massachusetts, 1724–1782," in *House and Home: Annual Proceedings of the Dublin Seminar for New England Folklife, 1988*, ed. Peter Benes (Boston: Boston University, 1990), 48–57; and Beales, "The Reverend Ebenezer Parkman's Farm Workers."

26. Laurel Thatcher Ulrich has characterized this process as a gradual transition period followed by a sharp break. The time between posting marriage banns and "going to housekeeping" could be several months in duration. But once her daughters had left to live in their own households, there was an insuperable break, symbolized by Martha Ballard's unfailing insistence in now referring to them in her diary by their married name. Ulrich, *A Midwife's Tale*, 138–42. The commonalties and differences in the case of the Parkmans are instructive. Like Ballard, Ebenezer Parkman joined in the process in which the series of new relations created by marriage were named: his daughter Molly, who married Eli Forbes, was now referred to as his "daughter Forbes," or, one step further removed, "Mrs. Forbes"; and when Molly interacted with Parkman's unmarried children, they might be said to be in the company of their "sister Forbes." Yet unlike Martha Ballard, Parkman also continued to call his married daughters by their first name in his diary. One wonders whether this was the prerogative of a patriarch. Similarly, the kinds of exchanges between the houses of parents and their married children was sensitive to gender. A couple's married daughters were more likely to live further afield than their married sons, especially in the case of a couple's eldest sons,

who might be able to continue to live on the farm. Molly (Parkman) Forbes married the same year as her brother, but Ebenezer Jr. was able to stay at the old house while Molly went to live with her husband in Brookfield, a town some twenty-five miles to the west.

27. Ross W. Beales Jr. discusses the initial part of this incident in his "Nursing and Weaning in an Eighteenth-Century New England Household," in *Families and Children: Annual Proceedings of the Dublin Seminar for New England Folklife, 1985*, ed. Peter Benes (Boston: Boston University, 1987), 55, and makes the point that "implicit in these arrangements was an attempt to balance the mother's health against the possibility that her milk would dry up if her daughter were kept too long from her."

28. The possibility of Alexander staying with Ebenezer Jr. was discussed, but, as Parkman put it, "this was not ripened" (August 30, 1756). It is unclear if subsequent discussion took place, but it does appear that Alexander stayed at the old house for some time.

29. Beales, "'Slavish' and Other Female Work in the Parkman Household," 57, suggests that the family should be considered "net consumers" of labor; they hired women to do work in the household but never had their daughters do waged work for others. But if we consider the moments in which families at different points in their life cycle converged, some parts of the family, too, might be considered "net consumers," not of waged work, but of family capital.

30. Patty Dunlop's case poses some interesting problems to consider. After registering her "uneasiness to go home" (April 9, 1759), Dunlop took matters into her own hands the following day: "N.B. John Dunlop came with an Horse whilst I was in my Chamber writing the above [entry], and carryed off his sister without either of them saying one word to me" (April 10, 1759). Earlier in the day, Parkman had gone out in search of "a Maid or Nurse to be in Pattys Stead," and had been fortunate that Persis Rice answered the call. But when Hannah Parkman "had a strong Ague Fitt, was sick and reached to Vomit" that afternoon, she seems to have pleaded with Patty to stay. "She can't part with *Patty* though *Persis* is here," Parkman noted tensely (April 10, 1759). Although Patty Dunlop had the desire and the right to go—Parkman had found someone to replace her—she was clearly in an awkward position here. Dunlop left the scene of affliction uneasily, breaking codes of propriety and deference, leaving without a word. Personal desires and prerogatives vied with those of affliction and its demands, and both took place within the ambiguities of evolving market relations. What was a reasonable and responsible course of action within this matrix? Perhaps when Patty Dunlop came back and watched with Hannah the following week, she found an acceptable middle ground (April 15, 1759).

31. Billy's case of the measles was probably not responsible for Suse Parkman coming down with the distemper some weeks later in mid-May (not long after she returned from Brookfield). But the idea of the connection between family visits and the spread of disease is intriguing. First, there is the question of mechanics. There seems to have been the possibility that the families in Brookfield transferred illnesses between one another. Visiting daughter Molly in 1759, Parkman observed that her "Children have the hooping Cough so has my son Ebenezers Children all of them" (August 25, 1759). Was the minister merely reporting on the state of both families, or was he intimating

a connection? It is easy enough to imagine children congregating and communicating illnesses to one another in a family center like Brookfield. Then the constant family traffic between the two towns insured that anyone without immunities to these diseases could contract them in Westborough. The same family ties that eased affliction might have been responsible for the spread of illness.

32. Hannah (Breck) Parkman was only nine years older than the minister's eldest child. It may be that her children, the eldest of whom was twenty-five years her junior (her eldest surviving child, William, was born in 1741), may have felt like a younger generation more in need of her duty and care.

33. The theme of the lonely husband left to fend for himself while his wife tended others abroad was common, not only in New England but in England as well. Jane C. Nylander, *Our Own Snug Fireside: Images of the New England Home, 1760–1860* (New Haven, CT: Yale University Press, 1993), 26; Leonore Davidoff and Catherine Hall, *Family Fortunes: Men and Women of the English Middle Class, 1780–1850* (Chicago: University of Chicago Press, 1987), 324–25.

34. "Parkman Family Genealogy," compiled by Breck Parkman, and "A Genealogical Record of the Ancestors and Descendants of Alexander Parkman," compiled by Samuel Spaulding Parkman. Typescripts of both are part of the Read Collection at the Westborough Public Library, Westborough, MA.

35. Barry Levy, *Town Born: The Political Economy of New England from Its Founding to the Revolution* (2009; repr., Philadelphia: University of Pennsylvania Press, 2011), ch. 8.

36. See Rebecca J. Tannenbaum, *The Healer's Calling: Women and Medicine in Early New England* (Ithaca, NY: Cornell University Press, 2002), for a broad discussion of women's healing practices and, especially, ch. 3, exploring women's healing networks. Ulrich, *A Midwife's Tale*, chs. 1, 5; Marla R. Miller, *Rebecca Dickinson: Independence for a New England Woman* (Boulder, CO: Westview Press, 2014), 77, 102–9, 121–23, 134–43, 165–69.

CHAPTER FOUR

1. Jack P. Greene, *Pursuits of Happiness: The Social Development of Early Modern British Colonies and the Formation of American Culture* (Chapel Hill: University of North Carolina Press, 1988), 71, 98–99; William D. Pierson, *Black Yankees: The Development of an Afro-American Subculture in Eighteenth-Century New England* (Amherst: University of Massachusetts Press, 1988), appendix, tables 5, 6; Jared Ross Hardesty, *Unfreedom: Slavery and Dependence in Eighteenth-Century Boston* (New York: New York University Press, 2016), Kindle edition, locs 428, 528, 898, finds 800 slaves in Massachusetts in 1700 (around 200–300 in Boston), 1,600 slaves in Boston at midcentury, and 5,249 persons of African decent living in Revolutionary Massachusetts. On slavery in Rhode Island, see Joanne Pope Melish, *Disowning Slavery: Gradual Emancipation and "Race" in New England, 1780–1860* (Ithaca, NY: Cornell University Press, 1998), and John Wood Sweet, *Bodies Politic: Negotiating Race in the American North, 1730–1830* (Philadelphia: University of Pennsylvania Press, 2003).

2. For the dialectic between the continuing presence of slaves and the enduring legacies of slavery, on the one hand, and the politics of erasure and effacement of that past, on the other, see Melish, *Disowning Slavery*.

3. On runaway slaves and self-fashioning, see David Waldstreicher, "Reading the Runaways: Self-Fashioning, Print Culture, and Confidence in Slavery in the Eighteenth-Century Mid-Atlantic," *William and Mary Quarterly* 56 (April 1999): 243–72. On sickness as a ploy to avoid sale, see Massachusetts Archives Collection, vol. 9: 171, September 5, 1714, Massachusetts State Archives, Boston, MA (cited hereafter as MAC); and Hardesty, *Unfreedom*, locs. 2803–24. On sickness as an excuse to absent oneself from work, see Philip D. Morgan, *Slave Counterpoint: Black Culture in the Eighteenth-Century Chesapeake and Lowcountry* (Chapel Hill: University of North Carolina Press, 1998), 195.

4. Prince Hoare, *Memoirs of Granville Sharp*, excerpted in Elizabeth Donnan, ed., *The Eighteenth-Century*, vol. 2 of *Documents Illustrative of the History of the Slave Trade to America* (Washington, DC: Carnegie Institution, 1931), 555–57.

5. Elizabeth Donnan, ed., *New England and the Middle Colonies*, vol. 3 of *Documents Illustrative of the History of the Slave Trade to America* (Washington, DC: Carnegie Institution of Washington, 1932), 135–36, 377, 385.

6. MAC, 9: 201, October 4, 1727, for petition; *The Acts and Resolves, Public and Private, of the Province of the Massachusetts Bay*, 21 vols. (Boston: Wright and Potter Printing, 1869–1922) 1: 578–79, for original legislation (cited hereafter as *Mass AR*); Pierson, *Black Yankees*, 4–5; Morgan, *Slave Counterpoint*, 444–45, for mortality rates.

7. *Mass AR*, 1: 213–16, 614–16.

8. Phrases taken from David Thomas Konig, ed., *Plymouth Court Records, 1686–1859* (Wilmington, MA: Michael Glazier, 1978), 5: 350, 381, Litchfield v. Cowing and Stertevant v. Howland, Common Pleas, 1702–1736 (hard-copy volumes cited hereafter as *PCR*, followed by volume, page, litigants, and court); Charles Phelps Jr., contract for slave Cesar, 1770, box 4, folder 15, Porter-Phelps-Huntington Family Papers, Amherst College Archives and Special Collections, Amherst, MA. On "soundness," see Sharla M. Fett, *Working Cures: Healing, Health, and Power on Southern Slave Plantations* (Chapel Hill: University of North Carolina Press, 2002), ch. 1.

9. *PCR*, 5: 366, 381, 382, Stertevant v. Howland, Common Pleas, 1702–1736.

10. *PCR*, 5: 350, 361, Litchfield v. Cowing, Common Pleas, 1702–1736.

11. Helen Tunnicliff Catterall, ed., *Cases from the Courts of New England, the Middle States, and the District of Columbia*, vol. 4 of *Judicial Cases Concerning American Slavery and the Negro* (New York: Octagon Books, 1968), 155, 197, 365 (the latter from New York). Saffin in MAC 9: 152, May 6, 1703. On this case, see Mark A. Peterson, "The Selling of Joseph: Bostonians, Antislavery, and the Protestant International, 1689–1733," *Massachusetts Historical Review* 4 (2002): 1–22; and Wendy Warren, *New England Bound: Slavery and Colonization in Early America* (New York: Liveright, 2016), ch. 7.

12. Extensive excerpts of the diary can be found in Thomas Eliot Andrews, ed., "The Diary of Elizabeth (Porter) Phelps, 1763–1805," *New England Historical and Genealogical Register* (*NEHGR*), 118 (1964): 3–30, 108–27, 217–36, 297–308; 119 (1965): 43–59, 127–40, 205–23, 289–307; 120 (1966): 57–63, 123–35, 203–14, 293–304; 121 (1967): 57–69,

95–100, 296–303; 122 (1968): 62–70, 115–23, 220–27, 302–9. A list compiled by Phelps of "Births and Deaths in Hadley from 1794–1816" is published in *NEHGR* 123 (1969): 16–32. I am indebted to Elizabeth Carlisle who generously shared her knowledge of the life histories of the servants and slaves at Forty Acres. Although I am calling Phillis a slave in these passages, her legal status was probably more ambiguous. Phillis's grandmother had been a free woman before selling herself into slavery, and although a series of legal challenges issued on the basis of the Massachusetts Constitution of 1780 eventually ended slavery as a legal practice, the institution continued in various guises (including long-term indentures) for years to come. Melish, *Disowning Slavery*, ch. 2.

13. William Buchan, *Domestic Medicine*, 2nd ed. (London, 1772), 687–91; Kenneth Kiple, ed., *The Cambridge World History of Human Disease* (Cambridge: Cambridge University Press, 1993), 978–80.

14. Buchan, *Domestic Medicine*, 505–9; Kiple, *The Cambridge World History of Human Disease*, 998–1000.

15. Morgan, *Slave Counterpoint*, 322. Lorenzo Greene, *The Negro in Colonial New England, 1620–1776* (New York: Columbia University Press, 1942), 225–29, argues that New England slaves were "well cared for," and Sylvester Judd notes that medical accounts for slaves could constitute a family's largest bills. "Selected Papers from the Sylvester Judd Manuscript," ed. Gregory H. Nobles and Herbert L. Zarov (Forbes Library, Northampton, MA, 1976, photocopy), 433, 436, 437, 439. The latter bill details visits made to Forty Acres while Phelps's father, Moses Porter, was still alive. On doctors' visits to enslaved persons in Boston, see Hardesty, *Unfreedom*, locs. 1599–608.

16. The latter term seems to have included both servants and slaves—everyone within the family household were part of "our people."

17. Richard B. Morris, *Government and Labor in Early America* (New York: Columbia University Press, 1946), 18nn8–9 (on West Indies and New Haven); John Demos, *A Little Commonwealth: Family Life in Plymouth Colony* (Oxford: Oxford University Press, 1970), 109; William Waller Henning, ed., *The Statutes at Large, Being a Collection of All the Laws of Virginia, from the First Session of the Legislature, in the Year 1619* (1810), 2: 450. Christopher L. Tomlins, *Law, Labor, and Ideology in the Early American Republic* (Cambridge: Cambridge University Press, 1993), 331–41, discusses the place of injury, and, to a lesser extent, illness, within seventeenth- and eighteenth-century law in Britain and America.

18. *Records and Files of the Quarterly Courts of Essex County, Massachusetts* (Salem: Essex Institute, 1911–75), 2: 275–76.

19. Helena M. Wall has drawn on incidents like these to illustrate the "wavering lines of responsibility and affection that linked parents, masters, and children" in seventeenth-century America. Wall, *Fierce Communion: Family and Community in Early America* (Cambridge, MA: Harvard University Press, 1990), 124.

20. These stock phrases, including the master's provision "in sickness as in health," appear routinely in a large collection of indentures. See, for example, Indenture Documents, 1692–1834, Ship. Mss. 23, Phillips Library, Peabody Essex Museum, Salem, MA.

21. Wall, *Fierce Communion*, 113–14.

22. Margaret Pelling, *The Common Lot: Sickness, Medical Occupations and the Urban Poor in Early Modern England* (London: Longman, 1998), ch. 6.

23. Barry Levy, *Town Born: The Political Economy of New England from Its Founding to the Revolution* (2009; repr., Philadelphia: University of Pennsylvania Press, 2011), 249–50, discusses Storey as an instance of orphan household placement.

24. The February 11, 1783, indenture between Charles Phelps Jr. and Elisha and Rachel Searl of Northampton for their son David can be found in box 4, folder 32, Porter-Phelps-Huntington Family Papers, Amherst College Archives and Special Collections, Amherst, MA. Phelps included the same provision regarding health in his agreement with Henry Fraser for his son Robert on January 12, 1807, box 4, folder 32.

25. Providence Town Papers, 1: 51, May 20, 1735, Rhode Island Historical Society, Providence, RI.

26. Ross W. Beales Jr., "The Reverend Ebenezer Parkman's Farm Workers, Westborough, Massachusetts, 1726–1782," *Proceedings of the American Antiquarian Society* 99 (1989): 121–49. Beales has usefully compiled a list of farm workers and their contracts and ages at the end of the article.

27. Consider the case of Phineas Forbush, who worked two weeks after his time was out in October 1772. Some of his extra time might be attributed to days lost to the violent rainstorms deluging Westborough that spring, and at least one day might have been added to make up for Forbush's participation in training-day exercises. But one suspects that some of this time was to compensate for several days that Forbush missed in August, when he, along with Parkman's daughter and wife, were all ill.

28. When Reuben Bellows inexplicably left Parkman after a month of work, Parkman subjected the young man to "pleading, urging, expostulating, offers to him, [and] pitying," "representing the Injustice, breach of promise, unhandsomeness, unsteddiness, [and] disgrace" of the action (December 25, 1772).

29. There appear to have been no hard feelings between the minister and the injured worker. Ebenezer Maynard stayed at the parsonage for the next week and was daily attended by the doctor. After returning home early in May, the young man was welcomed to dinner at the parsonage the following month—this a day after his replacement at the minister's farm had been injured while plowing with Parkman's mare (June 12–13, 1769).

30. Ross W. Beales Jr., "'Slavish' and Other Female Work in the Parkman Household, Westborough, Massachusetts, 1724–1782," in *House and Home: Annual Proceedings of the Dublin Seminar for New England Folklife, 1988*, ed. Peter Benes (Boston: Boston University, 1990), 48–57. Parkman's female workers were a more varied lot than those who worked at the Ballard household, who were almost entirely life-cycle servants. Laurel Thatcher Ulrich, *A Midwife's Tale: The Life of Martha Ballard, Based on Her Diary, 1785–1812* (1990; repr., New York: Vintage, 1991), 81–82.

31. I take "Capt. Ward" of Shrewsbury to be Nahum Ward. For information on the family, see Charles Martyn, *The William Ward Genealogy* (New York: A. Ward, 1925), 87–88.

32. As one of the wealthier men in the area, Ward may have had surplus laborers to hire out. On the same day he secured the services of Silence Bartlett, Parkman also hired one of Ward's farmhands.

33. Ulrich, *A Midwife's Tale*, 81.

34. For a parallel theme in treating servants accused of sexual indiscretions, see

M. Michelle Jarrett Morris, *Under Household Government: Sex and Family in Puritan Massachusetts* (Cambridge, MA: Harvard University Press, 2013), 49.

CHAPTER FIVE

1. Alfred W. Crosby, "Smallpox," in *The Cambridge World History of Human Disease*, ed. Kenneth F. Kiple (Cambridge: Cambridge University Press, 1993), 1008–9; Elizabeth A. Fenn, *Pox Americana: The Great Smallpox Epidemic of 1775–82* (New York: Hill and Wang, 2001), 16–20. Fenn's chart on communicability, symptoms, and pathogenesis is especially useful (19).

2. Donald R. Hopkins, *Princes and Peasants: Smallpox in History* (Chicago: University of Chicago Press, 1983); John Duffy, *Epidemics in Colonial America* (Baton Rouge: Louisiana State University Press, 1953), ch. 2; John B. Blake, *Public Health in the Town of Boston, 1630–1822* (Cambridge, MA: Harvard University Press, 1959), chs. 4, 5, 9; Ola Elizabeth Winslow, *A Destroying Angel: The Conquest of Smallpox in Colonial Boston* (Boston: Houghton Mifflin, 1974); Fenn, *Pox Americana*; Patricia Cline Cohen, *A Calculating People: The Spread of Numeracy in Early America* (Chicago: University of Chicago Press, 1982), 86–108; David S. Jones, *Rationalizing Epidemics: Meanings and Uses of American Indian Mortality since 1600* (Cambridge, MA: Harvard University Press, 2004), chs. 1–2; Joyce E. Chaplin, "Natural Philosophy and an Early Racial Idiom in North America: Comparing English and Indian Bodies," *William and Mary Quarterly* 54 (January 1997): 237–52; Margo Minardi, "The Boston Inoculation Controversy of 1721–1722: An Incident in the History of Race," *William and Mary Quarterly* 61 (January 2004): 47–76; Cristobal Silva, *Miraculous Plagues: An Epidemiology of Early New England Narrative* (Oxford: Oxford University Press, 2011), and the forum centered on the book: *William and Mary Quarterly* 70 (October 2013): 813–48. I have found the following approaches to the plague particularly suggestive: Giulia Calvi, *Histories of a Plague Year: The Social and the Imaginary in Baroque Florence*, trans. by Dario Biocca and Bryant T. Ragan Jr. (1984; repr., Berkeley: University of California Press, 1989); and Colin Jones, "Plague and Its Metaphors in Early Modern France," *Representations* 53 (Winter 1996): 97–127.

3. The other major source of infection was soldiers returning from abroad, which I discuss in chapter 7.

4. Paul Slack, *The Impact of Plague in Tudor and Stuart England* (London: Routledge, 1985), ch. 8 (on the elaboration of regulations), 261–66 (on Puritan magistrates as being on the vanguard of enforcement).

5. Duffy, *Epidemics in Colonial America*, ch. 2 (for the comparisons), 43–69 (on New England).

6. Blake, *Public Health in the Town of Boston*, 109–12; Simon Finger, *The Contagious City: The Politics of Public Health in Early Philadelphia* (Ithaca, NY: Cornell University Press, 2012), chs. 1–2; Duffy, *Epidemics in Colonial America*, 51.

7. Daniel Vickers, "An Honest Tar: Ashley Bowen of Marblehead," *New England Quarterly* 69 (1996): 531–53; *The Autobiography of Ashley Bowen, 1728–1813*, ed. Daniel Vickers (Peterborough, ON: Broadview Press, 2006), 11–30; Daniel Vickers with Vince Walsh, *Young Men and the Sea: Yankee Seafarers in the Age of Sail* (New Haven, CT:

Yale University Press, 2005), ch. 4. Andrew Wehrman, "The Siege of 'Castle Pox': A Medical Revolution in Marblehead, Massachusetts, 1764–1777," *New England Quarterly* 82 (September 2009): 385–429, discusses the 1773 outbreak in Marblehead (393) and the inoculation riots that followed.

8. Samuel Eliot Morison, *A Maritime History of Massachusetts, 1783–1860* (Boston: Houghton Mifflin, 1921), 23.

9. The memorandum is reprinted in *The Journals of Ashley Bowen (1728–1813) of Marblehead*, 2 vols., ed. Philip Chadwick Foster Smith, Publications of the Colonial Society of Massachusetts, vols. 44 and 45 of *Collections* (Boston: Colonial Society of Massachusetts, 1973), 2: 344–45 (cited hereafter as *ABJ*).

10. Bowen did his best to illustrate the relationships between the infected, noting, "It is to be understood that this Mrs. Sarah Mathews was daughter to Mrs. Sarah Shaw, widow, sister to Mr. Ebenezer Stacey, deceased, and I married James Shaw's widow, [he being a] son [-in-law] to said Sarah Shaw and that Mary Ingalls was [another] daughter to Mrs. Shaw." But even with Bowen's genealogy (and the parenthetical notes added by the editors), discerning the exact relation between the women involved is a difficult task. This much can be said with relative certainty: Sarah (Stacey) (Ingalls) Shaw had eight children with her second husband, Eleazar Ingalls; her eldest daughter from the marriage was Mary ("Mol") Ingalls; and Ashley Bowen's wife, Mary (Beal) (Shaw) Bowen, was daughter-in-law to the elderly Sarah Shaw through her second marriage. An Ingalls genealogy maintains that Mary Ingalls married Lawrence Bartlett. One assumes that the genealogy is either incorrect, or that Mary remarried an Ingalls after the death of Bartlett, something that is not implausible. The exact relation between Mary Ingalls and Sarah Mathews is unclear. Bowen calls the two sisters, but it seems unlikely that Sarah was the daughter of Sarah Shaw, as her daughter Sarah married Thomas Gould, and one Sarah Gould appears to have been infected in the outbreak. My assumption is that Sarah Mathews is sister to Mol Ingalls through marriage. See the "Ingalls Genealogy" at the Marblehead Historical Society, Marblehead, MA; and *Vital Records of Marblehead, Massachusetts, to the End of the Year 1849*, 3 vols. (Salem, MA: Essex Institute, 1903, 1904, 1908), vols. 1–2, under births, marriages, and deaths of the Beal, Bowen, Ingalls, Shaw, and Stacey families.

11. Ashley Bowen says that his sisters were called, and it is possible that one of his four living sisters came to his aid. More likely, given the arrival of his wife's sister the following day, is that all of the women who arrived were her relations, though this cannot be said with certainty.

12. Daniel Vickers, *Farmers and Fishermen: Two Centuries of Work in Essex County, Massachusetts, 1630–1850* (Chapel Hill: University of North Carolina Press, 1994), 168–70; T. H. Breen, *The Marketplace of Revolution: How Consumer Politics Shaped American Independence* (Oxford: Oxford University Press, 2004), chs. 2–5. On soap, see Jane C. Nylander, *Our Own Snug Fireside: Images of the New England Home, 1760–1860* (New Haven, CT: Yale University Press, 1993), 135–39; and R. W. Mitchell, *Castile Soap: A Monograph Covering the Origin, History and Significance of the Term* (Boston: printed by the author, 1927). Advertised by merchants in Boston beginning in the early eighteenth century and by Salem merchants beginning in the 1760s, the soap

may have been difficult to procure in Marblehead itself, and so a logical commodity for fishermen to purchase directly through shipboard exchange. Mitchell emphasizes that a major use of the soap was medical, something supported by a variety of advertisements that list the soap among other medicines and surgical instruments.

13. Vickers and Walsh, *Young Men and the Sea*, 111, finds that "among locally born sailors three in ten never reached the age of thirty." Bowen's genealogical notes, cited above, illuminate the complexity of these relations.

14. *ABJ*, 2: 351, July 24, 1773. The rest of the narrative comes from Bowen's day-book, smallpox journal, and almanacs, all of which have been usefully compiled and placed in chronological order in *ABJ*.

15. Blake, *Public Health in the Town of Boston*, 32–36 and ch. 5, offers an overview of these measures. On laws of concealment, see *The Acts and Resolves, Public and Private, of the Province of the Massachusetts Bay*, 21 vols. (Boston: Wright and Potter Printing, 1869–1922), 2: 621–22, 3: 35–37 (cited hereafter as *Mass AR*).

16. *ABJ*, 2: 351, July 24, 1773.

17. *ABJ*, 2: 351–53. Quote from journal on July 24. The editors have included excerpts from the local *Essex Gazette* that detail the town's efforts (352–53). See Marblehead Town Meeting Records, July 26, 1773, conveniently bound in WPA transcripts, Abbot Hall, Marblehead, MA, 112–13.

18. *ABJ*, 2: 353, July 31, 1773.

19. On education and labor markets, see Barry Levy, *Town Born: The Political Economy of New England from Its Founding to the Revolution* (2009; repr., Philadelphia: University of Pennsylvania Press, 2011); William J. Novak, *The People's Welfare: Law and Regulation in Nineteenth-Century America* (Chapel Hill: University of North Carolina Press, 1996), ch. 6, draws on colonial precedent to discuss such public protections in the nineteenth century.

20. *Essex Gazette* reprinted in *ABJ*, 2: 351–53.

21. Town officials were cautious in granting permissions for persons to move into and out of pesthouses. Attending nurses were regularly required to stay in infected houses until the sick either recovered or died. At a minimum, if Bowen had been able to enter the pesthouse, he would have faced the onerous task of shifting and cleansing his clothes, something that he does not mention in the diary.

22. The degree to which the sick could be accessed may have depended on the course of any given epidemic. Measures were slack enough in the initial days of the outbreak in Marblehead that Bowen was able to see his son Nathan "about the street barefooted," presumably in the immediate vicinity of the pesthouse. Later, as more became ill in the town, Bowen noted the tightening of measures. When he rode to the Ferry, where many of the ill had been transferred, he could only "inquire of Nathan" but "Could not see him." *ABJ*, 2: 353, 358, August 4, 1773, September 6, 1773.

23. *ABJ*, 2: 331–33, January 19–February 4, 1773, notes measles. Bowen and his wife most likely were struck with something other than measles, though the clustering of sickness within families was common. *ABJ*, 1: 271–80, April 14–August 17, 1771, records the sickness and death of his first wife, Dorothy.

24. Bowen had served the town in past epidemics and would do so again in the

future: he served as a guard at Marblehead's watch house at the entrance to the town in 1764 and manned a smokehouse in 1792. In both capacities, he was to prevent infected persons and objects from entering the town. *ABJ*, 1: 142; 2: 582–91.

25. Vickers, *Farmers and Fishermen*, ch. 4.

26. Consider Bowen's need to make up for the work of Nathaniel Dennin, one of his regular hired hands who had been absent. *ABJ*, 2: 338–39, April 2–12, 1773. Dennin himself secured employment during the epidemic. He was hired (for an unspecified task and for an unnamed amount) by Glover and Gerry from July 27–November 20. See "Debts Contracted and Persons Employed," no date [1773], Smallpox file, Abbot Hall, Marblehead, MA.

27. On Humphreys, see *ABJ*, 2: 355, August 12–18, 1773.

28. The one surviving bill during the early stages of the epidemic covered here lists Ashley Bowen as due for sundry "labor," but does not specify a sum. The bill makes clear that many persons were involved with care, noting tasks such as "Cloutman house clear'd" or "sent 10 persons to the ferry" (one of the primary pesthouses in the epidemic) that likely required the services of several persons. "Smallpox folder," Vault, Abbot Hall, Marblehead, MA. Long after his family had recovered from the pox, Bowen continued to perform occasional labor for the town. On November 9, 1773, he noted in his diary, "I assisted the Selectmen in gathering Mr. Dixey's corn." It was not a gesture performed within the framework of neighborly exchange; Bowen saw himself as doing a civic duty and could expect to be compensated. See *ABJ*, 2: 361.

29. On total numbers of sick and dead, see Wehrman, "The Siege of 'Castle Pox,'" 396n34. Boston's smallpox epidemic of 1721 afflicted more than half of the population: of 10,670 in the town, 5,980 were stricken and 844 died. See Duffy, *Epidemics in Colonial America*, 51. I want to thank Barry Levy for suggestion that the elderly Shaw's vulnerability was a measure of public health success.

30. In the months following the initial outbreak discussed here, the town became embroiled in a controversy over inoculation. I treat that incident briefly below. For a full discussion of the inoculation controversy, see Wehrman, "The Siege of 'Castle Pox.'"

31. On rituals of repentance and renewal, see David D. Hall, *Worlds of Wonder, Days of Judgment: Popular Religious Belief in Early New England* (Cambridge, MA: Harvard University Press, 1989), ch. 4. On the dramaturgy of epidemics, see Charles E. Rosenberg's "What Is an Epidemic? AIDS in Historical Perspective," in his *Explaining Epidemics and Other Studies in the History of Medicine* (Cambridge: Cambridge University Press, 1992), ch. 13.

32. Fenn's *Pox Americana* uses the pandemic of 1775–83 as a way to investigate the range of possible motion and human contact throughout North America.

33. John Adams to Abigail Adams, July 27, 1776, in *Adams Family Correspondence*, 2 vols., ed. L. H. Butterfield et al. (Cambridge, MA: Harvard University Press, 1963), 2: 63.

34. I elaborate on these themes in chapter 6.

35. On money, see, for example, Richmond Town Council, 1: 312, 316, June 2, 1760. My sincere thanks to Ruth Herndon, who has generously shared some of her transcrip-

tions of smallpox in Rhode Island towns. References to her transcripts will be noted with HT, followed by town meeting or town council record, volume, and date.

36. Jane Kamensky, *Governing the Tongue: The Politics of Speech in Early New England* (New York: Oxford University Press, 1997), 21, 48, 57–63, 125, 155–57, discusses rumor and gossip.

37. On laws of concealment, see *Mass AR*, 2: 621–22 and 3: 35–37.

38. HT, Richmond Town Council, 1:163–65, 169, 173, June 24, July 12, September 2, and December 2, 1754; HT, Richmond Town Meeting, 1: 461, June 3, 1755.

39. Herndon surmises that the £30 might have been the entirety of Harvey's savings. We don't know what became of Harvey and his family in the immediate aftermath of his case. Five years after his settlement with town officials, however, it appears that Harvey was still residing in Richmond. His name surfaces in another incident involving suspicion of the smallpox. This time, however, Harvey served as an appointed inspector for the town. HT, Richmond Town Council, 1: 276–77, January 16, 1760, likely in the case of the Holloway family, below.

40. HT, Richmond Town Council, 1: 275–77, January 9, 11, 16, 18, 1760. It is possible that John Holloway was sick at his father's house and that others of the family were not allowed back into it, but this seems unlikely because Nicholas Holloway would not have been allowed to move freely in town if he had been in contact with the infected.

41. New Englanders were not naive about the possible dangers carried on ships arriving from foreign ports. Beginning in the seventeenth century, acts to contain infectious disease borne of commerce were put into place. These laws were much like the rules regarding persons infected with the pox onshore that we have seen operating in Marblehead: infection was to be identified and isolated, and violations were to be met with hefty fines. Ships suspected of virulent distempers were made to anchor in harbors. Persons and goods were forbidden to land. Inspections were performed and fines issued. Exemptions were granted by special license and certificates. Over the course of the century, large centers of trade like Boston constructed "hospitals" on outlying islands—Spectacle Island in 1717 and later Rainsford Island in 1737—that both held quarantined persons and goods from abroad and provided permanent buildings to house the infected walking about the city. In short, eighteenth-century New England had devised a wide range of measures to protect the healthy from persons or objects bringing infection into its ports. Blake, *Public Health in the Town of Boston*, chs. 2, 5.

42. *Records of Boston Selectmen, 1716 to 1736* (Boston: Rockwell and Churchill, 1885), 13: 76, 142 , 242, 245 (hereafter BSR).

43. Bowen's poem may be found in *ABJ*, 2: 343–44. Roy Porter, "Diseases of Civilization," in *Companion Encyclopedia of the History of Medicine*, 2 vols., ed. W. F. Bynum and Roy Porter (London: Routledge, 1993), 1: 585–600. On earlier epidemics in Marblehead, see Christine Leigh Heyrman, *Commerce and Culture: The Maritime Communities of Colonial Massachusetts, 1690–1750* (New York: Norton, 1984), 304–5, and ch. 9 generally for the inoculation riots of 1730. Boston's epidemics and their spread can be found in Blake, *Public Health in the Town of Boston*, chs. 4, 5, 9.

44. *BSR*, 13: 87–89, 92, 96; *Journals of the House of Representatives of Massachusetts, 1721–1722* (Boston: Massachusetts Historical Society, 1922), 144.

45. See, for example, *The Diary of John Comer*, ed. by C. Edwin Barrows, vol. 8 of Rhode Island Historical Society, *Collections* (Rhode Island Historical Society, 1893), 20–25. Douglas L. Winiarski, *Darkness Falls on the Land of Light: Experiencing Religious Awakenings in Eighteenth-Century New England* (Chapel Hill: University of North Carolina Press, 2017), Kindle edition, is especially sensitive to the place of illness in conversion. See locs. 1308–480 (in "The Loud Calls of Divine Providence") and locs. 1403–32 on Comer.

46. For smallpox as an instrument of war, see Elizabeth A. Fenn, "Biological Warfare in Eighteenth-Century North America: Beyond Jeffrey Amherst," *Journal of American History* 86 (March 2000): 1552–80. Benjamin Lynde of Salem, Massachusetts, discovered that the pox could become a weapon of local squabbles as well. During the epidemic raging along New England's coast in 1752, Lynde was aghast to find "a small pox letter enclosing scabs and a plaster" placed in his kitchen window. After Lynde informed the lieutenant governor, a proclamation was issued to alert the public that "some Evil-minded Person or Persons" had a design to "communicate the Small-Pox to the Family," and Lynde offered a reward of £500 to discover the perpetrator. *The Diaries of Benjamin Lynde, Jr.*, ed. Fitch Edward Oliver (Boston: privately printed, 1880), 175–76; "A Proclamation," by Spencer Phips, May 28, 1752, Broadside Collection, American Antiquarian Society, Worcester, MA.

47. Charles J. Hoadly et al., comps., *Public Records of the Colony of Connecticut*, 15 vols. (Hartford, 1850–90), 6: 288–303 (for entire incident), 290 (for possible others at the house). See Allegra di Bonaventura, *For Adam's Sake: A Family Saga in Colonial New England* (New York: Norton, 2013), for Rogerenes (ch. 2) and a narrative of the illness of John Roger Sr. (215–18). Bonaventura finds thirty persons sickened. Joshua Hempstead, a sometime selectman from New London and a man with a keen ear for town affairs, noted that one of the victims of the pox at Roger's had been a "stranger." Robert Jackson, a "free Negro," lived on the compound with his family as well. *Diary of Joshua Hempstead of New London, Connecticut . . . from September, 1711, to November, 1758*, in New London County Historical Society, *Collections*, vol. 1 (New London: New London Historical Society, 1901), 114–15. The Boston epidemic of 1721 spread to a range of towns in Massachusetts (Martha's Vineyard, Sandwich, Roxbury, Brookline, Medford, and Cambridge) and Connecticut and Rhode Island. Duffy, *Epidemics in Colonial America*, 51–52.

48. *Public Records of the Colony of Connecticut*, 6: 294. The records noted that the "Blacks" on the property were especially loath to accept medical treatment, given their preference for faith healing. Bonaventura, *For Adam's Sake*, 216.

49. HT, South Kingston Town Council, 5:80–82, January 4 & 19, 1760.

50. HT, Middletown Town Council, 2: 120, December 27, 1783.

51. HT, East Greenwich Town Council, 3: 33, 33a, 35a, December 9–10, 1757, January 23, 1758. It is possible that Wever was taken to yet another house, that of William Jenckes, who lived in Cumberland, though this could have been the initial house in which Wever was placed. See HT, East Greenwich Town Council, 3: 43, 46, 47a, July 29, October 7, and November 25, 1758.

52. HT, Providence Town Council, 4: 193–94, September 16, 1759.

53. HT, Providence Town Council, 4: 192–93, September 6 & 8, 1759. I am indebted to Ruth Herndon for her notes on the social composition of visitors. On Obadiah Brown

and the Brown family, see James B. Hedges, *The Browns of Providence Plantations: The Colonial Years* (Providence, RI: Brown University Press, 1968), and 10 for assessment of Obadiah's importance in the 1750s.

54. Duffy, *Epidemics in Colonial America*, 23–42, provides an overview of colonial mainland British North America. On the inoculation controversy that roiled Boston in 1721, see Blake, *Public Health in the Town of Boston*, ch. 2; Minardi, "The Boston Inoculation Controversy," 47–76; Silva, *Miraculous Plagues*, ch. 4; and Amalie M. Kass, "Boston's Historic Smallpox Epidemic," *Massachusetts Historical Review* 14 (2012): 1–51. On a comparison of inoculation in Boston and Philadelphia, see Roslyn Stone Wolman, "A Tale of Two Colonial Cities: Inoculation against Smallpox in Philadelphia and in Boston," *Transactions and Studies of the College of Physicians of Philadelphia* 45 (1978): 338–47. Wehrman, "The Siege of 'Castle Pox,'" explores the connection between the inoculation riot in Marblehead and other like actions during the imperial crisis. Fenn, *Pox Americana*, ch. 3, and Finger, *The Contagious City*, locs. 2136–2169, examine the controversial decision to inoculate the Continental army.

55. Blake, *Public Health in the Town of Boston*, 77 (twenty-family rule), 80–81 (laws in 1730s–40s), 94 (town as hospital). On Philadelphia, see Duffy, *Epidemics in Colonial America*, 34–35; Blake, *Public Health in the Town of Boston*, 82, 91–92, 110; Fenn, *Pox Americana*, 39–40, 83–86.

56. Blake, *Public Health in the Town of Boston*, 94–96.

57. Blake, 77, 94–95.

58. On Philadelphia, see Blake, 110; Wolman, "A Tale of Two Colonial Cities," 343; Fenn, *Pox Americana*, 82–84. Blake, *Public Health in the Town of Boston*, 77, 94–95, discusses provision for the poor. On percentage of inoculees relative to those who took the infection the natural way in Boston, see Blake, 113, 115, and Duffy, *Epidemics in Colonial America*, 36 (for overall numbers).

59. Wehrman, "The Siege of 'Castle Pox,'" treats the incident in detail. I am indebted to his narrative and to his argument that the mob actions represent an episode in the emergence of "radical egalitarian justice," a larger sense that townsfolk should not be excluded from medical care. The proprietors were Azor Orne, John Glover, Jonathan Glover, and Elbridge Gerry. On the initial plans, see 393–95.

60. Wehrman, 397–98, 400.

61. Wehrman, 409, 411–13.

62. Wehrman, 427–28.

63. Blake, *Public Health in the Town of Boston*, 134–35, 138–40.

64. *BSR*, 13: 82–83, May 24, 1721.

65. *Mass AR*, 1: 606–7. Refusal to work on the highways and other services equivalent to militia services would be met with fines, and if these were not paid, imprisonment, discipline at the house of correction, and hard labor would follow. On the other hand, as Jared Ross Hardesty has suggested, while slave mobility in the streets was sharply limited in law, with curfews and restrictions on public gatherings, in practice slaves exercised some degree of freedom in roaming, gathering, and engaging in an underground economy, part of their accommodation of a world of unfreedom. See Hardesty, *Unfreedom: Slavery and Dependence in Eighteenth-Century Boston* (New York: New York University Press, 2016), ch. 3.

66. "Number of Inhabitants of Ratable Polls, and the Number Sick with Small Pox," Miscellaneous Bound Volumes, July 24, 1752, Massachusetts Historical Society, Boston, Massachusetts (MHS). Early bills of mortality published in Boston's *News-Letter* had begun to categorize deaths by race. See Cohen, *A Calculating People*, 88–89, and ch. 3 generally for the role of statistics in quantifying and assessing disease and epidemic, including the famed inoculation debate surrounding Boston's smallpox epidemic of 1721. Minardi, "The Boston Inoculation Controversy," argues that the debate between Cotton Mather and William Douglass witnessed the inception of "racialist" thought.

67. *BSR* 13: 87, September 11, 1721.

68. Gloria L. Main and Jackson T. Main have taken historians of New England to task for painting a stark picture of the region's economic fortunes in the eighteenth century. Far from being crushed by a Malthusian crisis, the people of the region were living "better and longer," say the authors. Even if one grants their position, longer lives should not be confused with healthier lives. Indeed, the longer persons lived, the more likely it was that they would face affliction. Living through the crisis did not mean that they would avoid the snares of affliction's costs. See Main and Main, "The Red Queen in New England?" *William and Mary Quarterly* 54 (January 1999): 121–50.

69. *Mass AR*, 16: 99.

70. *Mass AR*, 19: 562.

71. *Mass AR*, 14: 646. The General Court apparently recognized that selectmen and overseers had to be monitored in some cases so that they would not slight the vulnerable. When the North Precinct of Easton, Massachusetts, petitioned the Court in 1747/48, for example, the selectmen were given a sum to be "distributed to the several Familys, that have been Visited with the small Pox . . . (the Indians to be included) in proportion to the Number that had that distemper in their respective Families." See *Mass AR*, 14: 97, Resolve passed February 26, 1748. The assumption behind the order was that members of Indian families might not be reimbursed at the same rate as others. Instances as these suggest that disbursement had the potential to be part of a highly charged politics of social identification.

72. Duffy, *Epidemics in Colonial America*, 237–39. Duffy adds that the "loathsome nature" of the pox contributed to its terror.

73. *ABJ*, 2: 343–44.

CHAPTER SIX

1. There is a vast literature on warfare in New England. I have found the following works most useful: Fred Anderson, *A People's Army: Massachusetts Soldiers and Society in the Seven Years' War* (Chapel Hill: University of North Carolina Press, 1984); Harold E. Selesky, *War and Society in Colonial Connecticut* (New Haven, CT: Yale University Press, 1990); Richard Buel Jr., *Dear Liberty: Connecticut's Mobilization for the Revolutionary War* (Middletown, CT: Wesleyan University Press, 1980); William Pencak, *War, Politics, and Revolution in Provincial Massachusetts* (Boston: Northeastern University Press, 1981); and Jill Lepore, *The Name of War: King Philip's War and the Origins of American Identity* (1998; repr., New York: Vintage, 1999). The wars prior

to the Revolution were King William's War (1689–97), Queen Anne's War (1702–13), Governor Dummer's War (1722–25), King George's War (1744–48), and the Seven Years' War (1754–63).

2. In addition to the works cited above, see John Shy, *A People Numerous and Armed: Reflections on the Military Struggle for American Independence* (New York: Oxford University Press, 1976); Charles Royster, *A Revolutionary People at War: The Continental Army and American Character, 1775–1783* (Chapel Hill: University of North Carolina Press, 1979); Mary Beth Norton, *Liberty's Daughters: The Revolutionary Experience of American Women, 1750–1800* (Glenview, IL: Scott, Foresman, 1980); and Holly A. Mayer, *Belonging to the Army: Camp Followers and Community during the American Revolution* (Columbia: University of South Carolina Press, 1996), which examines the society created in and through the army.

3. Joy Day Buel and Richard Buel Jr., *The Way of Duty: A Woman and Her Family in Revolutionary America* (New York: Norton, 1984); Gary B. Nash, *The Urban Crucible: Social Change, Political Consciousness, and the Origins of the American Revolution* (Cambridge, MA: Harvard University Press, 1979); Allan Kulikoff, "The War in the Countryside," in *The Oxford Handbook of the American Revolution*, ed. Edward C. Gray and Jane Kamensky (Oxford: Oxford University Press, 2013), 227; Daniel Blackie, "Disability, Dependency, and the Family in the Early United States," in *Disability Histories*, ed. Susan Burch and Michael Rembis (Urbana: University of Illinois Press, 2014), ch. 1.

4. The benefits of reimbursement should not be exaggerated, however. Massachusetts still had to pay three-fifths of its wartime expenses. Anderson, *A People's Army*, 14–16.

5. Joseph Plumb Martin, *Private Yankee Doodle: Being a Narrative of Some of the Adventures, Dangers and Sufferings of a Revolutionary Soldier*, ed. George F. Scheer (Boston: Little, Brown, 1962), 170. Martin's memoir was first published in 1830.

6. Anderson, *A People's Army*, 98 (cities in the wilderness), 95–107 (on disease and camp life); Selesky, *War and Society*, 190–91; Royster, *A Revolutionary People*, 59–61; Philip Cash, *Medical Men at the Siege of Boston* (Philadelphia: American Philosophical Society, 1973), ch. 3; Sylvia R. Frey, *The British Soldier in America: A Social History of Military Life in the Revolutionary Period* (Austin: University of Texas Press, 1981), ch. 2; Erica Charters, *Disease, War, and the Imperial State: The Welfare of the British Armed Forces during the Seven Years' War* (Chicago: University of Chicago Press, 2014).

7. Selesky, *War and Society*, 191, calls camps the "deadliest places in colonial America." The tone of reports from areas besieged with disease, their resigned weariness and dispassionate counting of bodies, speaks to the routine nature of death. Consider the letter from William Pepperrell and Peter Warren to Governor William Shirley of Massachusetts, reporting on the state of affairs at Louisbourg in the winter of 1746: "Your Excelly on your departure from hence was so well acquainted with the state of this garrison that we have only to advise you the sickness which you left among us has continued to rage to such a degree that from the last of Nov. to this date we have buried 561 men, and have at this time 1100 sick. We flatter ourselves from the burials of three or four days past not amounting to more than 3, 4, and 5 a day, when before were gener-

ally from 14 to 17, that the distemper abates." William Pepperrell and Peter Warren to William Shirley, January 28, 1746, in *Correspondence of William Shirley*, 2 vols., ed. Charles Henry Lincoln (New York: Macmillan, 1912), 1: 303.

8. Anderson, *A People's Army*, 101; Selesky, *War and Society*, 190–91; Howard H. Peckham, ed., *The Toll of Independence: Engagements and Battle Casualties of the American Revolution* (Chicago: University of Chicago Press, 1974), 130–33. Peckham's mortality figures include 6,824 deaths in battle, 10,000 deaths in camp of wounds and infections, and 8,500 deaths in prison, for a total of 25,324 men.

9. A notable exception is Charters, *Disease, War, and the Imperial State*, which argues that the continuous and often overwhelming presence of disease in all theaters of the war was the occasion for the military command, leading politicians and an increasingly vocal public to voice their concerns about the welfare of soldiers. See, too, Cornelia H. Dayton and Sharon V. Salinger, *Robert Love's Warnings: Searching for Strangers in Colonial Boston* (Philadelphia: University of Pennsylvania Press, 2014), 141, 146, 150–54, which finds poor, ill, and disabled soldiers as a significant presence in Boston.

10. John Dent's petition in Nathaniel Bouton et al., eds., *Documents and Records Relating to New Hampshire*, 40 vols. (Concord and Manchester, 1867–1940), 12: 343 (cited hereafter as *NHDR*).

11. Anderson, *A People's Army*, 107n; Selesky, *War and Society*, 190.

12. Anderson, *A People's Army*, table 26, p. 239. See Charles H. Lesser, ed., *The Sinews of Independence: Monthly Strength Reports of the Continental Army* (Chicago: University of Chicago Press, 1976), xxix–xxxi, for a brief summary of their findings and a tally of morbidity rates of the rank and file of the Continental army by month and year. For individual companies, see, for example, "Return for the 3rd Massachusetts Brigade of Foot, January 26, 1782," in the United States Revolutionary War Collection, oversized miscellaneous, folder 6, American Antiquarian Society, Worcester, MA. These rates are, in general, consonant with what Erica Charters has found in her study of British soldiers during the Seven Years' War, though morbidity in the West Indies, especially, could be particularly high. In the Havana campaign in 1762, for example, July had 5,043 sick out of a total of 11,203 (45%) and August had 5,232 sick out of 10,804 (48%). Charters, *Disease, War, and the Imperial State*, 75.

13. On hospitals, see Anderson, *A People's Army*, 105; Cash, *Medical Men at the Siege of Boston*; and Harvey E. Brown, *The Medical Department of the United States Army from 1775 to 1873* (Washington, DC: Surgeon General's Office, 1873), 4–69.

14. Martin, *Private Yankee Doodle*, 54–55; *The Diary of Josiah Atkins*, ed. Steven E. Kagle (New York: New York Times and Arno Press, 1975), 41–42.

15. On the conception of the "perpetual motion of the American soldier's life" and its relation to sickness, see Buel, *Dear Liberty*, 101. For a detailed account of the everyday life of a soldier, see Anderson, *A People's Army*, ch. 3.

16. Robert C. Bray and Paul E. Bushnell, eds., *Diary of a Common Soldier in the American Revolution, 1775–1783* (Dekalb: Northern Illinois University Press, 1978), 16–18.

17. John C. Dann, *The Revolution Remembered: Eyewitness Accounts of the War for Independence* (Chicago: University of Chicago Press, 1980), 11–12.

18. It was common for the army to rely on the healing services of women in war, whether they be hired nurses, locals, or camp followers pressed into service, or those like Dimond, who appears to have been experienced in nursing men like Larabee. Cash, *Medical Men at the Siege of Boston*, 53–54, 76–77; Mayer, *Belonging to the Army*, 142–43, 222–23; Carol Berkin, *Revolutionary Mothers: Women in the Struggle for America's Independence* (New York: Vintage, 2005), ch. 4.

19. Anderson, *A People's Army*, 104–5.

20. Martin, *Private Yankee Doodle*, recounts several of these sorts of incidents, which he characterizes as a kind of necessary mischief performed in the name of survival.

21. John Duffy, *Epidemics in Colonial America* (Baton Rouge: Louisiana State University Press, 1953), 63.

22. "A Narrative of Henry Hallowell, of Lynn, Respecting the Revolution in 1775 . . . to January 17, 1780," in Howard Kendall Sanderson, comp., *Lynn in the Revolution*, part 1 (Boston: W. B. Clarke Company, 1909), 156–58.

23. *NHDR*, 11: 224–25. I am speculating that Obadiah was living in the vicinity of Smith's home town of Brentwood, New Hampshire.

24. *NHDR*, 11: 225.

25. *NHDR*, 11: 227–28.

26. *NHDR*, 12: 341 (Prescott); *NHDR*, 12: 230–31 (Bean).

27. Fred Anderson argues that the provincial forces from Massachusetts serving during the Seven Years' War were largely made up of young men who were temporarily poor, what Daniel Scott Smith has called the "life-cycle poor." Harold Selesky finds that over the course of the eighteenth century, soldiers in Connecticut's forces were increasingly likely to be marginal members of the community, if not the abject poor. Anderson relies heavily on figures from 1756, and, as Don Higginbotham has pointed out ("The Early American Way of War: Reconnaissance and Appraisal," *William and Mary Quarterly* 44 [April 1987]: 240), calculations from even a few years later might have revealed a military force drawn from "the bottom of the barrel of human resources," and thus may have looked more like Connecticut's army. John Shy has argued that during the Revolution, short-term militia service relied upon large numbers of men of various social positions, but long-term service was filled by "hard-core" fighters, such as New Hampshire's "Long Bill" Scott, who were drawn from the lower tiers of society. On "surplus males," see Anderson, *A People's Army*, ch. 2. For a comparison of morbidity and mortality rates of these young men versus the older, more marginal soldiers they served with, see Anderson, table 29, p. 241. For hard-core fighters during the Revolution, see Shy, *A People Numerous and Armed*, ch. 7.

28. Massachusetts Archives Collection, vol. 105: 610–11. December 18, 1760, Massachusetts, SC1/series 45X, Massachusetts Archives, Boston, MA (cited hereafter as MAC).

29. Martha Albertson Fineman, *The Neutered Mother, the Sexual Family and Other Twentieth-Century Tragedies* (New York: Routledge, 1995), 163.

30. I have in mind such things as the practice of coverture, in which a wife was legally subsumed into the person of her husband, or the practices of tax valuation, in which the entire productive efforts of the household were assessed on the head of household.

31. On "social medicine," see Laurel Thatcher Ulrich, *A Midwife's Tale: The Life of Martha Ballard, Based on Her Diary, 1785–1812* (1990; repr., New York: Vintage, 1991), 61. On the limits of that community's ability to respond to long-term misfortune, see ch. 2, above.

32. Royster, *A Revolutionary People*, 131–32.

33. John Duffy maintains that while smallpox was terrifying, diseases like dysentery and malaria were ultimately responsible for claiming more lives. *Epidemics in Colonial America*, 238–39.

34. *NHDR*, 11: 228–29.

35. *NHDR*, 11: 229–30.

36. *NHDR*, 11: 230.

37. Anderson, *People's Army*, 10, 145 (on "wagonloads"); *Mass AR*, 15:389. In December the General Court extended the aid to those traveling home who "are in health & Stand in need of relief & support till they shall arrive at their respective homes." *Mass AR*, 15: 409.

38. Anderson, 225 (wages and bounties). On petitions to the General Court, see *Mass AR*, 15: 419, 435, 438, 439, 446, 448, 449, 450, 452, 453, 455, 456, 460, 461, 471, 472, 480, 481, 483, 498, 500, 519, 544, 557, 584, 602, 607, 608, 615, 666, 691, 732, 736, 737, 740, 754, 757, 767, 770, 772. The number of petitions, and especially of individual claims, is likely much higher, if one were to add the "diverse" persons in need of reimbursement, including those who note "suffering" as a cause. For example, "An order allowing sundry amounts to divers persons" in response to Simon Davis and Others," soldiers on the Crown Point Expedition, in January 1756, lists six men (two of them captains, two esquires) for their care of eight men, presumably soldiers, including Davis. See *Mass AR*, 15: 654. Alison G. Olson, "Eighteenth-Century Colonial Legislatures and Their Constituents," *Journal of American History* 79 (September 1992): 556–57, argues that the Massachusetts General Court fielded far more petitions than other colonies from 1715 to 1765, averaging 95 a year between 1715 and 1720, and 257 a year between 1760 and 1765. This would mean that a substantial number of petitions during the war, in the wake of a campaign, were related to illness and injury. Along with Olson, legal scholars have been interested in the assembly's use of financial disbursements as a means of claiming public power over the course of the eighteenth century: Gregory A. Mark, "The Vestigial Constitution: The History and Significance of the Right to Petition," *Fordham Law Review* 66 (1998): 2153–231; and Christine A. Desan, "The Constitutional Commitment to Legislative Adjudication in the Early American Tradition," *Harvard Law Review* 111 (April 1998): 1381–446. Finally, one could argue that we see in such petitions—and in the broader scheme that had the Massachusetts government both organize its taxation system and arrange for social welfare accommodations, all in the name of prosecuting war—the incipient stages of a fiscal-military state. On the development of such a state in England, see John Brewer, *The Sinews of Power: War, Money and the English State, 1688–1783* (New York: Knopf, 1989). On the early American state, with a special focus on war, see Max M. Edling, *A Hercules in the Cradle: War, Money, and the American State, 1783–1867* (Chicago: University of Chicago Press, 2014). Only five of the petitions, as summarized in the Acts and Resolves, explicitly listed wounds as the sole cause for accommodation. But as we will see in the following

chapter, sickness and chronic disability became intertwined in this period. For a fuller
discussion, see chapter 7, below.

39. *The Journals of Ashley Bowen (1728–1813) of Marblehead*, 2 vols., ed. Philip
Chadwick Foster Smith, Publications of the Colonial Society of Massachusetts, vols.
44 and 45 of *Collections* (Boston: Colonial Society of Massachusetts, 1973), 1: 52–54, 2:
621–22 (cited hereafter as *ABJ*).

40. Bowen's petition to the General Court is reprinted in *ABJ*, 1: 104–5.

CHAPTER SEVEN

1. The word "disabled" was commonly used in eighteenth-century New England,
though, significantly, not to refer to a class of people. One does not find reference to
"the disabled." Rather, one was "disabled" or "disenabled" from various tasks, chiefly
from the physical labor necessary to support oneself and others. Following their lead,
I try below to uncover the social and economic contexts in which disability assumed
its significance, as well as the various parties that had an interest in the government's
recognition that veterans were disabled to the degree that they warranted a pension. In
treating "disability" as a contingent, socially constructed category, I am indebted to a
variety of writings in the new disability history and disability studies, cited above in
the introduction, note 15. On Revolutionary War pensions, see Laura Jensen, *Patriots,
Settlers, and the Origins of American Social Policy* (Cambridge: Cambridge University
Press, 2003), chs. 2–3; John Resch, *Suffering Soldiers: Revolutionary War Veterans,
Moral Sentiment, and Political Culture in the Early Republic* (Amherst: University
of Massachusetts Press, 2002); Daniel Blackie, "Disabled Revolutionary War Veterans
and the Construction of Disability in the Early United States, 1776–1840" (PhD diss.,
University of Helsinki, 2010), and Blackie, "Disability, Dependency, and the Family in
the Early United States," in *Disability Histories*, ed. Susan Burch and Michael Rembis
(Urbana: University of Illinois Press, 2014), ch. 1; Laurel Daen, "Revolutionary War
Invalid Pensions and the Bureaucratic Language of Disability in the Early Republic,"
Early American Literature 52, no. 1 (2017): 141–67; and Kim E. Nielsen, *A Disability
History of the United States* (Boston: Beacon Press, 2012), 53–56.

2. Jensen, *Patriots, Settlers, and the Origins of American Social Policy*, argues that
federal social provision has had a much longer history than has been formerly acknowledged in major studies of the subject, such as Theda Skocpol's *Protecting Soldiers and
Mothers: The Political Origins of Social Policy in the United States* (Cambridge, MA:
Belknap Press of Harvard University Press, 1992), reaching back to the early national
period when the federal government developed "programmatic entitlements," benefits
directed at groups of Americans deemed "worthy." Jensen gives light treatment to
disabled Revolutionary veterans, who were the first group to receive benefits, focusing
instead on pension legislation that, beginning in 1818, offered benefits to veterans in
"reduced" circumstances. Exploring in some depth the colonial and early Revolutionary pensions in this chapter throws the changes wrought in the 1790s into sharp relief.
Long before the development of categories of desert in 1818 and subsequent programs,
the federal government had fundamentally altered one of the key moral platforms of
governance: that personal ordeals, including tales of physical suffering, not only were

tolerated, but were the means by which the people's governors could determine worth and offer protection.

3. William H. Glasson, *Federal Military Pensions in the United States* (New York: Oxford University Press, 1918), ch. 1, quote on p. 10. Glasson is the most comprehensive source on early American pension legislation, but his history of pensions is biased, emphasizing the arrogance and graft and their burden on the state. See Resch, *Suffering Soldiers*; Jensen, *Patriots, Settlers, and the Origins of American Social Policy*, chs. 2–3; and Daen, "Revolutionary War Invalid Pensions," for updates.

4. *The Acts and Resolves, Public and Private, of the Province of the Massachusetts Bay*, 21 vols. (Boston: Wright and Potter Printing, 1869–1922), 1: 133–34, 175–76, 292–93, 398–400, 530–31 (cited hereafter as *Mass AR*).

5. Jill Lepore, *The Name of War: King Philip's War and the Origins of American Identity* (1998; repr., New York: Vintage, 1999), 88–89. On Baker, see *Mass AR*, 7: 248, 638–39.

6. *Mass AR*, 7: 638–39.

7. *Mass AR*, 7: 638–39. Richard L. Bushman, *King and People in Provincial Massachusetts* (1985; repr., Chapel Hill: University of North Carolina Press, 1992), 46–54 (on petitions); Roy Porter and G. S. Rousseau, *Gout: The Patrician's Malady* (New Haven, CT: Yale University Press, 1998). Bellomont had been awarded the position of Royal Governor of New Hampshire, New York, and Massachusetts in 1697 and arrived in the latter in 1699.

8. *Mass AR*, 7: 638–39.

9. Charles E. Rosenberg, "The Therapeutic Revolution: Medicine, Meaning, and Social Change in Nineteenth-Century America," in *The Therapeutic Revolution: Essays in the Social History of American Medicine*, ed. Morris J. Vogel and Charles E. Rosenberg (Philadelphia: University of Pennsylvania Press, 1979), 5; Roy Porter and Dorothy Porter, *In Sickness and in Health: The British Experience, 1650–1850* (1988; repr., New York: Basil Blackwell, 1989), chs. 2–5.

10. *Mass AR*, 7: 639. Under the hand of the doctor or surgeon, the patient's bills piled up, and the temptation to leave must have been great. But the General Court also seems to have entertained the notion (never explicitly stated in law, but nonetheless appreciable in the petitions) that one should try to obtain a "perfect cure," which might take months. The General Court's interest was in exercising restraint. Surgeons regularly complained that they had not been fully paid, patients were granted less than their medical bills, and some degree of skepticism was part of the negotiations around allotments for medical provision. That said, there was nothing formally along the lines of the contracts between patients and healers that Gianna Pomata has uncovered in Italy, in *Contracting a Cure: Patients, Healers, and the Law in Early Modern Bologna* (Baltimore: Johns Hopkins University Press, 1998).

11. *Mass AR*, 7: 638–39.

12. Lisa Wilson, *Ye Heart of a Man: The Domestic Life of Men in Colonial New England* (New Haven, CT: Yale University Press, 1999); Anne S. Lombard, *Making Manhood: Growing Up Male in Colonial New England* (Cambridge, MA: Harvard University Press, 2003); Thomas A. Foster, *Sex and the Eighteenth-Century Man* (Boston: Beacon Press, 2006); Thomas A. Foster, "Deficient Husbands: Manhood, Sexual Incapac-

ity, and Male Marital Sexuality in Seventeenth-Century New England," *William and Mary Quarterly* 56 (1999): 723–44.

13. Petition of Samuel Clark, Massachusetts Archives Collection, vol. 71: 6, 1703, SC1/series 45X, Massachusetts State Archives, Boston, MA (cited hereafter as MAC).

14. Petition of John Harvey, *Mass AR*, 7: 634, 1700; Petition of William Sutton, MAC, 71: 291–92, 1706/1707.

15. Petition of Thomas Philips, MAC, 71: 441–42, November 21, 1707; Petition of Josiah Jones, MAC, 72: 477, May 30, 1739; Petition of William Thayer, MAC, 80: 231, [c. 1762].

16. Petition of Hugh Pike, MAC, 71: 745, October 27, 1710.

17. Jack P. Greene, *The Quest for Power: The Lower Houses of Assembly in the Southern Royal Colonies, 1689–1776* (New York: Norton, 1963); Alison G. Olson, "Eighteenth-Century Colonial Legislatures and Their Constituents," *Journal of American History* 79 (September 1992): 543–67; Floyd D. Shimomura, *Louisiana Law Review* 45 (January 1985): 625–700; Gregory A. Mark, "The Vestigial Constitution: The History and Significance of the Right to Petition," *Fordham Law Review* 66 (1998): 2153–231; Christine A. Desan, "The Constitutional Commitment to Legislative Adjudication in the Early American Tradition," *Harvard Law Review* 111 (April 1998): 1381–446.

18. The numbers of petitions received by the Massachusetts House of Representatives are from Olson, "Eighteenth-Century Colonial Legislatures and Their Constituents," 556–57.

19. Petition of Benjamin Rockwood, MAC, 72: 622, November 4, 1742.

20. *Mass AR*, 13: 192; MAC, 72: 623–24, November 4, 1742, December 9, 1742. The shaky signatures bear the marks of old age. It is unclear who served as scribe for the petition, though it is not in the writing of William Man.

21. *Mass AR*, 13: 651–52.

22. Petitions of Peter Rich, MAC, 71: 623, June 7, 1710, and MAC, 73: 137 (no date). See also *Mass AR*, 14: 120. In 1710 Rich was awarded £4 "smart money" and £3 a year for two years. On April 15, 1748, Rich was awarded £5 for the present year in full consideration of his petition. On the money question and the problem of establishing different currencies, especially paper, as a measure of value and medium of exchange, see Margaret Ellen Newell, *From Dependency to Independence: Economic Revolution in Colonial New England* (Ithaca, NY: Cornell University Press, 1998), chs. 6–11; and Jeffrey Sklansky, *Sovereign of the Market: The Money Question in Early America* (Chicago: University of Chicago Press, 2017), chs. 1–2.

23. Petition of John Green, MAC, 72: 564, May 1741. On July 31, Green was awarded £10 in addition to the £5 he received until further order.

24. *Mass AR*, 21: 896, 969 (indexes that list pensioners): there were eleven pensioners from the French and Indian War and twenty-two from the Revolutionary War.

25. See *Mass AR*, 17: 9, 11, 21, 41, 72, 86, 88, 156, 167, 189, 190, 209, 255, 275, 285, 356, 488, 577. For individual cases, the court allowed anywhere from £3 to £20 for compensation. Some towns, such as Salem and Marblehead, simply wanted permission to erect fences, establish guards, and allow for examinations of all who would attempt to enter the town, which might include asking for an oath from the suspected that neither they nor their goods were infected. Other places, such as Swansea, which had been stricken

by a significant outbreak, asked for a whopping £300, which the General Court granted in the form of a loan: the town would annually add £50 to its province taxes until the loan was fully discharged. *Mass AR*, 17: 461, 470, 530. On symptoms of smallpox, see ch. 5, above.

26. Petitions of Daniel Druce, MAC, 80: 590–92, September 1765; MAC, 80: 663, March 12, 1770; MAC, 80: 702, June 12, 1772. Biography and quotations taken from the three petitions. The pastor signed his first petition, the selectmen his second. On January 31, 1766, Druce was awarded £3 for four years that was placed in charge of one of Grafton's selectmen. The petition was renewed at least two more times, each for an additional three years. See *Mass AR*, 17: 72, 18: 79, 448, 632.

27. Petition of William Clemens, MAC, 80: 9, 1761. On November 19, 1761, the House of Representatives granted Clemens £3 per year until further notice "on Account of His Suffering Mentioned in His Petition." The petition was evidently mislaid for two months before the council passed the resolve on February 16. See *Mass AR*, 17: 142.

28. Petition of Nathaniel Conant, MAC, 80: 667–68, 1770 [?]. On November 14, 1770, Conant was allowed £3 annually until further notice.

29. Petition of William Snell, MAC, 80: 621–22, [illegible]. On November 5, 1766, the council concurred with the House and agreed to £8 annually until further notice.

30. Karen Kupperman, "Fear of Hot Climates in the Anglo-American Colonial Experience," *William and Mary Quarterly* 41, no. 2 (April 1984): 213–40; Charles E. Rosenberg, "The Therapeutic Revolution: Medicine, Meaning, and Social Change in Nineteenth-Century America," and "Medical Text and Social Context: Explaining William Buchan's *Domestic Medicine*," reprinted in *Explaining Epidemics and Other Studies in the History of Medicine* (Cambridge: Cambridge University Press, 1992), chs. 1–2; Porter and Porter, *In Sickness and in Health*; Dorothy Porter and Roy Porter, *Patient's Progress: Doctors and Doctoring in Eighteenth-Century England* (Cambridge: Polity Press, 1989); Mary E. Fissell, *Patients, Power, and the Poor in Eighteenth-Century Bristol* (Cambridge: Cambridge University Press, 1991); Barbara Duden, *The Woman Beneath the Skin: A Doctor's Patients in Eighteenth-Century Germany* (Cambridge, MA: Harvard University Press, 1991). There is another possible medical angle here: the critique of medical provision for the provincial troops. The always provocative physician William Douglass, for example, had criticized Governor William Shirley, a major force promoting the intense involvement of Massachusetts troops in King George's War and the early years of the French and Indian War, for his lack of proper medical attention provided to soldiers after the taking of the fort at Louisbourg. Some nine hundred men died after taking the fort, and Douglass claimed that it was due to poor sanitation and want of proper discipline. There is resonance here with the later work of John Pringle, though his *Observations on the Diseases of the Army* (1752) was not published in America until Benjamin Rush brought out an edition in 1810. But the Douglass-Shirley debate was part of a larger sense that the often appalling morbidity and mortality rates of soldiers could in some degree be prevented with better organization and attention. And it may be that this strain of argument helped soldiers make their case that their wartime sickness and later debility were worthy of compensation. On the Douglass-Shirley incident, see the brief remarks in William Pencak, *War,*

Politics, and Revolution in Provincial Massachusetts (Boston: Northeastern University Press, 1981), 127, 143n57.

31. See chapter 6, above, and Marcia Schmidt Blaine, "The Power of Petitions: Women and the New Hampshire Provincial Government, 1695–1770," in *International Review of Social History* 46 (2001), supplement 9, ed. Lex Heerma van Voss, 57–77.

32. On state expansions, see Richard R. Johnson, *Adjustment to Empire: The New England Colonies, 1675–1715* (New Brunswick, NJ: Rutgers University Press, 1981); Fred Anderson, *A People's Army: Massachusetts Soldiers and Society in the Seven Years' War* (Chapel Hill: University of North Carolina Press, 1984), esp. 39–48.

33. *Journals of the Continental Congress, 1774–1789*, ed. Worthington C. Ford et al. (Washington, DC, 1904–37), 5: 702–5.

34. Richard Buel Jr., *Dear Liberty: Connecticut's Mobilization for the Revolutionary War* (Middletown, CT: Wesleyan University Press, 1980), 52 (assessment of Connecticut's troops); Lesser, *Sinews of Independence*, xxv, xxi (Washington's comments).

35. *Boston Evening Post*, November 16, 1761; John Adams to a friend in London, February 10, 1775, in *Letters of Delegates to Congress, 1774–1789*, 25 volumes, ed. Paul H. Smith et al. (Washington, DC: Library of Congress, 1976–2000), 1: 309. Resch, *Suffering Soldiers*, chs. 3–4 (on the politics of "pensioners").

36. Bernard Bailyn, *Faces of Revolution: Personalities and Themes in the Struggle for American Independence* (1990; repr., New York: Vintage, 1992), ch. 3, and Bailyn, *The Ordeal of Thomas Hutchinson* (Cambridge, MA: Belknap Press of Harvard University Press, 1974). Charles Royster, *A Revolutionary People at War: The Continental Army and American Character, 1775–1783* (Chapel Hill: University of North Carolina Press, 1979), 201–4 and ch. 8, discusses the debate over officers' pensions.

37. George Washington to John Hancock (circular), June 11, 1783, in the Washington Papers, http://gwpapers.virginia.edu/documents/george-washington-to-john-hancock -circular-11-june-1783/.

38. Washington to Hancock.

39. Washington to Hancock.

40. Joanne B. Freeman, *Affairs of Honor: National Politics in the New Republic* (New Haven, CT: Yale University Press, 2001); David Waldstreicher, *In the Midst of Perpetual Fetes: The Making of American Nationalism, 1776–1820* (Chapel Hill: University of North Carolina Press, 1997), ch. 2; Andrew Burstein, *Sentimental Democracy: The Evolution of America's Romantic Self-Image* (New York: Hill and Wang, 1999); Sarah Knott, "Sensibility and the American War for Independence," *American Historical Review* 109 (February 2004): 19–40.

41. Knott, "Sensibility and the American War for Independence."

42. Karen Halttunen, "Humanitarianism and the Pornography of Pain in Anglo-American Culture," *American Historical Review* 100 (April 1995): 303–34.

43. "Messieurs Printers," *Boston Gazette, and the Country Journal*, June 16, 1783.

44. "Messieurs Printers."

45. Christopher L. Tomlins, *Law, Labor, and Ideology in the Early American Republic* (Cambridge: Cambridge University Press, 1993), ch. 10.

46. *Acts and Laws of the Commonwealth of Massachusetts* (Boston: Adams & Nourse, 1895), 1782–83, ch. 91, 234; and 1784–84. ch. 134, 908–10. The *Mass AR* series continues after 1780 with *Acts and Laws* (cited hereafter as *Mass AL*).

47. *Mass AL*, 1782–83, ch. 91, 234; *Mass AL*, 1784–85, ch. 134, 908–10.

48. Robert F. Haggard, "The Nicola Affair: Lewis Nicola, George Washington, and the American Military Discontent during the Revolutionary War," *Proceedings of the American Philosophical Society* 146 (June 2002): 139–69.

49. *Journals of the Continental Congress, 1774–1789*, ed. Worthington C. Ford et al. (Washington, DC, 1904–37), 8: 485–86. In addition to securing new recruits wherever the corps was stationed and drilling the enlisted men, subaltern officers were expected to attend a "mathematical school," where they would "learn geometry, arithmetic, vulgar, and decimal fractions," and enjoy the fruits of a regimental library "of the most approved authors on tactics and petite guerre," to be purchased with the withholding of a day's pay every month. The privilege of being thus schooled was such that Congress felt it could be selective, cautioning that "no officers need apply but such as produce ample certificates of their having served with reputation, and having supported good characters, both as citizens and soldiers."

50. Haggard, "Nicola Affair," 148–56, provides a chronology of the Invalid Corps. For numbers of men in the Invalid Corps, see Charles H. Lesser, ed., *The Sinews of Independence: Monthly Strength Reports of the Continental Army* (Chicago: University of Chicago Press, 1976). The returns for the Invalid Corps start in 1778 and carry through 1783.

51. *Mass AR*, 21: 156 (Carlton petition); *Mass AL*, 1780: 707–8 (response); *Massachusetts: Society of the Cincinnati*, AmericanAncestors.org (online database, 2004), 434, https://www.americanancestors.org/DB187/t/11965175; *Massachusetts Soldiers and Sailors of the Revolutionary War*, vols. 1–17 (Boston: Wright & Potter Printing, 1896–1908), 3: 104, accessed through Ancestry.com. *Massachusetts Soldiers and Sailors in the Revolutionary War (Images Online*, online database (Provo, UT: Ancestry.com Operations Inc., 2004), https://www.ancestry.com/search/collections/ ma-revwarsoldiers/.

52. The overall number in the corps peaked in September 1779 at 465 men, split between Philadelphia and Boston; it never contained more than 400 men in 1780; and on average it had less than 300 men in 1781 and less than 200 men in 1782 and 1783. Boston's contingent was always less than Philadelphia's and reached its height in December 1779 at 175 men. Lesser, *Sinews of Independence*, 73, 114, 129, 133, 138, 145, 149, 153, 157, 169, 177, 181, 185, 189, 193, 200, 204, 210, 212, 214, 220, 224, 228, 230, 232, 234, 236, 238, 240, 242, 244, 246, 250, 252. For McFarland, see *Independent Ledger, and the American Advertiser*, July 2, 1781.

53. "Return of Recruits unfit for service, sent by the State of Massachusetts since Jan[ua]ry 1st, 1781," United States Revolutionary War Collection, oversized mss., folder 1, American Antiquarian Society, Worcester, MA.

54. Benjamin Lincoln quote in Haggard, "Nicola Affair," 160.

55. David P. Szatmary, *Shays' Rebellion: The Making of an Agrarian Insurrection* (Amherst: University of Massachusetts Press, 1980).

56. *Massachusetts Centinel*, November 10, 1787.

57. Quotations may be found in House unpassed legislation, #1842, June 16, 1785, SC1/series 230, Massachusetts Archives, Boston, MA. See also Senate unpassed legislation, #349, 1785; #512, 1786; #499, 1786, SC1/series 231, Massachusetts Archives, Boston, MA. The question of a unified pubic—the public entitled to equal justice with the pensioners—was belied here by a recognition that there were, in fact, at least two publics to consider: the body of citizens of the state and those of the towns. The draft legislation provided that towns that did not conduct certifications of their invalids and submit them to the General Court would have the invalids struck from the list—a comment on the self-interest of towns in continuing to receive funds from the state government that paid, in many cases, for veterans who were also part of the town's poor. There was a presumed local allegiance to town affairs and town coffers that trumped allegiance to the state and its treasury.

58. *Mass AL*, 1784–85, February session, 908–10. The resolve empowered John Lucas to examine claims of officers, soldiers, and seamen living in Massachusetts who had served in the army or navy of the United States or in the militia, and asked that they produce a certificate from either their commanding officer, surgeon of the regiment or company, a physician or surgeon of a military hospital, or someone who could offer "good and suficient testimony" that would document their disability that could be traced to their service. Lucas was to determine the validity of the claim and the pay justified, and to transmit a copy of his findings to the secretary of the commonwealth. The governor and council were thereafter empowered to form invalids who were deemed fit for garrison duty into a corps. Invalid soldiers were then compelled each year to find a justice of the peace in the county in which they lived to certify their examination. The resolve was passed on March 17, 1786.

59. Lucas's examinations can be found in Certificate book for Revolutionary War disability pensions SC1/series 2565X, Massachusetts Archives, Boston, MA (cited hereafter as Lucas Certificates). The bulk of these are from 1786 to 1787.

60. Lucas certificates, 8 (Hinds), 20 (Angier), 25 (Moore), 4 (Rumrill). While the compensation facing invalid veterans was complicated by the transfer of pensions from the federal government to the states, it appears that soldiers stationed at the garrison would earn wages in addition to whatever pension to which they were entitled, an issue that needed to be clarified in 1787. See *Mass AL*, 1786–87, ch. 105, 796–97.

61. Lucas certificates, 77 (Moses White). The word could also be "harnaptal."

62. Kenneth R. Bowling et al., eds., *Petition Histories: Revolutionary War-Related Claims*, vol. 7 of *Documentary History of the First Federal Congress of the United States of America* (Baltimore: Johns Hopkins University Press, 1997), 334.

63. Noah Brooks, *Henry Knox: A Soldier of the Revolution* (1900; repr., New York: De Capo Press, 1974); North Callahan, *Henry Knox: General Washington's General* (New York: Rinehart, 1958); Alan Taylor, "From Fathers to Friends of the People: Political Personas in the Early Republic," in *Federalists Reconsidered*, ed. Doron S. Ben-Atar and Barbara Oberg (Charlottesville: University Press of Virginia, 1998), ch. 11.

64. Taylor, "From Fathers to Friends of the People," 239. Gordon S. Wood, *The Americanization of Benjamin Franklin* (New York: Penguin, 2004), argues for the radicalism of Franklin's ability to move from commoner to gentleman. David Waldstreicher, *Runaway America: Benjamin Franklin, Slavery, and the American Revolu-

tion (New York: Hill and Wang, 2004), cautions that we must see in Franklin's rise the bounded labor and web of dependencies that made his independence possible.

65. Invalid pension legislation during the early years of the republic performed the delicate task of transferring oversight of state pension programs to Congress, and the laws changed many times during these years to make this transition as smooth as possible. Glasson, *Federal Military Pensions*, chs. 2–3; Robert Mayo and Ferdinand Moulton, *Army and Navy Pension Laws, and Bounty Land Laws of the United States: Including Sundry Resolutions of Congress, from 1776 to 1852: Executed at the Department of the Interior* (1852; 4th ed., Washington, DC: W. H. & O. H. Morrison, 1861), lxxviii–lxxxvii for an analytical summary; Bowling et al., *Petition Histories*, 332–35. In general, federal pensions came to encompass larger groups over time, eventually extending to volunteers, militia, and state troops.

66. Bowling et al., *Petition Histories*, 254–56 (for Roberts's case). As early as 1780, the Continental Congress had recommended that the widow and orphans of an officer receive benefits, usually half pay for five years. Individual bills continued this trend during the First Federal Congress.

67. Bowling et al., *Petition Histories*, 254–56. The severing of the tie between sympathy and governmental money must be seen in the larger context of an emerging culture of sensibility in the eighteenth- and early nineteenth-century Atlantic world. Resch, *Suffering Soldiers*, argues that more generous pension regulations devised in 1818 were the result of a surge in moral sentiment in favor of veterans, by exploring writings from around 1815 onward describing the sufferings of soldiers during the Revolution as demanding humility and gratitude. I think that it is suggestive, however, that the moral sentiment is focused on the wounds and sufferings of battle (especially Valley Forge), and less able to confront the ongoing social strain and physical pain in the decades that followed such recognized valor. As Karen Halttunen, "Humanitarianism and the Pornography of Pain in Anglo-American Culture," 303–34, suggests in another context, there is social distancing that accompanies even the warmest humanitarian impulses.

68. Saul Cornell, *Anti-Federalism and the Dissenting Tradition in America, 1788–1828* (Chapel Hill: University of North Carolina Press, 1999), ch. 2.

69. John Fea, "The Way of Improvement Leads Home: Philip Vickers Fithian's Rural Enlightenment," *Journal of American History* 90 (September 2003): 462–90.

70. Waldstreicher, *In the Midst of Perpetual Fetes*, ch. 3.

71. Bowling et al., *Petition Histories*, 375–78.

72. Elizabeth A. Fenn, *Pox Americana: The Great Smallpox Epidemic of 1775–82* (New York: Hill and Wang, 2001), 92–103. Another possibility was "secret disease," which referred to venereal diseases.

73. Charles E. Rosenberg, "Medical Text and Social Context: Explaining William Buchan's *Domestic Medicine*," *Bulletin of the History of Medicine* 57 (Spring 1983): 22–42.

74. Quote from Brooks, *Henry Knox*, 253–54. Knox wrote to Cobb in 1800, shortly after the book was reprinted in Boston: A. F. M. Willich, *Lectures on Diet and Regimen: Being a Systematic Inquiry into the Most Rational Means of Preserving Health and Prolonging Life* (Boston, 1800).

75. *George Cheyne: The English Malady (1733)*, ed. Roy Porter (repr., London: Routledge, 2013), esp. intro; Roy Porter, *The Creation of the Modern World: The Untold Story of the British Enlightenment* (New York: Norton, 2000), ch. 6, discusses trends in secularization in eighteenth-century England that touch on new conceptions of insanity.

76. Knox quoted in Callahan, *Henry Knox*, 296–97. The elite were thought especially susceptible to imaginative disease, less because of inhospitable surroundings, which might be managed, but because of active and delicate minds. Jacquelyn C. Miller, "An 'Uncommon Tranquility of Mind': Emotional Self-Control and the Construction of a Middle-Class Identity in Eighteenth-Century Philadelphia." *Journal of Social History* 30 (Fall 1996): 129–48.

77. Bowling et al., *Petition Histories*, 375–78 [Knox's initial suggestions). Mayo and Moulton, *Army and Navy Pension Laws*, 26–28, for Congressional Act of February 28, 1793, and revisions to first general regulations devised by Congress a year earlier, which had allowed wounds "or other known cause" as justification for claims.

78. Daen, "Revolutionary War Invalid Pensions," argues that we see in the new medical inspections and the elaboration of rules of evidence a new bureaucratic turn that facilitated the growth of the medicalized state. My argument here follows along similar lines, though it does not emphasize the medicalization of disability in the same fashion as Daen, for reasons I suggest below.

79. Bowling et al., *Petition Histories*, 371. The claim to have been so isolated that one was simply unaware of changes in laws was a common complaint. For extensions and exemptions granted at the state level to accommodate isolation, see Nathaniel Bouton et al., eds., *Documents and Records Relating to New Hampshire*, 40 vols. (Concord and Manchester, 1867–1940), 21: 72, 281, 322, 385. 457 (cited hereafter as *NHDR*). Knox had less patience with missed deadlines, regularly denying pensioners who failed to file applications on time. For a special exemption, see Knox's report on Jeremiah Ryan in Walter Lowrie and Walter S. Franklin, eds., *American State Papers: Documents, Legislative and Executive of the Congress of the United States*, vol. 9 [36], *Claims* (Washington, DC: Gales and Seaton, 1834), 8 (cited hereafter as *ASP Claims*).

80. Jeremiah Smith to Josiah Bartlett, February 24, 1792. in *The Papers of Josiah Bartlett*, ed. Frank C. Mevers (Hanover: New Hampshire Historical Society, 1979), 370, reveals the problem of repeated physical examinations. The number of applicants who were unable (or unwilling) to have their claims authenticated by surgeons is another indication of the difficulty in obtaining new examinations. *ASP Claims*, 83–172, includes the War Department's annotated list of claimants.

81. See brief comments attached to the case of Benjamin Fowler in *ASP Claims*, 91. Blind in one eye from smallpox, with a leg amputated after the war, Fowler was subsisting on charity and was unable to secure "any certificates from reputable freeholders, on account of his wandering and unsettled life." I take up poverty and transiency in chapter 8, below.

82. Royster, *A Revolutionary People*, 200–204, 333–51, discusses battles over service pensions for officers and New England's strong objections to half pay for officers, 345–46. See Bowling et al., *Petition Histories*, 345, 407, for witnesses who testified against officers. Officers also protested that they had been given lesser invalid pensions by

states than they deserved. See the case of Thomas Simpson, a lieutenant captain from New Hampshire who complained that he was awarded only a quarter pension by the state legislature for the loss of an eye due to smallpox and several serious wounds, including a musket ball still lodged in his body. *NHDR*, 20: 171, 174, 202, 206, 277; and Bowling et al., *Petition Histories*, 342–43. Knox denied Simpson's petition on the same grounds that he had denied Ruth Roberts—local decisions were to be upheld by the national government. But Knox did appear to have special sympathy for officers invalided in war. In order to receive an invalid pension, officers first had to return the amount they had received as commutation for their service pension, or five years' full pay at the salary they had received while in the service. For officers awarded only partial disabilities in their invalid pensions, this could mean a substantial decrease in income. Invalid officers, like other invalid pensioners, could receive a maximum of half pay for life, and lesser disabilities were given proportionally smaller amounts. Knox eventually supported the return of the amount of commutation inversely proportional to the invalid pension received, e.g., an officer allowed an invalid pension of one-third his monthly wage for life would have to return two-thirds of his commutation. See Knox's report on the subject, in Bowling et al., *Petition Histories*, 336–38, 395–98.

83. The phrase "wounds or other known cause" can be found in the Congressional Act of March 23, 1792. Mayo and Moulton, *Army and Navy Pension Laws*, 22–24.

84. *ASP Claims*, 86 (Airs), 90 (Dunham), 92 (Charlesworth), 91 (Fowler), 137 (Moore). These approvals and denials by the War Department were subject to consent by Congress.

85. The documents here are reports that list in columns a soldier's name, a brief account of the wartime cause of his impairment, and the degree of his disability that was recommended by physicians. There is no direct record of the interactions between the patients and physicians, only the determination of the latter that patients were or were not entitled to a pension and in what degree. One has to infer from the descriptions of the soldiers' disabilities, which read like summaries of petitions, that these are the stories brought to the physicians, who then had to determine if they aligned with the physical exam.

86. *ASP Claims*, 136 (Newton), 90 (Grose), 136 (Morse).

87. Disability from "wounds" or "known wounds" were the operative phrases in the dominant acts of the late eighteenth and early nineteenth centuries. Acts that allowed sickness through such phrases as "wounded or disabled" or "disabled by wounds or otherwise" were almost always followed by acts that restricted claimants to wounds only. Benefits for widows and orphans stemmed exclusively from soldiers killed by wounds. One can trace the phraseology of disability in the reprints of the acts in Mayo and Moulton, *Army and Navy Pension Laws*.

88. Mayo and Moulton, *Army and Navy Pension Laws*, 336–39. See, for example, the claim of Jacob Purkill, who asked for the loss of his slave, Archy, who was impressed into service in 1814. The government maintained that despite the fact that Archy had worked in dreadful conditions in the name of the public, it was impossible to determine whether his subsequent illness and death were the result of that service or the consequence of the sustained brutality of enslaved life: "such property is at all times held subject to those casualties which destroy health and life." *ASP Claims*, 668–69.

89. Glasson, *Federal Military Pensions*, 64.

90. Resch, *Suffering Soldiers*, 153. Alfred A. Young, *Masquerade: The Life and Times of Deborah Sampson, Continental Soldier* (New York Knopf, 2004), 227–37, for a vivid portrait of just how hard it was for one (admittedly somewhat unusual) veteran to receive back pay, an invalid pension, and general service pension.

91. Jensen, *Patriots, Settlers, and the Origins of American Social Policy*.

92. K. Walter Hickel finds, for example, that by 1924, some 485,000 of 940,000 adjudicated invalid pensions of World War I veterans had been denied on the basis of insufficient medical evidence. Physiological diseases were much more common cause for disability claims, but were more difficult to authenticate than anatomical damage. Hickel, "Medicine, Bureaucracy, and Social Welfare: The Politics of Disability Compensation for American Veterans of World War I," in *The New Disability History: American Perspectives*, ed. Paul K. Longmore and Lauri Umansky New York: New York University Press, 2001), 244.

CHAPTER EIGHT

1. *Massachusetts Gazette*, July 25, 1788. On other articles by Juvenis from 1788, see May 9 (gambling), May 16 (religion), May 30 (idleness), June 13 (prostitution), June 27 (reform), and July 18 (matters deserving public attention).

2. *Massachusetts Gazette*, July 25, 1788.

3. Cornelia H. Dayton and Sharon V. Salinger, *Robert Love's Warnings: Searching for Strangers in Colonial Boston* (Philadelphia: University of Pennsylvania Press, 2014), offers a recent and comprehensive overview of the poor laws in Massachusetts, tracing British antecedents and colonial departures. Dayton and Salinger are distinctive in arguing that Boston's poor relief was built on a two-tiered system, one directed toward those with residency in Massachusetts and the other, the province poor accounts, directed toward the many "strangers" (non-residents) and "sojourners" who moved most often from other areas of New England. Laurel Daen, "'To Board & Nurse a Stranger': Poverty, Disability, and Community in Eighteenth-Century Massachusetts," *Journal of Social History* (2020): 1–26, offers a social history of the Pauper Accounts that focuses on the cultural politics of state poor law accommodation, caregiving, and disability. While Daen suggests that more research is necessary, she has compiled county, province, and state poor law provision regarding strangers without legal settlement that could be found in other New England colonies and states (20n4). It is possible that future research will yield a picture of a more robust poor law provision for strangers throughout New England and beyond.

4. I have not undertaken a full count of the state paupers, and more work needs to be done on the total population in the program, both those receiving indoor and outdoor relief. Laurel Daen's work has been the most exacting, finding a total of 831 unique adults boarding in homes in the program from 1786 to 1799. Daen notes that this number is surely an undercount, since she excludes children from her tally and notes other incidental omissions. Given the large numbers of state paupers at the almshouses and workhouses in Boston, Salem, and elsewhere in port towns, the overall number of state paupers could be extended further still. See Daen, "'To Board & Nurse a Stranger,'" 4–7

and n. 15 for overall numbers; fig. 5 (7) for a breakdown of gender, race, age, nationality, military service, and cognitive capacity; and fig. 6 (8) for country of origin. Whatever the final tallies, the crucial point here is that while the numbers of state paupers were never a large percentage of the overall population, the program as a whole comprised a significant portion of the recurring allocations of the state budget. There is an important difference between a regular part of the budget and the budget as a whole for any given year. The person trying to determine the entire state budget for any given year faces a daunting task. There are numerous warrants listed without reference to the projects to which they are directed (including warrants for large sums); there are debts and credits that are carried over from year to year; and even the relatively orderly system of pauper accounts contributed to the confusion because not every town claimed its money in the year it was rewarded. The statement that the pauper accounts claim a *regular* part of the state budget is a commentary on how loosely organized state finance was in the period. The total costs of the paupers can be compared to the total costs for militia, sheriffs, coroners, printing, and "miscellaneous" in the digests offered at the end of each "roll" submitted by the Committee on Accounts (discussed below) to the General Court and published in the *Massachusetts Acts and Resolves* for each legislative session beginning in 1786. The population in Massachusetts in 1800 can be found in *Return of the Whole Number of Persons within the Several Districts of the United States* [for the year 1800] (New York: Norman Ross Publishing, 1801), 12.

5. Kunal M. Parker, "State, Citizenship, and Territory: The Legal Construction of Immigrants in Antebellum Massachusetts," *Law and History Review* 19 (Fall 2001): 583–643. I am indebted to Parker's pathbreaking work on state paupers and its connection between settlement laws, citizenship requirements, and the ways in which both domestic and immigrant populations were construed as "foreign." My term "foreign settlement" follows from Parker's approach, though in focusing on illness and problems of extremity, I argue that even marginalized populations received care, however spare. In addition to Parker, see chapter 2, above, for the elaboration of the poor laws.

6. On the law of 1675, see *The Colonial Laws of Massachusetts* (Boston, 1887), 238. See chapter 2, notes 12 and 29, for full references to province poor and Acadians.

7. Account Rolls, Pauper Accounts, C06/series 2268X, Massachusetts Archives, Boston, MA (cited hereafter as PA, followed by volume, town, and year). The finding aid for Committee on Accounts and Account Roll Submissions offers a concise and quite useful legislative history. I am indebted to Stephanie Dyson, archivist at the Massachusetts State Archives, for her generous help in sorting through the accounts and their tortuous history.

8. See Daen, "'To Board & Nurse a Stranger,'" fig. 1 (5), for 1786 and 1790. The counts for 1798 and 1800 are mine.

9. Parker, "State, Citizenship, and Territory," 595–605.

10. Sandisfield had 1,581 persons in 1790 (with another 161 in an adjoining parcel of land of 11,000 acres to the south) and 1,637 persons in 1800. See *Heads of Families at the First Census of the United States Taken in the Year 1790* (Baltimore: Genealogical Publishing Company, 1966), 9; and *Return of the Whole Number of Persons . . . of the United States,* 12.

11. Most committee work revolved around single-issue problems, the hastily

convened and dissolved committee serving as a quite modest form of bureaucracy. The Committee on Accounts was a rare standing committee, and it was rarer still to have its members receive a salary. Pegged at around 50 cents a day, it was more of a gesture of goodwill than a significant source of income (though the work grew steadily over the years, and by the turn of the century, members might well spend sixty to seventy days reviewing accounts). The senators on the committee typically served for several years, the House members for at least a few sessions. It comes as no surprise that committee members were not marginal characters: established farmers, militia captains, lawyers, and judges make up the majority.

12. PA, 39, Sandisfield, 1798.

13. PA, 40, Salem and Boston, 1798.

14. Ann Fabian, *The Unvarnished Truth: Personal Narratives in Nineteenth-Century America* (Berkeley: University of California Press, 2000).

15. James Bowdoin, "Address to the Convention, March 1780," in *The Popular Sources of Political Authority: Documents on the Massachusetts Constitution of 1780*, ed. Oscar Handlin and Mary Handlin (Cambridge: Belknap Press of Harvard University Press, 1966), 437.

16. Returns from the towns reprinted in *Popular Sources of Political Authority*: Petersham (860). Alexander Keyssar, *The Right to Vote: The Contested History of Democracy in the United States* (New York: Basic Books, 2000), 12–14, 18–19, gives the context of early limitations on the franchise.

17. *Popular Sources of Political Authority*: Belchertown (538); Richmond (487); Northampton (584).

18. David P. Szatmary, *Shays' Rebellion: The Making of an Agrarian Insurrection* (Amherst: University of Massachusetts Press, 1980), 57, 96.

19. Daen finds that "Blacks comprised about 12% of those boarded out, a huge number considering that only 1.4% of Massachusetts inhabitants were black according to the 1790 census." And she finds immigrants and those identified as "foreigners" to be 28% and 7%, respectively. Daen, "'To Board & Nurse a Stranger,'" 7, fig. 5 (7).

20. On the ambiguities of emancipation in post-Revolutionary New England, see Joanne Pope Melish, *Disowning Slavery: Gradual Emancipation and "Race" in New England, 1780–1860* (Ithaca, NY: Cornell University Press, 1998), 88, 97.

21. *The Laws of the Commonwealth of Massachusetts . . . In Two Volumes* (Boston: Manning & Loring, 1801), 1: 411–13. Linda K. Kerber, *No Constitutional Right to Be Ladies: Women and the Obligations of Citizenship* (New York: Hill and Wang, 1998), 54–55.

22. Marilyn C. Baseler, *"Asylum for Mankind": America, 1607–1800* (Ithaca, NY: Cornell University Press, 1998), 233n72 (on naturalizations).

23. Baseler, *"Asylum for Mankind,"* 270–85, argues that while Federalists initially supported immigration as part of mercantilist development, their interest in aliens declined in the 1790s and they supported the Alien Enemies Act and Naturalization Act extensions. James M. Banner Jr., *To the Hartford Convention: The Federalists and the Origins of Party Politics in Massachusetts, 1789–1815* (New York: Knopf, 1970), 89–99, discusses nativism in the early Federalist Party, which he argues was increasing over time and had continuity with next waves in the 1820s, the 1840s, and post–Civil War.

See also the constitutional amendment that the Massachusetts General Court circulated to other states in 1798 urging that no person be eligible for election to the United States Congress unless a "Natural Born Citizen of the United States," which was a way to combat "Foreign Influence on our National Councils. . . ." (Massachusetts General Court, July 12, 1798) [Early American Imprints, First Series, #48514]. On the alien property disabilities, see Parker, "From Poor Law to Immigration Law," 598. On John Hancock, see *Acts and Laws of the Commonwealth of Massachusetts* (Boston: Adams & Nourse, 1895), 1790–91, May Session, 549. The *Mass AR* series continues after 1780 with *Acts and Laws* (cited hereafter as *Mass AL*).

24. David Waldstreicher, *In the Midst of Perpetual Fetes: The Making of American Nationalism, 1776–1820* (Chapel Hill: University of North Carolina Press, 1997), 251–62.

25. Articles of Confederation, article 4. In keeping with the active erasure of slavery, not only in New England, but in the nation as a whole, the Articles did not refer specifically to fugitive slaves, but rather construed the matter as one of "not preventing the removal of property, imported into any State."

26. Congress made one attempt to provide a hospital for invalids in the wake of the war. A committee consisting of Alexander Hamilton, Richard Peters, and Daniel Carroll recommended in May 1783 that officers who "have lost a limb or been otherwise equally disabled" should be allowed full pay for life. Non-commissioned officers and soldiers who found themselves "strangers in the country and having been disabled in service" were "proper subjects for a Hospital," and should be supported there for the duration of their lives. The fear for these men was that as "strangers" without legal settlement in any town or state, they might be bounced from town to town, removed from localities that wished to avoid tapping into their public coffers to provide poor relief. While officers would be given the means to avoid hospitals, which, during the war, were considered death traps, fit for no gentleman, enlisted men could, at least, not meet the fate of strangers—Indians, free blacks, foreign nationals, loyalists returning home, and others. *Journals of the Continental Congress, 1774–1789*, ed. Worthington C. Ford et al. (Washington, DC, 1904–37), 24: 321–22. Caroline Cox, *A Proper Sense of Honor: Service and Sacrifice in George Washington's Army* (Chapel Hill: University of North Carolina Press, 2004), ch. 4, discusses the ability of officers to avoid regimental hospitals.

27. Bernard Bailyn, ed., *The Debate on the Constitution* (New York: Library of America, 1993), 1: 1103; *Western Star*, March 23, 1790.

28. John W. Thrask, *The United States Marine Hospital, Port of Boston* (Washington, DC: Federal Security Agency, Public Health Service, 1940), and Richard Thrum, *For the Relief of the Sick and Disabled: The U.S. Public Health Service Hospital in Boston, 1799–1969* (Washington, DC: Government Printing Office, 1972), discuss the early history of the Marine Hospital in Charlestown and later Boston that resulted from the legislation.

29. *Annals of Congress, House of Representatives, 5th Congress, 2nd Session*, 1385–92.

30. *Annals of Congress, House of Representatives, 5th Congress, 2nd Session*, 1385–92. Waldstreicher, *In the Midst of Perpetual Fetes*, 251–62, discusses New England as a nation.

31. Baseler, *"Asylum for Mankind,"* 271, 274–79.

32. PA, 39, Marblehead, 1798. Christine Leigh Heyrman, *Commerce and Culture: The Maritime Communities of Colonial Massachusetts, 1690–1750* (New York: Norton, 1984), 245–46, chronicles the early history of immigrants who came to Marblehead from the island of Jersey.

33. Bernard Bailyn, *The Peopling of British North America: An Introduction* (New York: Vintage, 1986), 18. On increased "warnings out" in the 1760s, see Douglas Lamar Jones, "The Strolling Poor: Transiency in Eighteenth-Century Massachusetts," *Journal of Social History* 8 (1975): 28–54.

34. Douglas Lamar Jones, "The Transformation of the Law of Poverty in Eighteenth-Century Massachusetts," in *Law in Colonial Massachusetts, 1630–1800,* ed. Daniel R. Coquillette, vol. 62 of *Collections* (Boston: Colonial Society of Massachusetts, 1984), 153–90. *Laws of the Commonwealth of Massachusetts, Passed from the Year 1780, to the End of the Year 1800* (Boston: Manning & Lorning, 1801), 2: 619–30 (poor law of 1794), 2: 607 (law of inhabitancy of 1794). Parker, "State, Citizenship, and Territory," 595–605, has linked the liberalization of the poor law with the increase in years of inhabitancy necessary for legal settlement.

35. In the Revolutionary era, migration in New England can be placed in the expansive frame of a much larger peopling of an inland arc stretching from Maine through Florida. In addition to citations in chapter 3, n. 24, see Bernard Bailyn, *Voyagers to the West: A Passage in the Peopling of America on the Eve of the Revolution* (New York: Knopf, 1986); and David Jaffee, *People of the Wachusett: Greater New England in History and Memory, 1630–1860* (Ithaca, NY: Cornell University Press, 1999).

36. PA, 36, Deerfield, 1796. The bulk of the manuscript accounts concerning the paupers lies between 1786 and 1799. Although the program continued to grow in intensity, the manuscript materials in the nineteenth century are thin. The discussion below focuses on the years between 1796 and 1798 for two reasons: the former is the first date at which towns reliably sent in detailed settlement histories (as per a resolve of the General Court in 1795); the latter date is the final year at which the manuscripts are nearly complete. The year 1805 is the last in which pauper accounts and certificates exist in any number.

37. Robert M. Calhoon, *The Loyalist Perception and Other Essays* (Columbia: University of South Carolina Press, 1989), 195–215; David Edward Maas, *The Return of the Massachusetts Loyalists* (New York: Garland, 1989), chs. 10, 11; Stephanie Kermes, "'I wish for nothing more ardently upon earth, than to see my friends and country again': The Return of Massachusetts Loyalists," *Historical Journal of Massachusetts* 30 (Winter 2002): 30–49.

38. If narratives of the "liberal age" in the years after the Revolution are dominated by the kinds of men whom Joyce Appleby has found moving outward without looking backward, the pauper rolls afford a view of persons who seem to have failed in such endeavors or to have had second thoughts. Compare Joyce Appleby, *Inheriting the Revolution: The First Generation of Americans* (Cambridge, MA: Belknap Press of Harvard University Press, 2000), 64–68, with Ruth Wallis Herndon, *Unwelcome Americans: Living on the Margin in Early New England* (Philadelphia: University of Pennsylvania Press, 2001).

39. PA, 39, Billerica, 1798. The Committee on Accounts agreed to the legitimacy of the claim, though they deducted the account by one-third with no explanation, one suspects because the trip to Boston was not considered the state's responsibility. They reduced the total bill by $6.63, and cost of conveyance was $5.43. If one takes away some candles that may not have been allowed as excessive, and deducts by half one night's board, the numbers add up. Ultimately, of course, it is impossible to know exactly what was going through the committee's mind unless they note the specific items that are being reduced or not allowed.

40. PA, 40, Danvers, 1798 (Wooden); PA, 39, Attleboro, 1798 ("Black Catherine," Hannah Jane); PA, 40, Attleboro, 1798 (Hannah Jane). Daen finds that 12% of her sample of boarders were elderly: "'To Board & Nurse a Stranger,'" fig. 5 (7).

41. PA, 36, Boylston, 1796; PA, 19, Topsfield, 1790.

42. PA, 39, Hardwick, 1798.

43. PA, 36, New Gloucester, 1796 (Judith Royal); PA, 36, Andover, 1796 (John Dunlop); PA, 39, Williamstown, 1798 (Rachel Galusha). Cornelia H. Dayton, "'The Oddest Man That I Ever Saw': Assessing Cognitive Disability on Eighteenth-Century Cape Cod," *Journal of Social History* 49, no. 1 (Fall 2015): 77–99, discusses guardianships and contested wills. Daen finds that 6% of boarders in her sample were labeled "insane" or "idiot": "'To Board & Nurse a Stranger,'" fig. 5 (7).

44. The first regular clinical practice at the almshouse appears to have been undertaken later, after Boston's almshouse had moved to Leveret Street, when faculty at Harvard's Medical School successfully petitioned in 1810 to bring their students into the institution. There was, in addition to the almshouse, the Boston Dispensary (established in 1796) and the Marine Hospital in Charlestown (opened in 1804). Henry R. Viets, *A Brief History of Medicine in Massachusetts* (Boston: Houghton Mifflin, 1930), 108–9, 113; Leonard K. Eaton, *New England Hospitals, 1790–1833* (Ann Arbor: University of Michigan Press, 1957), 10. For the resolve in 1784, see House unpassed legislation, #113, March 23, 1784, SC1/series 230, Massachusetts Archives, Boston, MA. For Warren's service, which was not repaid for several years, see *Mass AL*, 1785, February Session, 916.

45. The Nathaniel Appleton Notebook can be found in Boston Almshouse Physicians Accounts, 1779–1786, Massachusetts State Archives, Boston, MA.

46. PA, 36, Groton, 1796. James Delbourgo, "Common Sense, Useful Knowledge and Matters of Fact in the Late Enlightenment: The Transatlantic Career of Perkins's Tractors," *William and Mary Quarterly* 61 (October 2004): 643–84; Delbourgo, *A Most Amazing Scene of Wonders: Electricity and Enlightenment in Early America* (Cambridge, MA: Harvard University Press, 2006); Peter Benes, "Itinerant Physicians, Healers, and Surgeon-Dentists in New England and New York, 1720–1825," in *Medicine and Healing*, ed. Peter Benes, vol. 15 of *Annual Proceedings of the Dublin Seminar for New England Folklife* (Boston: Boston University Press, 1990), 95–112. Oliver Prescott Jr. was no fringe character. His grandfather had been a member of the General Court. His father, Oliver Sr. (1731–1804), was a prominent figure in the military, medical, and civic life of the state. On Prescott, see Howard A. Kelly and Walter L. Burrage, *Dictionary of American Medical Biography* (New York: D. Appleton, 1928), 989, and *Dictionary of American Biography* (New York: C. Scribner's Sons, 1935), vol. 15, 194–95. On lectures

and published work on electricity, see Raymond Phineas Stearns, *Science in the British Colonies of America* (Urbana: University of Illinois Press, 1970), 508–9, and Brooke Hindle, *The Pursuit of Science in Revolutionary America, 1735–1789* (Chapel Hill: University of North Carolina Press, 1956), 344.

47. At the age of thirty-eight, Bartlett was already an outstanding figure in Boston's medical circles. Born in Charlestown, he had served an apprenticeship with a local physician and later gained extensive medical experience when his master was appointed to the medical department of the American army at Cambridge. Kelly and Burrage, *Dictionary of American Medical Biography*, 67. Martin S. Pernick, "The Calculus of Suffering in 19th-Century Surgery," in *Sickness and Health in America: Readings in the History of Medicine and Public Health*, ed. Judith Walzer Leavitt and Ronald L. Numbers (Madison: University of Wisconsin Press, 1985), 98–112, discusses "therapeutic nihilism," which he uses to refer to debates in the antebellum period.

48. PA, 36, Charlestown, 1796. There is a strikingly congruent situation with a bill submitted to the Marine Hospital in Charlestown in 1804. The Navy Department accountant wrote to a Boston Customs officer that he had referred one "Joseph" Bartlett's account out to a "Medical Gentleman, for his propriety of the Charges," and had been assured that Bartlett's "mode of charging each patient prescribed for, with a visit, is not only a very unusual thing—but a very unjust, and a very unreasonable charge." The National Archives Project, Comp., *U.S. Marine Hospital Chelsea, Mass. Letters 1796 to 1832* (Boston, 1940), I, 26. A doctor who dispensed few medicines might also have a sense of entitlement; his visits alone, his learning and unique ability to understand changes in the patient's condition, warranted the charges. Charles E. Rosenberg, "The Therapeutic Revolution: Medicine, Meaning, and Social Change in Nineteenth-Century America," and "Social Class and Medical Care in Nineteenth-Century America: The Rise and Fall of the Dispensary," reprinted in his *Explaining Epidemics and Other Studies in the History of Medicine* (Cambridge: Cambridge University Press, 1992), chs. 1, 6.

49. Nursing may have been a problem with a far greater potential impact on town finances than doctoring. One dimension of the problem discussed below: namely, the seamless way in which towns added nursing and doctoring costs to bills for the elderly that had formerly been for boarding alone. More subtle, and worthy of closer scrutiny, are the ways in which nursing might be applied to a wider array of persons than the aged. A few days here or there during times of extremity did not make much of a difference. But when nursing became a matter of weeks and even months, the committee was faced with a difficult problem. If one did not overcharge for the weekly costs of nursing, which ran anywhere from $1.50 to $2.25 at the turn of the century, then the decision would have been reached about the point at which nursing was no longer necessary. Every state pauper was entitled to board, including yearly board, which was by far the largest expense in each account unless there was some kind of acute condition. By adding nursing to the mix, towns may have found a way to inflate their requests for compensation without seeming to make an outlandish demand. Daen, "'To Board & Nurse a Stranger,'" discusses nursing throughout, including the possibility that it was often done in conjunction with other medical care (though was also considered cheaper than other medical care), that it might be done by family members and both women and

men (the latter for heavy lifting and restraining), and that it might be a means whereby families could have the state pay for onerous caregiving (9, 11–13).

50. Daen finds a bi-modal pattern of boarding in her sample, with the greatest numbers either boarding less than one year or more than ten years: "'To Board & Nurse a Stranger,'" fig. 7 (11). For those who stayed for many years, Scudmore's case makes it is possible to see the ways in which health care would become a matter of routine in petitioning. For Scudmore, see PA for town of Westborough from 1796 to 1805 and rolls in *Mass AL*, 1796–1805:

> 1796: Roll 36. January Session: for "supporting" @ $83.18
> 1797: Roll 37. May Session: "supporting in full" @ $30.80
>   Roll 38. January Session: "supporting" @ $68.16
> 1798: Roll 39. May Session: "supporting" "including Extra Nursing & Medicines" @ $30.29
>   Roll 40. January Session: clothing, nursing, and doctoring @ $59.83
> 1799: Roll 42. January Session: boarding, clothing, and nursing @ $98.90
> 1800: Roll 44. January Session: boarding, clothing, and nursing @ $85
> 1801: Roll 45. May Session: boarding, clothing, doctoring, and nursing @ $37
>   Roll 46. January Session: boarding and clothing @ $74.31
> 1802: Roll 47. June Session: boarding, nursing, and doctoring @ $32.75
> 1803: Roll 48. March Session: boarding, clothing, doctoring, and nursing @ $76.23
>   Roll 49. June Session: boarding, clothing, nursing, and doctoring @ $32.92
> 1804: Roll 50. March Session: boarding, clothing, and doctoring @ $79.22
>   Roll 51. June Session: boarding, clothing, nursing, and doctoring @ $39.98
> 1805: Roll 52. March Session: boarding, clothing, doctoring, funeral @ $89.92

51. PA, 39, Franklin, 1798; PA, 18, Newburyport, 1790; PA, 39, Freeport, 1798.

52. Pauline Maier, "The Revolutionary Origins of the American Corporation," *William and Mary Quarterly* 50 (January 1993): 56; Conrad Edick Wright, *The Transformation of Charity in Postrevolutionary New England* (Boston: Northeastern University Press, 1992), 5; Peter Dobkin Hall, *The Organization of American Culture, 1700–1900: Private Institutions, Elites, and the Origins of American Nationality* (New York: New York University Press, 1982).

53. Maier, "The Revolutionary Origins of the American Corporation," 51–84, traces the unlikely rise of the corporation in the wake of the Revolution and the precocious development of the corporate form in Massachusetts.

54. House unpassed legislation #2550, March 28, 1788.

55. House unpassed legislation #2635, November 17, 1787. On John Manning, see Joseph B. Felt, *History of Ipswich, Essex, and Hamilton* (Cambridge, MA: C. Folsom, 1834), 188–89.

56. Senate unpassed legislation, #1198, February 25, 1790, March 1790.

57. House unpassed legislation #3239, January 14, 1790.

58. *Boston Town Records, 1784–1796* (Boston, 1903), 31: 238 (hereafter BTR).

59. BTR, 31: 239. Michael Meranze, *Laboratories of Virtue: Punishment, Revolution, and Authority in Philadelphia, 1760–1835* (Chapel Hill: University of North

Carolina Press, 1996), ch. 3, discusses "mimetic corruption," which could spread through observation.

60. BTR, 31: 251.

61. *Independent Chronicle and the Universal Advertiser*, June 30, 1791. Senate unpassed Legislation, #1759, which includes proposals from all of the towns, the bulk of which fall between 1792 and 1793. For town populations, see *Return of the Whole Number of Persons . . . of the United States*, 8–12.

62. Senate unpassed legislation, #1759/18, January 17, 1792 (Woburn); #1759/21, January 18, 1792 (Holliston); #1759/20, December–January 1791–92 (Stowe).

63. Senate unpassed legislation, #1759/12, February 9, 1792 (Boston).

64. John L. Brooke, *The Heart of the Commonwealth: Society and Political Culture in Worcester County, Massachusetts, 1713–1861* (Amherst: University of Massachusetts Press, 1989), 221–22, 189–91.

65. Barry Levy, *Town Born: The Political Economy of New England from Its Founding to the Revolution* (2009; repr., Philadelphia: University of Pennsylvania Press, 2011), discusses town responsibility for education and labor markets.

66. Senate unpassed legislation, #1759/6, February 29, 1792 (New Braintree).

67. *The Argus*, June 5, 1792.

68. *The Argus*, June 5, 1792.

69. *The Argus*, June 5, 1792. It was a position in keeping with Gardiner's long-standing interest in advancing a spirit of "liberality" in Boston's public culture. He had pushed to liberalize the liturgy of King's Chapel, moving the church in the direction of Unitarianism, and had fought to end a long-standing ban on the theater in Boston. In the debate over state paupers, Gardiner found a way to make even poor relief, with its roots in the Elizabeth Poor Laws, a potential means of personal and civic advancement. Like the sophisticated elite to which all might aspire to join, paupers should be given the means to avail themselves of the improvements that country life uniquely afforded. T. A. Milford, "Boston's Theater Controversy and Liberal Notions of Advantage," *New England Quarterly* 72 (March 1999): 62–88; Milford, *The Gardiners of Massachusetts: Provincial Ambition and the British-American Career* (Hanover: University of New Hampshire Press, 2005), 45–171.

70. Senate unpassed legislation, #1759/11, June 7, 1792 (Boston).

71. Senate unpassed legislation, #1759/11, June 7, 1792 (Boston).

72. Senate unpassed legislation, #1759/11, June 7, 1792 (Boston).

73. On the fear of imperium in imperio, see Maier, "The Revolutionary Origins of the American Corporation," 62, and Forrest McDonald, *States' Rights and the Union: Imperium in Imperio, 1776–1876* (Lawrence: University of Kansas Press, 2000), chs. 1–4.

74. Boston's initial plan was to care for the poor for 6s. per week for three years. It agreed finally to 5s. per week for five years. House unpassed legislation, #3752, June 27, 1792; *Western Star*, March 3, 1793.

75. Parker, "State, Citizenship, and Territory," 615n84 (for restrictions). Quotation from *The Overseers of the Poor of the City of Boston, to Their Constituents* (Boston, 1823), 21.

EPILOGUE

1. This section recapitulates arguments made in depth in the prior chapters, where the reader may find full references.

2. For a brief moment, then, New Englanders had an expansive view of the new national government as a protective body that would hear and respond to their intimate stories of suffering. In this sense, the national government was not "hidden in plain sight," but something that could be more directly accessed. That citizens were rapidly disabused of that idea in the early republic speaks to later developments in the nineteenth century and the more common sorts of state and federal partnerships that formed the associational state. On the latter, see Brian Balogh, *A Government Out of Sight: The Mystery of National Authority in Nineteenth-Century America* (Cambridge: Cambridge University Press, 2009).

3. [Josiah Quincy], *Report of the Committee on the Pauper Laws of this Commonwealth* (1821), reprinted in *The Almshouse Experience: Collected Reports*, ed. David J. Rothman (New York, 1971), 1–3 (cited hereafter as Quincy Report, followed by original pagination that is reprinted in the edited collection); *Columbian Centinel*, March 3, 1821; *New Bedford Mercury*, March 16, 1821.

4. Quincy Report, 3. The discourse on pauperism—a term that made a steady appearance in the public prints beginning in the 1810s in sermons, newspaper editorials, and reports on charitable organizations in the Bay State and further afield—went beyond a discussion of the misfortune and misdeed of individual paupers; it was concerned with exposing the social pathologies that fueled a stark, dangerous, and seemingly immutable sort of poverty that was deemed unacceptable in the new republic. Raymond A. Mohl, *Poverty in New York, 1793–1825* (New York: Oxford University Press, 1971), ch. 15.

5. Quincy Report, 4.

6. Quincy Report, 4.

7. Quincy Report, 5.

8. Quincy Report, 9.

9. Quincy Report, 23.

10. Quincy Report, 32–34.

11. Quincy Report, 16–17.

12. Quincy Report, 15. While the returns in the report do not frame the issue in this way, one might read these anecdotes as demonstrating a creative use of social welfare resources by the poor, including seasonal and temporary use of the almshouse. See Seth Rockman, *Scraping By: Wage Labor, Slavery, and Survival in Early Baltimore* (Baltimore: Johns Hopkins University Press, 2009), ch. 7, and Simon P. Newman, *Embodied History: The Lives of the Poor in Early Philadelphia* (Philadelphia: University of Pennsylvania Press, 2001), ch. 1.

13. *The Overseers of the Poor of the City of Boston, to Their Constituents* (Boston, 1823), 2 (cited hereafter as *Overseers to Constituents*). The conflict between Josiah Quincy and Boston's overseers of the poor over the proposed new House of Industry is traced in Robert A. McCaughey, *Josiah Quincy, 1772–1864: The Last Federalist* (Cambridge, MA: Harvard University Press, 1974), 115–17, which McCaughey frames as part

of a larger argument over control of the new city government and the promise and peril of urban reform.

14. *Overseers to Constituents*, 3.

15. *Overseers to Constituents*, 15.

16. Harold Kirker and James Kirker, *Bulfinch's Boston, 1787–1817* (New York: Oxford University Press, 1964), 97–98, plates 10–11.

17. A report on medical conditions at the almshouse had been scathing: "The Almshouse in Boston, is perhaps the only instance known where Persons of every description and disease are lodged under the same roof and in some instances in the same or Contiguous Apartments, by which means the sick are disturbed, by the Noise of the healthy, and the infirm rendered liable to the Vices and diseases of the diseased, and profligate." *Boston Town Records, 1784–1796* (Boston, 1903), 31: 239.

18. Letter draft from James Jackson to the Boston Overseers of the Poor, no date (c. 1805), James Jackson Papers, Massachusetts Historical Society, Boston, MA.

19. Letter draft from James Jackson to the Boston Overseers of the Poor. J. M. Opal, *Beyond the Farm: National Ambitions in Rural New England* (Philadelphia: University of Pennsylvania Press, 2008), and Joyce Appleby, *Inheriting the Revolution: The First Generation of Americans* (Cambridge: Belknap Press of Harvard University Press, 2000), both describe cultural ambition, though the former notes many failures along the way. For resounding stories of failure, see Ann Fabian, *The Unvarnished Truth: Personal Narratives in Nineteenth-Century America* (Berkeley: University of California Press, 2000); Scott A. Sandage, *Born Losers: A History of Failure in America* (Cambridge, MA: Harvard University Press, 2005); and Bruce H. Mann, *Republic of Debtors: Bankruptcy in the Age of American Independence* (Cambridge: Harvard University Press, 2002).

20. On this sort of moral corruption, see Michael Meranze, *Laboratories of Virtue: Punishment, Revolution, and Authority in Philadelphia, 1760–1835* (Chapel Hill: University of North Carolina Press, 1996), ch. 3.

21. Gordon Wood, *Empire of Liberty: A History of the Early Republic, 1789–1815* (Oxford: Oxford University Press, 2009), 486. Wood draws on Conrad Edick Wright's definitive treatment of the topic, *The Transformation of Charity in Postrevolutionary New England* (Boston: Northeastern University Press, 1992), 63.

22. Karl Haglund, *Inventing the Charles River* (Cambridge, MA: MIT Press, 2003), 34, provides the view of Massachusetts General Hospital (MGH). The voluntary hospital, an institution "founded by individuals and groups, rather than the state," came relatively late to Massachusetts. London had five major hospitals founded by philanthropy and bequest between 1720 and 1745; various specialized institutions followed suit in the provinces, including foundling hospitals for "abandoned babies, lying-in hospitals, 'lock' hospitals for venereal diseases and 'Magdalene' institutions for prostitutes," along with outpatient services offered by dispensaries. In the British North American colonies, Pennsylvania had established a hospital in 1751 (with considerable promotion from Benjamin Franklin) to treat the poor and insane, and the New York Hospital (or City Hospital) was founded in 1771. Massachusetts developed several institutional means of care for the sick over the course of the eighteenth century; in addition to almshouses, there were quarantine hospitals established in Boston Harbor on Spectacle Island (1717)

and Rainsford Island (1737); a military hospital created in Cambridge during the Revolution; and the Marine Hospital in Charlestown (1804) provided by "An Act for the Relief of Sick and Disabled Seamen" (1798), which funded the hospital through a deduction in seamen's wages (see chapter 8, above). But New England's first voluntary hospital, comparable to those established in Philadelphia and New York, was the Massachusetts General Hospital, and it was not established until many decades after the others. The relatively weak development of charities in New England prior to the Revolution compared to the Mid-Atlantic (Pennsylvania's Quaker community was notable for early charitable development), a far lesser number of immigrant arrivals in Massachusetts prior to the Revolution and a lesser-perceived problem with "foreign" immigrants in need of care in eighteenth-century New England (again, a major issue in the founding of the Pennsylvania Hospital, with Philadelphia fielding many immigrants), and the fact that New England's "town state" had found a mechanism to provide social welfare that was unusually robust in comparison to other colonies all help to explain the somewhat later appearance of the voluntary hospital in New England. There may well have been lesser need for the hospital in the earlier period.

On hospitals in Europe, see Mary Lindemann, *Medicine and Society in Early Modern Europe* (Cambridge: Cambridge University Press, 1999), ch. 5, and 136 (for definition of volunteer hospital); and Roy Porter, *The Creation of the Modern World: The Untold Story of the British Enlightenment* (New York: Norton, 2000), 207 (for London and provincial hospitals). On the Pennsylvania hospital, see Thomas G. Morton, *The History of the Pennsylvania Hospital, 1751–1895* (1895; repr., New York: Arno Press, 1973); Newman, *Embodied History*, ch. 3; and Simon Finger, *The Contagious City: The Politics of Public Health in Early Philadelphia* (Ithaca, NY: Cornell University Press, 2012), Kindle ed., locs. 1380–600. For an overview of New England hospitals, see N. I. Bowditch, *A History of the Massachusetts General Hospital* (2nd ed., 1872; repr., New York: Arno Press & The New York Times, 1972); Leonard K. Eaton, *New England Hospitals, 1790–1833* (Ann Arbor: University of Michigan Press, 1957), ch. 2 (on MGH); John Harley Warner, *The Therapeutic Perspective: Medical Practice, Knowledge, and Identity in America, 1820–1885* (Princeton, NJ: Princeton University Press, 1997); and Catherine L. Thompson, *Patient Expectations: How Economics, Religion, and Malpractice Shaped Therapeutics in Early America* (Amherst: University of Massachusetts Press, 2015), which discusses classes of patients, treatments, and leading physicians as a part of a larger discussion of therapeutics and healing in New England. See also Barry Levy, *Town Born: The Political Economy of New England from Its Founding to the Revolution* (2009; repr., Philadelphia: University of Pennsylvania Press, 2011), 290–91, who coins the term "town state."

23. Warren and Jackson Address in 1810 is reprinted in Bowditch, *A History of the Massachusetts General Hospital*, 3–9 (cited hereafter as Jackson and Warren [1810]).

24. *Address of the Trustees of Massachusetts General Hospital* (1813), 3.

25. Samuel May, *A History of the Boston Dispensary* (Boston, 1869), 51, 57, 218, 219.

26. "An Act to incorporate Samuel Parker and others, into a Society by the name of The Boston Dispensary" (1801), 7.

27. "An Act to incorporate Samuel Parker and others," 7.

28. On the problem of nursing, see Jackson and Warren (1810), 4, and John G. Coffin,

An Address Delivered before the Contributors of the Boston Dispensary at Their Seventeenth Anniversary, October 21, 1813 (Boston, 1813), 12.

29. Jackson and Warren (1810), 4.

30. Female Humane Society of Cambridge (hereafter FHSC), vol. 1, folder 1, Annual Meeting, August 14, 1818, pp. 51–52, Schlesinger Library, Harvard University, Cambridge, MA.

31. For a list of items, see FHSC, vol. 1, folder 1, Annual Meeting, First Monday in September 1816, pp. 25–30. An early restriction in the FHSC, which was later loosened, held that members needed to provide bond for loaned items.

32. On bathing tubs, First Church (Watertown, MA) Records, Watertown Female Society for the Relief of the Indigent Sick (hereafter WFS), box 34, folder 4, special meeting, May 31, 1817, and July 7, 1817, Massachusetts Historical Society, Boston, MA.

33. John E. Crowley, *The Invention of Comfort: Sensibilities and Design in Early Modern Britain and Early America* (Baltimore: Johns Hopkins University Press, 2003). An "easy chair" provided by the societies nicely captures a change in the practices and discourse of comfort. Originally part of the sick chamber, its use migrated to the parlor in the nineteenth century. Jane C. Nylander, *Our Own Snug Fireside: Images of the New England Home, 1760–1860* (New Haven, CT: Yale University Press, 1993), 39; Richard L. Bushman, *The Refinement of America: Persons, Houses, Cities* (New York: Vintage, 1992), 272.

34. Kathleen M. Brown, *Foul Bodies: Cleanliness in Early America* (New Haven, CT: Yale University Press, 2009), chs. 7–9.

35. Brown, *Foul Bodies*, 133–35, 192–94, 200–211, argues that bathing and washing were part of a larger campaign to promote the cleanliness and refinement of the middle class. Lori Ginzberg, *Women and the Work of Benevolence: Morality, Politics, and Class in the Nineteenth-Century United States* (New Haven, CT: Yale University Press, 1990), discusses women's charitable societies as an entry point into matters of governance. John Duffy, *The Sanitarians: A History of American Public Health* (Urbana: University of Illinois Press, 1990), chs. 1–8, and Charles E. Rosenberg, *The Cholera Years: The United States in 1832, 1849, and 1866* (1962; repr., Chicago: University of Chicago Press, 1987), chs. 1–9, reveal the limits of public health in the early nineteenth century.

36. See Duffy, *Sanitarians*, 96–97; Ginzberg, *Women and the Work of Benevolence*; and Nancy Tomes, *The Gospel of Germs: Men, Women, and the Microbe in American Life* (Cambridge, MA: Harvard University Press, 1998).

37. See the WFS case of "a Black Man & his Wife," considered worthy poor but, according to some, best comprehended through funds for state paupers. WFS, box 34, February 7, 1818, monthly meeting.

38. See the FHSC case of the widow Norton, a "respectable member of the society" who was aged and infirm. The FHSC supported her for over a decade, finally increasing aid to include an attendant from 1830 to 1834, but feared that such care would allow little funds for others. FHSC, vol. 1, meetings on November 7, 1823; May 19, 1824; September [n.d.] 1824; February 18, 1825; May 8, 1826; May [n.d.] 1828; May 14, 1834; September 30, 1834; May 20[?], 1835.

39. On the Massachusetts Hospital Life Insurance Company (MHLIC), see Robert F.

Dalzell Jr., *Enterprising Elite: The Boston Associates and the World They Made* (Cambridge, MA: Harvard University Press, 1987), 135–37; and Tamara Plakins Thornton, "'A Great Machine' or a 'Beast of Prey': A Boston Corporation and Its Rural Debtors in an Age of Capitalist Transformation," *Journal of the Early Republic* 27 (Winter 2007): 567–97. Oscar Handlin and Mary Flug Handlin, *Commonwealth: A Study of the Role of Government in the American Economy, Massachusetts, 1774–1861* (Cambridge, MA: Belknap Press of Harvard University Press, 1969), emphasize the partnership that had corporations awarded charters as a means of advancing the public good; Pauline Maier, "The Revolutionary Origins of the American Corporation," *William and Mary Quarterly* 50 (January 1993): 51–84, emphasizes the early fear that corporations represented the threat of imperium in imperio. Johann N. Neem, *Creating a Nation of Joiners: Democracy and Civil Society in Early National Massachusetts* (Cambridge, MA: Harvard University Press, 2008), 63–64, illuminates the ways in which the politics of association became part of a larger struggle for power between Federalists and Republicans in early national Massachusetts. The hospital conveniently met the priorities of both. Josiah Quincy's address is reprinted in Bowditch, *A History of the Massachusetts General Hospital*, 43.

40. John B. Blake, *Public Health in the Town of Boston, 1630–1822* (Cambridge, MA: Harvard University Press, 1959), provides population figures in appendices, 249, 251.

41. *Address of the Board of Trustees of the Massachusetts General Hospital to the Public* (1814), 11.

42. Robert A. Gross, "Giving in America: From Charity to Philanthropy," in *Charity, Philanthropy, and Civility in American History*, ed. Lawrence J. Friedman and Mark D. McGarvie (Cambridge: Cambridge University Press, 2003), ch. 1.

43. "Copy of a Letter sent to Salem, Newbury, Marblehead, Beverly, Plymouth, and New Bedford," December 1816, AC4, folder 159, Massachusetts General Hospital Archives (hereafter MGH Archives), Boston, MA. Perkins was not only a key supporter of MGH and what became McLean Hospital, but also the Boston Athenæum, the Boston Museum of Fine Arts, and, most prominently, the Perkins School for the Blind, which was founded in 1829. On Perkins and others amassing new mercantile and industrial fortunes in this period and devoting themselves to philanthropy, see Mark Peterson, *The City-State of Boston: The Rise and Fall of an Atlantic Power, 1630–1865* (Princeton, NJ: Princeton University Press, 2019), 452–78, 523–39.

44. The Trustees made a special pitch for the provision for the "insane," envisioning two institutions that might be built. The asylum for the insane would serve towns "by the liberality which they trust will characterize the contributions to it, [and] will, at no distant period, relieve, not only many individuals, labouring under this heaviest of human calamities, but also all the towns of the Commonwealth of a great part, if not the whole of the burden, to which they are at present subject for their superintendence and support." Printed circular of May 1816, MGH Archives, AC4, box 9, folder 159.

45. See Bowditch, *A History of the Massachusetts General Hospital*, 432–33, and the convenient summary in Dalzell, *Enterprising Elite*, 128.

46. See responses by spokespersons from Worcester, Bolton, Andover, Marlborough,

and Fitchburg in the MGH Archives, AC4, box 9, folder 159. See similar points made by Dedham, Leighton, and Chelsea.

47. On town state, see Levy, *Town Born*. These sorts of critical responses to the fundraising efforts might be seen as evidence of the separation of rural New England from the metropole in this period that Mark Peterson has recently described. Whatever the immediate issues raised in the responses, the larger context for discontent with Boston arose as part of the reorientation of a political economy that had formerly united Boston, the ports, and the hinterland in a larger Atlantic commerce through the eighteenth century, which was now giving way to the rise of new mercantile and industrial fortunes forged in the 1810s. The enriching of the Boston Associates and others around commodities such as cotton that had little part in rural New England had meant the slow unraveling of the prior integrated order. And the philanthropic efforts of new Boston elites "marked another step in the growing divide between rich and poor, and the emergence of a new Boston in which the institutions of charity and philanthropy were dominated by a wealthy elite, and understood as an ornament of their power." Peterson, *The City-State of Boston*, 525, and note 43, above.

48. *Columbian Centinel*, December 3, 1817.

49. Jeanne Boydston, *Home and Work: Housework, Wages, and the Ideology of Labor in the Early Republic* (New York: Oxford University Press, 1990); Brown, *Foul Bodies*, chs. 7–10.

50. Dalzell's *Enterprising Elite*, 135–37, highlights the use of the MHLIC as conservative means used by the Boston Associates to administer their trusts. Thornton's "A Great Machine" uses MHLIC's records to recover a particular strand in the social relations of capitalism in the New England countryside, which pitted corporation administrators, who demanded punctuality in interest payments, against rural landholders, who had mortgaged their property to pay debts. On the darker edge of philanthropy, which was used as a means of class separation by the new elites of Boston (and, increasingly, in luxurious homes in the countryside), see Peterson, *City-State of Boston*, 523–30.

51. On comparable institutions and practices in nineteenth-century New England that were part of remaking communities in this fashion, see Mary Babson Fuhrer, *A Crisis of Community: The Trials and Transformation of a New England Town, 1815–1848* (Chapel Hill: University of North Carolina Press, 2014). I thank Robert A. Gross for his help in thinking through a range of issues that attended such a transformation, which could happen quietly and subtly in New England towns.

52. *Address of the Trustees of the Massachusetts General Hospital to the Subscribers and to the Public* (1822), 8, 10.

53. *Address of the Trustees* (1822), 7–8. On the theme of early national social welfare institutions being unable to resist the forces outside their walls, see David J. Rothman, *The Discovery of the Asylum: Social Order and Disorder in the New Republic* (1971; repr., Boston: Little, Brown, 1990).

54. On the failures of the antebellum hospital, see Charles E. Rosenberg, *The Care of Strangers: The Rise of America's Hospital System* (New York: Basic Books, 1987), chs. 2–3. Margaret Gerteis, "The Massachusetts General Hospital, 1810–1865: An Essay on the Political Construction of Social Responsibility during New England's Early

Industrialization" (PhD diss., Tufts University, 1985), traces the trials of the hospital, including struggles to fund free beds, and charts a longer trajectory that had MGH retreat from its mission as a public institution to one that was more akin to a private charitable institution.

55. A few representative examples include Richard L. Bushman, *From Puritan to Yankee: Character and the Social Order in Connecticut, 1690–1765* (Cambridge, MA: Harvard University Press, 1967); Helena M. Wall, *Fierce Communion: Family and Community in Early America* (1990; repr., Cambridge, MA: Harvard University Press, 1995); T. H. Breen, *The Marketplace of Revolution: How Consumer Politics Shaped American Independence* (Oxford: Oxford University Press, 2004); and Bushman, *The Refinement of America.*

56. Portions of the last two paragraphs appear in an earlier op-ed piece published in the *Oregonian*: Ben Mutschler, "A Public Option: Health Care in the American Grain," *Oregonian*, August 31, 2009, https://www.oregonlive.com/opinion/2009/08/a_public _option_health_care_in.html.

Parkman, OH, 92

Partridge, Sarah, 246

paternalism, 102, 117, 202, 233

patriarchy, 7, 37, 103, 139, 143, 174, 189, 197, 278. *See also* matriarchy

paupers: and extremity, claims of, 240–45; and foreign settlement, 226–31, 244–45, 260; limits on claims for relief, 9; and localities, 235–40; medical charities for, 275–87; medical negotiations for, 245–49; and migration, 240–45; and moral contagion, 269; numbers, 226–31; obstacles faced, 232; and public health, 152, 259; as refugees, 242; relief, evolution of, 225, 231–36; relief, limits on claims for, 9; relief for, and failure of corporations, 249–51; relief for, and poor laws, 9, 239–40, 251–60, 268–75, 307n12; relief for, evolution of, 231–36; and settlement laws, 240–45; and smallpox, 257–58; and social suffering, 231; as state patients, 8, 223–60, 266; taint of, 277; warning-out system, 17, 240, 307n12. *See also* beggars; malingerers; poverty; sick poor; vagrants/vagrancy

Peckham, Howard, 161

Pelling, Margaret, 106

Penn, William, 123

pensioners/pensions. *See* colonial pensioners/pensions

perils. *See* community of perils

Perkins, Thomas Handasyd, 283

Perry, Simeon, 138

pesthouses, 34, 122, 129–31, 133–34, 145, 148, 158, 176, 254, 264, 321n21–22, 322n28

Phelps, Charles, Jr., 30, 101–2, 106

Phelps, Elizabeth (Porter), 13, 29–32, 33, 36, 46, 100–103, 263–64

Philadelphia: smallpox in, 33, 123, 149–50; yellow fever in, 216

Philips, Thomas, 189

Phillips family, 283

phlebotomy, 25

Pierson, William, 98

Pitt, William, 160

plague, 17, 122–23

political economy: of New England, 4, 53, 250–51

politics: of corporeal identity, 122; and illness, 41; of localism, 212; of poor relief, 52–53; and sick poor, 59; of

smallpox, 40–46, 141, 142–55; of state pension relief, 210–11. *See also* local governance

poor. *See* paupers; poverty; sick poor

poorhouses, 113, 239, 247, 253, 271–72. *See also* almshouses; workhouses

Porter, Elizabeth. *See* Phelps, Elizabeth (Porter)

Potter, Alice, 138

Potter, James, 144

poverty: and affliction, 245; assistance and protection for, 46; as chronic problem in Boston, 45; and debility of body, 46, 275; and disease, 122; and dislocations, 17, 64; and idleness, 9, 42–43, 45–46, 60, 202, 223, 233, 235, 271–72; and illness, 269; and mobility, 266; and negligence, 286–87; objectified and adjudicated, 221; *vs.* physical suffering, 221; and protection, 46; relief, and reformation of poor laws, 9, 17, 60–61, 66, 225, 268–75; relief, politics of, 52–53; and sickness, 32, 259, 267; social relations of, 52; and warfare, 176. *See also* paupers; sick poor

power, social, 56–57, 89

Pratt, Edward, 188

Prescott, Joshua, 170–71

Prescott, Oliver, Jr., Dr., 246–47

prescriptions, 3

Primitive Physick (Wesley), 26

protection: commitment to in New England, 16–18; covenant, 255, 299n27; monarchical, 8–9, 18, 198, 200, 212, 221; and poverty, 46; and province of affliction, 8, 14; and public health, 130; and social relations, 17; and social suffering, 14–18. *See also* extremity; local governance; locality

Protestantism, *vs.* providentialism of daily life, 4

Providentialism, *vs.* work ethic Protestantism, 4

province, as place and metaphor, 10–13

province of affliction, 18–20, 23–48, 272–73, 276, 279–83, 286–88; costs of as considerable, 288; in daily/everyday life, 1–2, 46, 70, 156, 287–88; enduring patterns in, 261–67; extremity and power, 15; perseverance and forbearance of, 28; social and political implications, 5–8, 11, 13–19, 35, 122, 124, 127, 135–41, 159,